A Desk Reference to

Personalizing Patient Care

Dearest Kathy,
Wishing you the
very best in 2015!
Continue to touch
people's lives with
all the gifts God
has given you!
Love,
Anvera
1 Jan 2015

The Essential Guide for Physicians, Nurses, and Other Healthcare Professionals

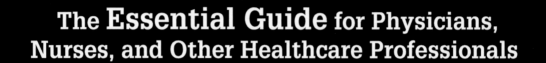

General Editor	Aurora Realin, MBA, CDM
Contributing Editors	Marie C. Ruckstuhl, BSN, MBA, RN, CPHQ, CHRM
	Louis R. Preston JR, MDiv, CDM
	Candice S. Ricketts, BA, MBA (Candidate)

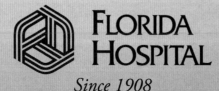

FLORIDA
HOSPITAL
Since 1908

A Desk Reference to

Personalizing Patient Care

A Guide for Compassionate
Healthcare Professionals on
Enhancing the Patient Experience
by Understanding Differences in:

Cultures

Religions

Disabilities

Generations

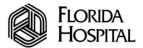

FLORIDA HOSPITAL

PERSONALIZING PATIENT CARE
Copyright © 2012 Florida Hospital
Published by Florida Hospital Publishing
900 Winderley Place, Suite 1600
Maitland, Florida 32751

TO EXTEND *the* HEALTH *and* HEALING MINISTRY *of* CHRIST

EDITOR-IN-CHIEF	Todd Chobotar
MANAGING EDITOR	David Biebel, DMin
EXTERNAL PEER REVIEW	Tia Hughes, MBA
	Steve Paquet, MS, RN
INTERNAL PEER REVIEW	John Guarneri, MD, FACOG
	Mary Halstead, RN, CCRN-CMC, CSC
	Sandra Randolph, FACHE, MBA, PT
	Karen Marcarelli, RN, JD, MSN, MS
	Sylvia Taylor, RN, BSN, CCRN
	Melissa Carollo, RN, BSN
	Laurie Levin, JD
PROMOTION	Laurel Dominesey
PRODUCTION	Lillian Boyd
COPY EDITORS	Barbara Trombitas
	Pamela Nordberg
COVER DESIGN	Jones Creative
PHOTOGRAPHY	Spencer Freeman
INTERIOR DESIGN	Tim Brown

For volume discounts please contact special sales at:
HealthProducts@FLHosp.org | (407) 303-1929

Cataloging-in-Publication Data for this book
is available from the Library of Congress.
Printed in the United States of America.
FP 12 11 10 9 8 7 6 5 4 3 2 1
ISBN 13: 978-0-9820409-3-5

For Whole Person Health resources visit:
FloridaHospitalPublishing.com
Healthy100Churches.org
CreationHealth.com
Healthy100.org

Share With Us

This book is a work in progress. In fact, we view it as more of a dialogue than a monologue. We will be updating this guide from time-to-time as new information or research becomes available. Please join us in making this resource the best it can be. If you have comments or suggestions, please submit them—along with supporting references and documentation—to the contact information listed below. If your idea or information is used, you will be given credit (if you wish to have your name listed) as a contributor in the next updated edition of the book.

We would also like to hear your stories of how this guide has proven useful to you or your team. Please share your story with us in as much detail as you can. Thank you in advance for helping us to improve this important resource. You may submit stories, suggestions, or feedback to:

Personalizing Patient Care

c/o Florida Hospital Department of Diversity and Inclusion
900 Winderley Place, Suite 1300, Maitland, FL 32751
PersonalizingPatientCare@FLHosp.org

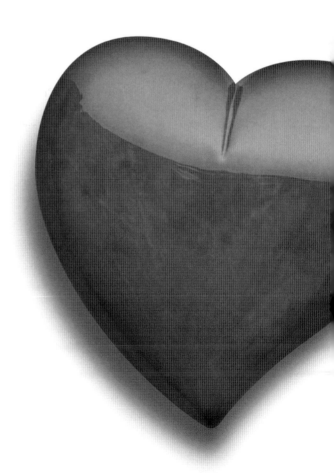

Contents

Editor's Introduction

"THE REASON I GOT INTO HEALTHCARE WAS TO HELP HURTING PEOPLE. BUT I DON'T want to just treat their symptoms, I want every patient to know how much I care for them as a person." The look on Susan's face spoke to me as clearly as her voice. Like many physicians, nurses, and other caregivers I talk to, she was earnest and passionate about her patients. She wanted each to know that they weren't some nameless widget in an impersonal healthcare assembly line. Each of her patients was special. Each was unique.

This guide exists for caregivers like Susan. It was researched and written for healthcare professionals who want to give both quality care and personalized care. How can you do that? Providing personalized patient care requires an awareness of the physical, psychological, social, spiritual, and cultural needs of the patient. To do this, it is helpful to have an awareness of the religious and cultural background of the patient. It is also useful to have an understanding of disability and generational information that might relate to a particular patient's care. Knowing even a few of these unique differences can facilitate a more personalized patient care experience during a health crisis.

If you are a caregiver, imagine how much better you might be able to provide appropriate care if you have a little extra knowledge of the perceptions, practices, needs, and expectations of your patients. That knowledge may offer opportunities for conversation where patients reveal more information about their personal beliefs and practices. Such conversations could provide insights into culturally sensitive ways to provide quality care that treats the patient as an individual rather than just a member of a particular group.

While no book will be able to give you information to perfectly match every situation you will face, these pages do provide a solid starting point for your journey to personalizing patient care. So use it. Interact with it. And please, give us feedback on how we can improve it.

Our goal for this guide is to help you and your team become the best, most compassionate caregivers you can be.

Todd Chobotar
Publisher and Editor-in-Chief

Foreword

I REALLY WISH THAT A BOOK LIKE PERSONALIZING PATIENT CARE HAD BEEN AVAILABLE when I was in training. It would have helped me deliver more personalized care to a broader spectrum of my patients through the years.

But of course there was no book like that, then. And to my knowledge, there never has been a book like this ... UNTIL NOW! So, it should go without saying that this book should become required reading for every doctor in training.

In addition, I believe that every doctor's office or nurses' station will benefit from having this reference right there on the shelf, available when any member of the healthcare team needs to know more about the needs, preferences, or expectations of members of various religious or cultural groups, different generations, or persons with disabilities – or even a combination of these characteristics.

Many times patients come under our care whose backgrounds or practices differ widely from those of anyone we've ever treated or even known, personally. Consequently, even though we want to provide the most compassionate care possible, we may not be aware, for example, that a Sikh wears five symbols, referred to as "five Ks" of dress: kesh, kangha, kara, kirpan, and kach ... and that none of these should be removed without permission and only after washing one's hands. That's where this book can help.

While this reference has facilitated a wholistic approach (body, soul, and spirit) within our hospital, its applicability goes far beyond our eight campuses, 17,000 employees, and one million patients per year who receive treatment. Its usefulness extends even beyond faith-based healthcare to all healthcare setting that are experiencing, as we have, a significant increase in the diversity of patients seen.

On a more personal level, this compendium will serve as a resource to help each of us understand and help each other in this journey of life that we share.

God made us different, not to divide us, but to delight us. Kindness is not regional; it doesn't matter whether you say "Y'all" or "Youse guys" or "Tutti ragazzi." He has made our hearts, minds, and spirits multilingual and that is one more thing to love about being together.

It is my hope that you will use this text to understand, help, and heal.

John D. Guarneri, MD, FACOG
Director and Chairman
Department of Healthcare and Spirituality, Florida Hospital
Past President - Medical Staff, Florida Hospital

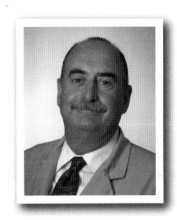

Personalizing Patient Care

CONSIDER THIS SCENARIO. A HINDU HAS BECOME ONE OF YOUR PATIENTS. A DAILY bath is required; but it is not acceptable to add cold water to hot in preparing for bath. Furthermore, a patient may refuse bath after a meal. Personal care is done with left hand. Prayer and "ritual cleansing" of left hand is very important. Hindus of either gender prefer to wear clothing under hospital gowns; for procedures, clothing covers private areas. Many Hindu diabetics do not take insulin made from animals, so explain what insulin contains before administering it.

In this unique book, you will find crucial patient care information like this related to twenty of the world's religions, twenty of the world's cultures, four generations, and seven of the most common disabilities—all in easy to read tabular form.

What you have in your hands is an extensive clinician's guide to providing individualized trans-cultural, multi-generational, whole-person patient care. Physicians, nurses, administrators – indeed, any caregiver – will come to view this resource as an invaluable reference to the special needs, preferences, and expectations of patients from widely diverse backgrounds.

Current and predicted demographics indicate that cultural diversity is growing. It is no longer unusual to encounter patients having different cultural and religious backgrounds quite different from our own. Other demographic differences such as age and disability are also important to understand because being aware of these differences is important to providing a personalized patient care experience.

HOW THIS GUIDE CAME TO BE

Florida Hospital, the largest admitting hospital in America, is a part of Adventist Health System, which operates the largest not-for-profit Protestant healthcare system in the nation. Over the past several decades, significant changes have occurred in the cultural and spiritual composition of the hospital's patient base. As a result, the decision was made to create a guide to assist caregivers in providing trans-cultural and spiritual patient care. This book, originally entitled The Florida Hospital Religion and Culture in Healthcare Caregivers Guide was developed by the Florida Hospital Nursing Department Patient Education Ad Hoc Committee and published internally. The first edition of the guide addressed basic topics within different religions and cultures including beliefs, birth, baptism, death, diet, health crisis, and healing environment.

Over a decade after it was first published, an effort was made to update and expand the guide. While the Nursing Department remained a key participant, sponsorship of the second edition was transitioned to the Florida Hospital Biomedical Ethics Committee. Under its auspices, the Nursing Department and the Diversity and Inclusion Department revised the publication for easier reading and included new information from the literature. Topics such as pregnancy, pain management, advance directives, DNR, blood, organ donation, and autopsy were added. The new edition, also published internally, was renamed the Guide to Religion and Culture.

Nearly five years after publication of the second edition, the committee chose to add two new sections to the guide to cover disabilities and generations. Additional emphasis was also made on enhancing the guide to help caregivers provide a better patient experience. Along with many suggestions and additional research, this revised and expanded third edition has been renamed to reflect the broader topic base and to emphasize its use in creating a more personal experience for every patient. The title of the third edition is A Desk Reference to Personalizing Patient Care.

During the development of this edition, one of our goals was to publish a reference guide that would be useful far beyond the Adventist Health System, since similar demographic and religious changes are occurring everywhere in this country and around the world. We trust the information and principles in this guide will prove helpful for all healthcare professionals and allied health professionals who wish to better understand the special needs or expectations of their patients or clients, in order to provide them the highest quality personalized care possible.

WHAT MAKES THIS GUIDE SO DISTINCTIVE

It's not often a unique resource appears at a time that is also unique. Over the past several decades the "face" of our society has changed in the areas of culture, religion, generations, and disabilities. The impact is especially evident in the area of healthcare delivery.

On any given day, a healthcare professional is likely to see not only a wide range of diseases from around the world—since so many people travel internationally—but is also likely to see individuals representing cultures and religions with which he or she may be unfamiliar. These patients have specific practices and beliefs that affect their needs and expectations when it comes to healthcare. It is incumbent, therefore, upon any professional who desires to provide excellent, personalized care to become as familiar as possible with these factors. That is where this guide can help.

A Desk Reference to Personalizing Patient Care presents a wide range of carefully researched, non-judgmental information on faith, culture and other subjects that could prove invaluable in relating to patients needs. While this information is especially important in a faith-based healthcare setting (such as Florida Hospital), it is also important to any hospital, physician practice, or healthcare facility wishing to provide personalized care.

The material in this book has been researched, compiled, and tested over the course of fifteen years. It has been accessed and utilized by thousands of caregivers (2,000 physicians and 4,000 nurses) at Florida Hospital as well as numerous other hospitals. The guide also contains over 3,000 reference notations and complete bibliography.

One of the primary reasons this book is unique is the composition of the team of contributing editors. Specifically, the blend of background, education, and professional experience of those closest to this publication speak to its distinctiveness. Contributors include: Aurora Realin, MBA, SLP, CDM, a specialist in the area of Diversity and Inclusion; Marie Ruckstuhl, BSN, MBA, RN, CPHQ, CHRM, a registered nurse with administrative and editorial experience; Louis Preston, MDiv, CDM, an ordained minister with experience in hospital leadership and administration; and Candice Ricketts, BA, MBA (candidate), a journalist with experience in writing for both consumer and professional audiences.

We believe that the combination of the following factors sets this guide apart as the best resource of its kind available today. Factors include:

- The diverse experience of the contributing editors.
- Over 3,000 notations including complete bibliography.
- Fifteen years of research and refinement of this publication.
- A broad base of healthcare professionals already utilizing the material.
- The foundation of a hundred-year-history of wholistic healthcare at Florida Hospital.

Yet, as thorough as this guide is, we view it as a work in progress, and invite reader feedback and suggestions as we seek to improve what is already a remarkable resource.

NON-JUDGEMENTAL OVERVIEWS

We realize that no short summary of any religious or cultural group, or a general overview of the values of multiple generations, or generalities about attitudes toward people with disabilities can possibly hope to exhaustively represent the beliefs, attitudes, or expectations toward healthcare of every person from every group mentioned.

We realize that even trying to create a resource like this may invite controversy, since individuals from any of the various groups described may hold views that differ from those presented as typical of their group. While every effort has been made to include information from primary sources, which are cited in the references, nothing contained in this book should be interpreted as a value judgment on anyone's beliefs or practices or expectations.

Our goal is simply to enhance understanding and improve patient care. Our focus is on how factors common to a particular group may be relevant to the healthcare setting and may affect a healthcare provider's ability to deliver the most appropriate and personalized patient care possible to a given individual whose background may differ from his or her own.

THE NATURAL LIMITATIONS OF THIS GUIDE

The stated purpose of this guide is to present factual information that has been verified. It is important to understand that care has been taken to research and confirm the accuracy of the information contained in this guide and to describe a number of core practices, values, and ideals based on religion, culture, disability, and generation. Even so, it has not been possible to describe every religion, culture, disability, and generation. Nor has it been possible to describe each and every difference or distinction within a particular religion, culture, disability, or generational group.

Complicating our task is the fact that multiple religions may be practiced within the same culture and multiple cultures may practice a particular religion in their own unique ways. Further, even within the same religion and culture, different people may have different perspectives, values, and beliefs, including their beliefs and practices in relation to persons with disabilities, and all of these perspectives, values, and beliefs may be affected as well by the generation of the person in question.

HOW TO USE THIS GUIDE

The information provided in this guide is basic and should not be strictly applied to everyone who is part of a particular religion, culture, generation, or who has a particular disability. In order to obtain religious, cultural, disability, or generational information so you can individualize care, it may be helpful to say to a patient, "I understand that some (name religion, culture, disability, or generation) may like to (name activity, e.g., pray in a quiet space). Would this be helpful for you?" By eliciting the information from the patient, individualized care can be provided, thereby enhancing the patient's experience and providing more personalized care.

This guide provides information in tabular form in order to facilitate its use as a quick reference. Entries in the first three sections of this guide (Religions, Cultures, and Disabilities) are listed alphabetically. Entries in the final section (Generations) are listed in descending age order.

In order to make the information easier and faster to access, we have designated subcategory information with a "▶" prior to the information. Suggestions that might be most relevant to healthcare professionals use a "✓" mark to highlight the information.

CULTURAL TRADITIONS AND PRIVACY CONCERNS

It is important to note that Western Medicine values patient autonomy. However, patients in many cultures may be accustomed to family group decisions. In some cultures the patient information is shared with the family leader (e.g., a senior member of the family) or spokesperson before the information is disclosed to the patient.

The Health Insurance Portability and Accountability Act (HIPAA) does not allow the caregiver to share patient health information with others unless the patient (or guardian) provides explicit permission to do so. Please be aware of this and obtain the appropriate patient permission if the patient would like to have information provided to designated individuals.

NON-ENDORSEMENT

We need to be clear that publishing and circulating this Guide does not imply an endorsement by Florida Hospital—nor by the editors—of any one point of view, set of values, or belief system. Rather, this guide is provided as a resource or compendium of information collected from the literature to help caregivers prepare to ask patients specific questions about their religious, cultural, disability, and generational practices.

It is beyond the scope of this guide to provide a detailed treatment of the subject matter. Information in this document is supported by references listed at the end. An extensive bibliography is also offered for those who wish to delve more deeply into the topics covered.

PROFESSIONAL RESPONSIBILITY

Please keep in mind that the information presented in this guide is presented as reference material only for healthcare providers offering services or treatment to patients. This guide is not intended as a substitute for discussions with YOUR patients concerning their healthcare needs. Each individual is affected by his or her own life experiences and continues to change over time. Depending on the patient's geographical area, number of years his or her family has been in the country, generation, and educational level, the patient may or may not believe or follow the information provided. Therefore, the application or use of this information in a particular situation remains the professional responsibility of the practitioner.

Religions

IN THIS SECTION, INFORMATION IS PROVIDED ON TWENTY OF THE MOST PREVALENT religions, explaining how an individual's religious background may affect his/her needs and expectations as a patient. The following table shows how Americans self-identified with religious identity in 2008.[1]

Religious Identity	% of Americans (2008)
Buddhist	0.6%
Christian	75.0%
Hindu	0.2%
Muslim	0.5%
Jewish	1.2%
Sikh	0.3%

Spirituality and religion have always been an essential component of health and well-being. Research supports this claim that patients who actively participate in a religion enjoy a longer life span and shorter stays in the hospital than those who do not.[2] In modern times, the role of spirituality and religion in medicine includes such practices as the use of meditation and prayer in healing, pastoral counseling, extending compassion, extending the need to forgive or to accept forgiveness, seeking to explain the mystery of death in end-of-life care, and the search for meaning in illness for patients and families, as well as the health professionals who work with them.[3] Integrative medicine recognizes and promotes the importance of making spirituality a part of the healing process. Today healthcare professionals are embracing and encouraging a whole-person or "holistic" approach to providing health care, one that addresses the mind, the body, and the spirit.

A 2004 survey by the National Center for Complementary and Alternative Medicine (NCCAM)[4] of more than 31,000 adults, found that prayer was the most commonly used practice among all the approaches mentioned in the survey:

Of those who responded, 45 percent had used prayer for health reasons, 43 percent had prayed for their own health, close to 25 percent had had others pray for them, and nearly 10 percent had participated in a prayer group for their health. Others reported approaches with a spiritual component that included meditation, yoga, tai chi, qi gong, and energy healing, such as Reiki.[5]

Addressing a patient's spiritual needs has become such an important aspect of healthcare provision that most hospitals now have Pastoral Care departments which help to facilitate patient access to religious leaders for counsel and prayer. In fact, two-thirds of the nation's 125 medical schools now include courses on spirituality and faith in their curricula, up from just three in 1992.[6]

In this section, twenty religions and Christian denominations are presented, outlining how each may impact the healthcare decisions made by the patient. For example, in the "Diet and Nutrition" section, information is based on choices a patient may make from a religious perspective, abstaining from all meat or only certain kinds of meat; in the "Blood" section, whether a patient may refuse a blood transfusion; or "Healing Environment," whether a patient may read Scripture or want to attend a religious service.

Some of the major world religions addressed in this guide include Buddhism, Christianity, Hinduism, Islam, Judaism, and Sikhism.

Buddhism

There are approximately 376 million Buddhists worldwide, accounting for 6 percent of the world's population.[7] Approximately 0.7 percent of the US population identify themselves as Buddhists. It is the fourth largest religion practiced in the US today.[8]

Buddhism teaches that suffering is the result of ignoring true human nature and being self-indulgent. Buddhism encourages harmony of mind, body, emotion, and spirit through meditation in order to achieve optimal health and happiness.

Christianity

Christianity is ranked as the largest religion in the world today with approximately 2 billion followers. It is the most dominant and widespread religion worldwide.[9] Thirty-three percent of the world's population is considered to be Christian, with about 38,000 Christian denominations worldwide. Today in America, about 75 percent of adults, or 159 million Americans, identify themselves as Christian. In comparison, the next largest religions in America are Islam and Judaism. Combined, they represent only about one to two percent of the United States population. In America, there are approximately 1,500 different Christian denominations.[10]

Christians center their lives around one true God who brought the universe into being and sustains it. Christians believe that God is revealed in nature, history, experience, reason, Scripture, and most decisively, in Jesus Christ. They are "people of the book" - the Bible. The Bible is a collection of people's experiences with God from different times and places, collectively telling how their lives should be lived day by day and that Jesus Christ was the incarnation of God on Earth.[11]

Hinduism

There are approximately 850 million Hindus in the world.[12] This represents 13 percent of the world population, making Hinduism the third largest world religion.[13] Eighty and one-half percent of Hindus reside in India. Other countries include Nepal, Bangladesh, Indonesia, Sri Lanka, Pakistan, Indonesia, and other Southeast Asian countries – Malaysia, Singapore, and Thailand. In 2001, the Graduate Center of the City University of New York estimated that there were 766,000 Hindus living in the United States, 0.4 percent of the population.[14]

Believers of the Hindu faith believe that optimal health is achieved through balance between mind, body, and spirit. Hindus believe that by pursuing this balance and wholeness in life they build positive "karma" for their next existence.[15]

Islam (Muslim)

There are approximately 1.57 billion Muslims in the world.[16] This represents 23 percent of the global population of 6.8 billion people. In May 2007, Pew Research Center estimated that there were about 2.35 million Muslims living in the US.[17] In post-9/11, many Muslims and Arab Americans saw erosion of their civil rights and became targets of negative stereotypes and discrimination.[18] To deal with some of these issues, Muslims have begun to establish national, regional, and local Muslim institutions such as the Muslim Public Affairs Council, the Council on American-Islamic Relations, Muslim Students Association, Islamic Society of North America, Institute of Religion and Civil Values, and Council of Religious Scholars.[19]

The Pew survey also indicated that overall Muslims have a positive evaluation of the American public and society, viewing the US as a place where actualizing one's potential with equity and fairness can be achieved. Practically all (99%) view random acts of terrorism against innocent civilians as not justifiable.[20] Unlike Christianity, there is no concept of original sin in Islam. It is believed that every human is born with an unadulterated conscience and a disposition to abide by universal moral and ethical values. However, everyone is tempted and can fall prey to sin and can seek forgiveness. Muslims revere their Islamic faith and its practices such as modesty, even in sickness. Healthcare professionals who respect the seriousness with which Muslims practice their faith will help to show the patient proper care.[21]

Judaism

Judaism is the oldest monotheistic religious system and the first textually-based religion in the Western world. It is primarily concerned with addressing issues of life, health, and healing.[22] In 2007, the Pew Institute estimated the worldwide Jewish population to be approximately 13.2 million persons. Nearly six million live in the State of Israel, while 40 percent, or 5.28 million, are said to live in the United States.[23]

Judaism professes values of sanctity of life and respect for the body. All but three commandments of the Torah (prohibiting murder, rape, and idolatry) may be violated for the sake of saving a life. Existing life has priority over potential life. The body is considered sacred and should not be defiled with tattoos or cuttings. Food considerations are also important within the Jewish faith. Healthcare considerations are central to Judaism and help patients make ethical decisions that impact life and death.

Sikhism

The worldwide Sikh population is estimated to be 20 million. Seventeen million Sikhs reside India, with 14 million in the Punjab region, which is the traditional Sikh homeland.[24] Approximately two million Sikhs live outside of India in such countries as Great Britain, the United States, Canada, East Africa, Malaysia, and Australia.[25] It is estimated that half a million Sikhs live in the United States.[26]

For the Sikh believer religion is central to the practice of health and wellness because health is an ultimate goal in life, in line with the path to the One True God, and disease and sickness is viewed as an attachment of ego.[27] Medical advancement is an instrument which should be used for extending compassion, a key principle for living a righteous life. A Sikh patient's treatment can benefit from an understanding of his/her religious beliefs and practices.[28]

The 20 Religions in this section are (alphabetically):

- Adventist, Seventh-Day

- Amish (Anabaptists)

- Baptist

- Buddhism

- Church of Christ, Scientist

- Church of the Nazarene

- Episcopalian

- Hinduism

- Islam (Muslim)

- Jehovah's Witnesses

- Judaism

- Lutheran

- Mennonite (Anabaptist)

- Methodist, United

- Mormons/Church of Christ of Latter-day Saints

- Pentecostal/Assemblies of God

- Presbyterian

- Roman Catholic

- Sikhism

- Unitarian

Adventist, Seventh–Day

Note: The following information is general. Specific beliefs and practices may vary. Details on page 12.

Legend: ✓ = Suggestions for Healthcare Professionals; ▶ = Significant Details or Exceptions.

CARE OF THE PATIENT

Beliefs	• Holy Scriptures are the Word of God revealing his infallible will, written by men, who were moved by the Holy Spirit[29] • Triune God: God the Father is a merciful, loving, forgiving God; God the Son became man; and God the Holy Spirit guided those who wrote the Bible and helps believers[30] • The Lord's Supper is observed every three months with grape juice; a rite of foot-washing is conducted before the Lord's Supper is served , which symbolizes "service to others"[31] • Plan of salvation centers on Jesus Christ as Savior[32] • Holistic care[33] • Promote prevention/wellness; health is from God[34] • Saturday is Seventh day or Sabbath, which is observed from sundown Friday until sundown Saturday[35] • Sabbath is set apart for worship, fellowship and deeds of mercy; secular activities are avoided[36] • Members value Bible promises, family, good works, nature, cleanliness, fresh air, sunshine, water, exercise and rest, and peaceful music[37, 38]
Blood	• Transfusion and donation may be acceptable[39]
Diet and Nutrition	• No alcohol or tobacco; caffeinated beverages limited by most; encourage vegetarian diet (about 50 percent are vegetarians) and avoidance of high-fat foods[40, 41] • Abstain from eating "unclean foods" as identified in the Old Testament, Leviticus 11:1-47 (i.e. pork, rabbit, carnivorous animals, shellfish, and fish without fins or scales)[42] • Meats are restricted to "kosher" meats as identified in Scriptures[43]
Healing Environment	• Chaplain, Pastor, or other Christians may pray with/for patient[44] • Prayer for sick is important in extending God's healing power[45] • May be comforted by healing prayers with healthcare workers or by "reading Scriptures, listening to religious music, watching televised worship services"[46] • Baptism, the Lord's Supper, or anointing of the sick may be requested[47] • May be anointed if patient or family requests[48] • Provide bright, clean, cheerful environment; express kindness, encouragement, and sympathy[49]

Pain Management	• Christians have responsibility to care for suffering and provide relief[50] • May be comforted by Scriptures and healing prayers[51]

END OF LIFE

Advance Directives	• Up to individual; no church teachings against use[52]
Autopsy	• May be acceptable[53]
Death – Body Care	• Family may wish to view body of deceased before removal from hospital room[54]
Death – Special Needs	• No last rites at death; dead are asleep until Christ returns[55]
Death Process	• Believe death is time of comfort until Second Coming of Jesus; resurrection of body will occur at the Second Coming[56]
DNR	• Follow medical procedures and/or treatments that sustain life;[57] believe individual does not have to accept treatments that only extend dying process[58]
End-of-Life Discussion	✓ Per HIPAA, healthcare professional must obtain patient's permission to disclose health information to third parties ✓ Healthcare professional may ask patient who will make healthcare decisions for them if not themselves ✓ Health professional may discuss patient's terminal illness if applicable
Organ Donation	• Promote organ donation and transplantation[59]
Withholding/Withdrawal	• Up to individual; does not go against church teachings[60]

PERINATAL CARE

Baptism/Birth Ceremony	• No rites of faith practiced at birth; may have baby dedication when child is still young[61] • May request baptism when child is old enough to embrace faith[62] • Baptism is by immersion[63]
Birth Process (Labor/C-Section/Vaginal Birth)	• No specific rituals or traditions for birth[64]
Circumcision	• Up to individual and/or family; no religious recommendations[65]
Contraception	• Birth control is up to individual; use of measures to prevent conception is generally accepted[66] • Barrier methods are acceptable; abortions are not[67]
Genetic Conditions	• If fetus has serious genetic defect, may consider abortion[68]

Neonatal/ Infant End of Life	• No special rites; may wish to have Pastor pray for the dying baby[69]
Post-Partum Care	• No special traditions
Prenatal Care	• No faith prescriptive for prenatal care[70] • For vegetarian mother, may need information on additional nutritional needs during pregnancy and supplements[71] • In vitro is acceptable[72]
Termination of Pregnancy	• In general, abortion not acceptable[73] ▸ May "be considered" in special cases such as rape, incest, "severe congenital defects," or if life of mother is in danger

Amish (Anabaptists)

Note: The following information is general. Specific beliefs and practices may vary. Details on page 12.

Legend: ✓ = Suggestions for Healthcare Professionals; ▶ = Significant Details or Exceptions.

❤ CARE OF THE PATIENT	

Beliefs	• Christian group; belief system stresses lifestyle and peace; Amish are "missionaries by example"[74]
	• Church is composed of adults who freely commit to disciplined lifestyle[75]
	• Amish beliefs include:[76]
	  ▶ Bible teachings
	  ▶ Separation between church and state
	  ▶ Peaceful living
	• As a reflection of belief that they are God's servants, frequently speech is slow and soft to express "humility and meekness"[77]
	• Religious meetings are in members' houses[78]
	• Lifestyle includes daily prayer, Bible reading, worship on Saturday or Sunday[79]

Diet and Nutrition	• Many live on farms where plenty of food is available; have no restrictions in diet[80, 81] • Not usually concerned about diet or weight loss; follow tradition for food preparation without additives; diet is high in "fats and carbohydrates"[82]
Communication	• May not show physical signs of affection; touch is limited[83] • It is important to respect personal space while providing kindness and support[84]
Healing Environment	• Accepts modern medicine to improve health, but understands that good health and healing are God's gift[85] • Believe when one eats well, appearance is good, and is able to work, that person has good health[86] • Families care for their elderly, who are well-respected and valued[87] • May use home remedies, including folk and alternative medicines, before seeking professional healthcare; may not be aware of disease etiology, disease transmission, and immunizations[88] • Extended family and community members may visit to show interest and caring for patient[89] • Amish women usually wear a hair covering at all times; this should not be removed unless necessary[90] • Might not carry medical insurance nor accept any kind of financial help from government; church will assist if unable to pay bills[91]

Healing Environment (continued)	• Schooling usually through elementary years; assessment of knowledge level of patient is important with regards to health care[92]
	✓ Patient may prefer healthcare professional to direct and give straightforward questions and explanations
	✓ Healthcare education should include the family, as appropriate
	✓ Per HIPAA must obtain patient's permission to disclose health information to third parties
	• Many Amish do not have telephones or motorized vehicles[93]
	• Education for the patient's family may include what to do in case of an emergency when there will be a delay in getting to medical help
Blood	• Transfusion and donation may be acceptable[94]
Pain Management	• Generally does not verbalize or express pain or emotion; children are generally very quiet in presence of unfamiliar person or place; may deny pain in presence of healthcare worker, although pain is severe[95]
	• Believes that suffering allows one to become closer to God[96]

END OF LIFE

Advance Directives	• Does not normally have advance directives[97]
Autopsy	• May be acceptable, if required by law[98]
Death – Body Care	• May accept hospital practices; no prescribed rite for preparation of body[99]
Death – Special Needs	• May prefer to die at home[100]
	• In certain communities patient may request anointing prior to death; anointing signifies forgiveness of sins[101]
Death Process	• Community will support and help individual deal with loss[102]
	• Family may not be emotional at death of patient since death is considered a step toward "eternal life with God"[103]
DNR	• Focus on quality of life; seldom consider heroics to extend life[104]
End-of-Life Discussion	✓ Per HIPAA, healthcare professional must obtain patient's permission to disclose health information to third parties
	✓ Healthcare professional may ask patient who will make healthcare decisions for them if not themselves
	✓ Health professional may discuss patient's terminal illness if applicable
Organ Donation	• May not agree to transplantation if outcome is uncertain for the recipient; otherwise, accept transplantation[105]
Withholding/Withdrawal	• Individual decision; delaying death is not encouraged; fatalistic attitude that death is "God's will" and consider the cost for extensive procedures and life prolonging treatments[106]

PERINATAL CARE

Adoption	• Adoption is supported[107]
Birth Process (Labor/C-Section/Vaginal Birth)	• Believe that having children is woman's highest goal; birth causes few changes in mother's life[108] • Since one must be able to reason to freely choose church, children are considered a part of God's kingdom until they reach "the age of reason"[109] • Amish may prefer home birth; Cesarean section is prohibited for Amish and may result in "excommunication from community"[110]
Breastfeeding	• Some mothers will breastfeed. May only breastfeed for 6 weeks so that mother can return to pre-pregnancy lifestyle[111]
Circumcision	• Up to individual, not a religious issue[112]
Contraception	• Traditionally do not support birth control[113] • Discussion of sex is prohibited in most Amish families[114] ✓Patient may prefer not to discuss sexual matters
Family/Father involvement	• Husband may be present for birth[115]
Genetic Conditions	• Many in a community are related by marriage; genetic issues may arise from intermarriages[116] • All infants, including those with serious birth anomalies, are integrated into the Amish lifestyle; each infant is a "gift from God"[117]
Neonatal Illness	• If newborn is ill, Amish consider it "God's will"[118]
Neonatal/Infant End of Life	• If newborn dies, Amish consider it "God's will"[119] • Life is gift from God; if infant is disabled by condition, family will care for infant at home[120]
Newborn Care	• Typically begin solid foods at six weeks when mother returns to routine duties; may increase likelihood of allergies[121]
Post-Partum Care	• May resume normal role in a few days post birth[122]
Prenatal Care	• Prenatal care may be minimal, late in gestation, or not at all, especially with subsequent pregnancies[123] • With uncomplicated first birth in hospital will probably have following pregnancies delivered at home[124] • In vitro: Generally do not practice[125]
Termination of Pregnancy	• Abortion not acceptable[126]

PEDIATRICS

Child/Teen Environment of Care	• Children are generally very quiet in presence of unfamiliar person or place; may deny pain in presence of healthcare worker, even when pain is severe[127] • Parents usually stay with children when hospitalized[128]

Baptist

Note: The following information is general. Specific beliefs and practices may vary. Details on page 12.

Legend: ✓ = Suggestions for Healthcare Professionals; ▶ = Significant Details or Exceptions.

[Note: There are more than sixty Baptist denominations in the USA, plus many other baptistic denominations not named in this document; though some doctrines may differ, most embrace the beliefs and practices listed below.]

♥ CARE OF THE PATIENT

Beliefs	• Christian, with each church independent but holding common beliefs[129] ▶ Bible provides guidance for life; Jesus Christ is Lord ▶ Individual freedom to communicate directly with God ▶ Salvation through faith in Christ • Ordinances: Baptism and Communion[130] • All life (including health and healing) comes from God[131] • Believe in responsibility to share faith and do mission work[132]
Blood	• Transfusion may be acceptable[133]
Diet and Nutrition	• No alcohol;[134] use of tobacco may be acceptable
Healing Environment	• Scripture reading, music, televised worship services[135] • May be comforted with healing prayers[136]

END OF LIFE

Advance Directives	• No church position, but up to individual[137]
Autopsy	• May be acceptable[138]
Death – Body Care	• Family may request to see body before removal from hospital room[139]
Death – Special Needs	• May consult Chaplain for assistance[140] • May request Lord's Supper, prayer for dying, readings of Scripture texts[141]
Death Process	• Belief in "life with God" after death[142]
End-of-Life Discussion	✓ Per HIPAA, healthcare professional must obtain patient's permission to disclose health information to third parties ✓ Healthcare professional may ask patient who will make healthcare decisions for them if not themselves ✓ Health professional may discuss patient's terminal illness if applicable
Organ Donation	• Transplant may be acceptable if it will improve life of recipient[143]
Withholding/Withdrawal	• In futile cases, withholding or withdrawal does not go against teachings; up to individual[144]

PERINATAL CARE	
Baptism/Birth Ceremony	• Baptism by immersion; no infant baptism[145] • Baby dedication: May present infant at church services where parents affirm their responsibility for raising the infant[146]
Circumcision	• Generally practiced, not a religious mandate[147]
Prenatal Care	• In vitro: Various opinions in different Baptist groups; generally discouraged, but is individual decision[148]
Termination of Pregnancy	• Abortion generally not acceptable[149]

Buddhism

Note: The following information is general. Specific beliefs and practices may vary. Details on page 12.

Legend: ✓ = Suggestions for Healthcare Professionals; ▶ = Significant Details or Exceptions.

♥ CARE OF THE PATIENT	
Beliefs	• No God, but Buddha is honored as having set a model lifestyle[150]
	• Does not prescribe means to reach ultimate goal of Nirvana; belief in re-incarnation; healing does not occur through faith alone[151]
	• Buddha provided four "Noble Truths":
	▶ Life includes suffering
	▶ Desire for sensual gratification leads to suffering
	▶ If one gives up worldly desires, can eliminate suffering and attain Nirvana
	▶ The path to Nirvana is "eight-fold"[152]
	• Believe that doing good deeds in this life will improve/raise the state that one is born into in the next life[153]
	• May use prayer beads to help meditate[154]
	• Promotes harmony; believe group benefit supersedes individual[155]
Blood	• Transfusion may be acceptable[156]
Communication	• Depending on the culture, touch may not be appropriate; clinician may want to wait to see if patient extends a hand[157]
	• May "chant out loud"[158]
Diet and Nutrition	• Food taken in moderation; may avoid eating some foods together[159]
	• Prohibits alcohol; some branches of Buddhism may require diets with no meat[160]
	• Generally, a healthy diet is recommended[161]
Healing Environment	• Family and community may support patient by visiting[162]
	• Illness is a result of action taken or events that occurred in this or previous life; may believe peace from Buddha's wisdom is factor in "healing and recovery process"[163]
Pain Management	• Suffering is part of living[164]
	• May refuse pain medication due to concern about effect of medication on thoughts and clarity of mind[165]
🏥 END OF LIFE	
Autopsy	• May be acceptable[166]

Death – Body Care	• Body should not be moved before Priest arrives[167] ✓ When moving the body, family may prefer staff to "avoid jostling" because of the belief that the spirit remains with body for some time after death[168]
Death – Special Needs	• No death ceremony[169] • May have rites with "chanting at bedside soon after death"[170]
Death Process	• When patient is dying, allow patient undisturbed times for meditation to mentally prepare for death; Buddhist Priest should be notified after patient's death in order to pray with body[171] • Patient may read Scripture to help prepare for passage to next life[172] • Patient desires a clear mind, especially at end of life[173]
DNR	• If recovery is possible, all support is encouraged[174]
End-of-Life Discussion	✓ Per HIPAA, healthcare professional must obtain patient's permission to disclose health information to third parties ✓ Healthcare professional may ask patient who will make healthcare decisions for them if not themselves ✓ Health professional may discuss patient's terminal illness if applicable
Organ Donation	• No religious position regarding organ donation; up to individual[175] • Religious values of compassion and helping others support concept of organ donation[176]

 PERINATAL CARE

Baptism/Birth Ceremony	• No baptism[177]
Contraception	• No restriction on birth control[178]
Genetic Conditions	• Condition may be considered "karma"[179]
Neonatal/ Infant End of Life	• Parents may seek special rituals by local leaders of their faith to counteract the lack of preparation by the baby/child for death[180]
Prenatal Care	• Woman who is expecting may not attend funerals; thought to be unlucky for fetus[181]
Termination of Pregnancy	• Abortion may be acceptable. Respect for life.[182] • Patient's health status and circumstances may be considered when making a decision about abortion[183]

PEDIATRICS

Child/Teen Environment of Care	• In case of child's death, parents may seek special rituals by local leaders of their faith to counteract the lack of preparation by the child for death[184]

Church of Christ, Scientist

Note: The following information is general. Specific beliefs and practices may vary. Details on page 12.

Legend: ✓ = Suggestions for Healthcare Professionals; ▶ = Significant Details or Exceptions.

❤ CARE OF THE PATIENT	
Beliefs	• Believe each person is inseparable from God who created everything; everything reflects God's goodness[185] • Belief based on Bible (King James) and text "Science and Health With Key to the Scriptures" by Mary Baker Eddy, founder of the Church of Christ, Scientist[186] • Doctrine: healing can be effected by prayers, therefore, they do not seek medical treatments; healing is natural result of becoming "closer to God"[187, 188] • Church has individuals with title of "Nurse" who have received training in the teachings of the church to provide non-medical care; a "Practitioner" is one who practices "Christian Science healing through prayer"[189] • Church teachings indicate that golden rule should be foundation of all actions; sin results when we "try to live apart from God"[190] • Each individual has "a unique relationship with God" and a unique spirituality[191] • Described as "religious teaching and practice based on words and works of Christ Jesus" who is called the "Way-Shower"[192] • Believe following the words of the Bible will lead to eternal Life[193] • Disease comes from mental state that can be remedied by practicing Christian discipleship and following what Jesus taught[194] • Church may have visiting/home nurse service[195] • Worship with "music, singing, and prayer and readings" on Sunday; meet on Wednesdays for similar service and individuals share experiences in healing[196]
Blood	• Transfusion not acceptable[197] [In cases of children of Christian Scientists needing transfusion, the law may intervene.]
Diet and Nutrition	• May avoid alcohol, tobacco, and drugs[198]
Healing Environment	• Individual choice is very important to members; each determines what is best after prayer[199] • May use prayer to seek a cure[200] • May request healthcare professional allow time for the patient to resolve health issue through his/her Christian Science faith[201] • Member who request medical treatment may ask to have drugs and therapy minimized[202] • Church may have visiting/home nurse service[203]

Healing Environment (continued)	• Will avoid most testing and medical care, which Christian Scientists "believe is in violation of their religious beliefs"[204] ✓ Patient may prefer to discuss acceptable treatment options • Believe that God can heal all conditions; however, may seek help from medical system for fractures[205]
Pain Management	• May use prayer[206]

🛏 END OF LIFE

Advance Directives	• Up to the individual[207]
Autopsy	• Up to individual or family[208]
Death – Body Care	• Recommend that when the deceased church member is female, the body be attended by women[209]
Death – Special Needs	• No ceremony at death of patient; believe death is but a phase of life[210] • Term "passed on" is used to indicate that this life has ended and that there is continuity for the deceased in another life [210]
Death Process	• Family may pray for patient's recovery until patient dies[211] • There are no church "last rites"[212]
DNR	• Pray for recovery but do not seek heroics or extending life through medical treatments[213]
End-of-Life Discussion	• Believe God can heal all conditions; do not generally take medications, agree to biopsies or exams; do not usually want to extend life[214] ✓ Per HIPAA, healthcare professional must obtain patient's permission to disclose health information to third parties ✓ Healthcare professional may ask patient who will make healthcare decisions for them if not themselves ✓ Health professional may discuss patient's terminal illness if applicable
Organ Donation	• There are no church restrictions on organ donation, up to individual[215] • Rely on spiritual healing, not physical; from that standpoint may not agree to transplant, donate, or receive organ[216]
Withholding/Withdrawal	• Up to individual or family[217]

👶 PERINATAL CARE

Baptism/Birth Ceremony	• Baptism is not practiced[218]
Birth Process (Labor/C- Section/ Vaginal Birth)	• May prefer home birth if possible[219] • No church rites at birth[220]

Circumcision	• Decided by parent or individual[221]
Contraception	• Birth control decided by individual[222] • Discourage use of oral contraceptives because they are drugs[223]
Prenatal Care	• Prenatal care is up to individual[224] • In vitro: no church position; up to individuals[225]
Termination of Pregnancy	• Abortion not acceptable[226]

PEDIATRICS

Child/Teen Environment of Care	• In some cases, parents have been taken to court to get authority to treat seriously ill minors[227]

Church of the Nazarene

Note: The following information is general. Specific beliefs and practices may vary. Details on page 12.

Legend: ✓ = Suggestions for Healthcare Professionals; ▶ = Significant Details or Exceptions.

♥ CARE OF THE PATIENT	
Beliefs	• Holy Scriptures are the Word of God revealing his infallible will, written by men, who were moved by the Holy Spirit[228] • Triune God: God the Father is a merciful, loving, forgiving God; God the Son became man; and God the Holy Spirit guided those who wrote the Bible and helps believers[229] • Local churches vary on how often Lord's Supper is observed. Only unfermented wine is used in this sacrament[230] • Plan of salvation centers on Jesus Christ as Savior[231]
Blood	• Transfusion and donation may be acceptable[232]
Diet and Nutrition	• Tend to abstain from habit-forming products like alcohol and tobacco[233]
Healing Environment	• Chaplain, Pastor or other Christians pray with/for patient[234] • Prayer for sick is very important in extending God's healing power[235] • Believe in the biblical doctrine of divine healing and believers are urged to seek and offer the prayer of faith for the healing of the sick[236] • Believe God heals through the means of medical science[237] • Baptism, the Lord's Supper, or anointing of the sick may be requested[238] • Anointing may be done if patient or family requests[239] • Provide bright, clean, cheerful environment; express kindness, encouragement and sympathy[240]
Pain Management	• No restrictions on use of pain medication[241] • Have a responsibility to care for the suffering and provide relief[242] • May be comforted by Scriptures and healing prayers[243]

🛏 END OF LIFE	
Advance Directives	• Up to individual; no church teachings against use[244]
Autopsy	• May be acceptable[245]
Death – Body Care	• Family may wish to view body of deceased before removal from hospital room[246]
Death – Special Needs	• No last rites at death; dead are asleep until Christ returns[247]

Death Process	• When death is imminent, either withdrawing or not originating artificial life-support systems is permissible within the range of Christian faith and practice[248] ▸ Applies to persons in a persistent vegetative state, where the application of extraordinary means for prolonging life provide no reasonable hope for a return to health[249] • Euthanasia (including physician-assisted suicide) is not permitted[250]
DNR	• Follow all medical procedures and/or treatments that sustain life, however, believe individual does not have to accept treatments that only extend dying process[251]
End-of-Life Discussion	• Trust in God's faithfulness and have the hope of eternal life, which makes it possible to accept death as an expression of faith in Christ, who overcame death on our behalf and robbed it of its victory[252] ✓ Per HIPAA, healthcare professional must obtain patient's permission to disclose health information to third parties ✓ Healthcare professional may ask patient who will make healthcare decisions for them if not themselves ✓ Health professional may discuss patient's terminal illness if applicable
Organ Donation	• Encourages its members who do not object personally to support donor/recipient anatomical organs through living wills and trusts[253]
Withholding/Withdrawal	• Up to individual; does not go against church teachings[254]

PERINATAL CARE

Baptism/Birth Ceremony	• No rites of faith practiced at birth[255] • Believe in child dedication where baby is brought into sanctuary and a prayer of dedication is offered to the Lord[256] • Baptism is requested when child is old enough to embrace faith[257] • Baptism is by sprinkling, pouring, or immersion, according to the choice of the applicant[258]
Birth Process (Labor/C-Section/Vaginal Birth)	• No specific rituals or traditions related to birth[259]
Breastfeeding	• Up to individual; no religious recommendations; encourage whatever is best for the baby[260]
Circumcision	• Up to individual, family; no religious recommendations[261]
Genetic Conditions	• Supports the use of genetic engineering to achieve gene therapy[262] • Recognizes that gene therapy can lead to preventing and curing disease, and preventing and curing anatomical and mental disorders[263]

Genetic Conditions (continued)	• Genetic engineering: Opposes any use that promotes social injustice, disregards the dignity of persons, or that attempts to achieve racial, intellectual, or social superiority over others (eugenics)[264] • DNA studies: Opposes any studies that might encourage or support human abortion as an alternative to term live birth[265]
Neonatal/ Infant End of Life	• No special rites; may wish to have Pastor pray for the dying baby[266]
Prenatal Care	• No faith prescriptive for prenatal care[267]
Termination of Pregnancy	• Responsible opposition[268] • Provide a support system with the initiation and support of programs designed to provide care for mothers and children[269]

Episcopalian

Note: The following information is general. Specific beliefs and practices may vary. Details on page 12.

Legend: ✓ = Suggestions for Healthcare Professionals; ▶ = Significant Details or Exceptions.

CARE OF THE PATIENT

Beliefs	• Bible (Old and New Testaments) provides all that is needed for salvation; it is the "ultimate standard of faith"[270]
	• People, guided by the Holy Spirit, wrote the Scriptures, which members are to use for guidance while making moral decisions[271]
	• Believe:[272]
	  ▶ Triune-based faith: one God in three - Father, Son, and Holy Spirit
	  ▶ Incarnation of Jesus, "fully human and fully divine"
	  ▶ Members are part of entire Body of Christ, which is all baptized individuals
	  ▶ With baptism, the Holy Spirit resides in the Christian, allowing growth in Christ
	• Two sacraments: Baptism and Lord's Supper[273]
	• Communal worship, on Sundays and at other times[274]
	• Believe God is "ultimate source of all life, health, and healing"[275]
	• Evangelism as well as mission work is important to many Episcopalians[276]
	• "Daughter" of the Church of England[277]

Blood	• Transfusion and donation may be acceptable[278]
Diet and Nutrition	• No religious restrictions; some fast before receiving Lord's Supper[279]
Healing Environment	• Comfort may be obtained from reading Scriptures or other religious material, listening to religious music, watching worship services, or from healing prayers[280]
Pain Management	• Promotes palliative care[281]

END OF LIFE

Advance Directives	• Encourages the use of advance directives[282]
Autopsy	• Individual decision[283]
Death – Body Care	• Family may request to see deceased before removal from hospital room[284]
Death – Special Needs	• Baptism may be requested; sprinkling is acceptable[285] • May request Lord's Supper[286]

Death Process	• Hospice care is acceptable[287] • Soul and spirit go to heaven at death; resurrection of body with reunion of "spirit, soul and body" will occur at Second Coming of Jesus"[288]
DNR	• Acceptable to decline heroics in futile case[289]
End-of-Life Discussion	• Discussion about care in terminal case should include patient/surrogate[290] ✓ Per HIPAA, healthcare professional must obtain patient's permission to disclose health information to third parties ✓ Healthcare professional may ask patient who will make healthcare decisions for them if not themselves ✓ Health professional may discuss patient's terminal illness if applicable
Organ Donation	• Acceptable, up to individual[291]
Withholding/Withdrawal	• Individual decision; no restrictions in medically futile cases[292]

PERINATAL CARE

Baptism/Birth Ceremony	• Sacrament of baptism by pouring water or immersion, conducted by Priest[293] • Family may request baptism; consult Chaplain or clergy[294]
Circumcision	• No religious indications; individual decision[295]
Contraception	• No restrictions regarding birth control[296]
Neonatal Illness	• Acceptable to decline heroics in a futile case[297]
Prenatal Care	• No restrictions regarding in-vitro fertilization[298]
Termination of Pregnancy	• Not acceptable as method of birth control[299] • Individual decision; acceptable to support mother's health, mental and physical[300]

Hinduism

Note: The following information is general. Specific beliefs and practices may vary. Details on page 12.

Legend: ✓ = Suggestions for Healthcare Professionals; ▶ = Significant Details or Exceptions.

CARE OF THE PATIENT	

Beliefs	• Hinduism is the belief system of the majority of East Indians[301]
	• Worship practice varies depending on community[302]
	• Religion "is a way of life"[303]
	• Basic teachings:[304]
	  ▶ Soul is divine
	  ▶ One "Reality" (Brahman); there is one God
	  ▶ One God, but many manifestations ("Truth is one; sages call it by various names")
	  ▶ All religions lead to same end goal
	• Individual interprets teachings, which is verified through personal life experience[305]
	• "Creation, preservation, and dissolution" are endless cycles as creation cannot occur from nothing[306]
	• Karma: Individual has accountability for thoughts, words and deeds; cause and effect gives individual incentive to act morally correct[307]
	• Reincarnation: Many cycles of life, striving for ultimate goal of raising consciousness to highest level[308]
	• Four goals of life:[309]
	  ▶ Dharma: Duty to self and society
	  ▶ Artha: Need for material goods
	  ▶ Kama: Desire for pleasure of the senses, legitimately
	  ▶ Moksha: Seeking the ultimate goal, "Liberation," in which one is freed from repeated life cycles
	• Rituals and prayers: Call upon divine presence[310]
	• Promote "ayurveda" ("life science") which is positive attitude to health and maintaining the balance between "body humors;" imbalance in these causes illness[311]
	• Practice mutual tolerance and believe all ways to God are acceptable[312]
	• There is no single belief system:[313]
	  ▶ Some believe in "faith" healing others
	  ▶ Some believe health problems are from God as punishment
	  ▶ Some believe in reincarnation, which depends on one's "moral behavior" in this life

Blood	• Transfusion may be acceptable[314]
	• Blood is viewed as precious; may refuse to have lab drawn and provide for blood donations[315]
Communication	• Greet with palms together and a bow of the head toward the person they are greeting to recognize the person and the person's soul[316]
	✓Patient may prefer healthcare professional to verbally greet patient's husband or oldest female present before greeting female patient[317]
	• Shaking hands is common but only between two people of the same sex[318]
	• Unless married, eye contact between two people of opposite sex is seen as disrespectful[319]
Diet and Nutrition	• Religious fasting is common; ill are not obliged to fast but may choose to fast to promote healing; special permission may be obtained to eat fruits, vegetables, etc., for fasting individuals with health issues[320]
	• May be lactose intolerant[321]
	• Consider a good digestive system essential to good health and place emphasis on diet[322]
	• Strict rules for food preparation[323]
	• Many eat no meat; those who eat meat usually eat no beef or pork [324]
	• Many do not take alcohol or caffeine[325]
	• During meals Hindus only use right hands to feed themselves[326]
	• Will clean his/her mouth "with water before and after meals"[327]
Healing Environment	• Daily bath is required; not acceptable to add cold water to hot in preparing for bath[328]
	• Patient may refuse bath after meal[329]
	• Personal care is done with left hand[330]
	• After toileting, may wish to bathe with water[331]
	• Prayer and "ritual cleansing" of left hand is very important[332]
	• Hindu female may prefer female doctor[333, 334]
	• Hindus of either gender prefer to wear clothing under hospital gowns; for procedures, clothing covers private areas[335]
	• Family may want to do hands-on care for patient; extended family may remain at hospital when member is admitted[336]
	• Family is very important; hierarchical system with father or oldest son at head; however decisions are result of vote by family members[337]
	• Include both husband and wife in conversations about medical information, then leave them alone to make a decision[338]
	✓Patient may prefer healthcare professional to ask questions or discuss issues with family spokesperson
	✓Per HIPAA, healthcare professional must obtain patient's permission to disclose health information to third parties

Healing Environment (continued)	• Many Hindu diabetics do not take insulin made from animals, so explain what insulin contains before administering it[339] • Prefer natural and homeopathic medicine to drugs and surgery. If drugs are given, explain what they're for and what effects they'll have[340] • May request injections. Believes that illness can only be cured if treatment includes injections[341]
Pain Management	• Patient may accept some interventions for relief[342] • May be concerned about possible addiction and consequently refuse pain medication or reduce the dosage[343] • Patient may refuse pain medication that does not allow for a clear mind at the time of death[344]

END OF LIFE

Advance Directives	• Encourages the use of advance directives[345]
Autopsy	• Autopsy is avoided unless required by law[346]
Death – Body Care	• Deceased's body is typically prepared by bathing, anointing with oil, and covering with white fabric. The family usually does the cleaning and dressing rather than leaving it to strangers.[347] • Items such as a piece of thread around the neck or wrist (signifying that Hindu Priest blessed the patient) or red mark on forehead should remain[348] • Arrangements for deceased are made by the oldest son[349] • Body must be cremated[350]

Death – Special Needs	• Small wishes of the dying patient for food should be fulfilled[351]
	• Family may desire to have sweet basil dipped in water from the Ganges or milk placed on lips of patient[352]
	✓ Patient may prefer to consult Hindu temple or Chaplain
	• Family may desire to place a picture of a "Personal Deity" near the patient[353]
	• Family may ask Hindu Temple Priest to provide spiritual support for patient when dying; support is provided by chanting mantras, songs, and encouraging patient to visualize the image of God[354]
	• Other support practices include:[355, 356]
	  ▸ Tying blessed thread around neck/wrist of dying patient
	  ▸ Sprinkling holy water
	  ▸ Basil leaf placed on tongue
	  ▸ Reminding dying that the real "Self" is immortal

Death Process	• May desire health care professional to discuss "terminal illness" only with family, not patient[357] • At death, the soul continues and will return in "another body"[358]

Death Process (continued)	• Soul reincarnates until all necessary karmas are created and resolved[359] • According to Scripture, the dying person obtains object of thinking at time of death; goal is to raise spiritual consciousness at time of death[360] • Prayers, chants for soul's passing from this life to next; ceremonies following death usually last for thirteen days[361]
DNR	• Artificially prolonging life viewed as interfering with karma[362]
End-of-Life Discussion	• Death passage is part of the life cycle, balancing out birth passage into life; deceased enters into another life[363] • Heroics to extend life are acceptable[364] ✓ Per HIPAA, healthcare professional must obtain patient's permission to disclose health information to third parties ✓ Healthcare professional may ask patient who will make healthcare decisions for them if not themselves ✓ Health professional may discuss patient's terminal illness if applicable
Organ Donation	• Not generally accepted, as it does not allow for completed release of the soul of the donor[365] • View varies as to whether the Hindu will receive an organ donation; may be acceptable if likely that there will be a good quality of life afterward. For some, heart transplant may not be acceptable because of the belief that the heart is "the seat of the soul"[366]
Withholding/Withdrawal	• Does not encourage prolonging death[367] ✓ Patient may prefer healthcare professional to discuss withdrawal of heroics with nearest kin or authorized representative before removing

👤 PERINATAL CARE

Birth Process (Labor/C-Section/ Vaginal Birth)	• May prefer female doctor and nurse for delivery[368] • Mother may practice tradition of rest for 40 days after birth; child remains with mother except for medical reasons[369] • For 10 days after birth, only midwife or MD touches mother and infant due to belief that they are impure[370] • Elders may take part in care for neonate[371] • Hindu ritual of welcoming may be performed at birth; mantras said for long and happy life[372]
Breastfeeding	• Breastfeeding is preferred—many times up to two or three years old; if must feed formula, ensure it has no animal byproducts except milk[373]
Circumcision	• Circumcision is not a religious tradition; up to parents[374]
Contraception	• All types of birth control are acceptable[375]

Family/Father Involvement	• Husband may attend delivery in hospital. May choose to not be present should the birth take place in the home[376]
Fetal/End of Life	• Parents may desire to bury deceased fetus[377]
Genetic Conditions	• Accept "genetic therapy and genetic screening"[378]
Neonatal/ Infant End of Life	• Parents may desire to bury deceased infant[379]
Prenatal Care	• Certain foods are avoided in belief that they may cause "miscarriage or fetal abnormalities"[380] • Hindus may offer prayers to protect unborn and to petition for a male child[381] • In vitro: acceptable when donors are husband and wife[382]
Termination of Pregnancy	• Abortion is prohibited in Hindu scriptures[383]

Islam (Muslim)

Note: The following information is general. Specific beliefs and practices may vary. Details on page 12.

Legend: ✓ = Suggestions for Healthcare Professionals; ▶ = Significant Details or Exceptions.

❤ CARE OF THE PATIENT	

Beliefs	• Believe in one God, Allah[384]
	• Believe there will be a "day of judgment" for all[385]
	• Individual communicates directly with Allah; no religious intermediary[386]
	• Imam guides faithful in religious and spiritual matters[387]
	• Faithful are called Muslims[388]
	• Most follow Sunni (90% of world's Muslims) or Shi'ite traditions[389]
	• Qur'an was revealed to Mohammad, prophet[390]
	• Fundamentals of faith in Qur'an include directions for daily life, marriage, economics, politics, and worship[391]
	• There are five "Pillars of Faith:"[392]
	  ▶ There is one God
	  ▶ Pray five times a day
	  ▶ Donate money to support poor
	  ▶ Fast in Ramadan
	  ▶ Make pilgrimage to Mecca, if possible
	• Prayer is very important[393]
	  ▶ Done after rite of cleansing
	  ▶ Personal cleanliness associated with purity of spirit
	• May use prayer mats, rug, or towel for prayer[394]
	• Prayer rug and Qur'an should not be touched by anyone "ritually unclean" (e.g., with blood or urine on hand); nothing should be placed on top[395]
	• May wear amulet (which should not be removed) with words from Qur'an in or on it[396]
	• Talismans are often used for the ill; should not be removed unless necessary and only after discussion with patient, or in the case of incapacitation or death, children, the parents[397]
	• Other:[398,399]
	  ▶ Children are duty-bound to take care of their parents
	  ▶ Premarital sex prohibited; abstinence expected of male and female until marriage

Blood	• Transfusion may be acceptable[400]

Communication	• Culture may dictate no handshakes or contact between opposite sexes[401]
	• There is no touching during casual conversation by non-family members from opposite gender (e.g., shaking hands); some avoid eye contact due to modesty[402]
Diet and Nutrition	• No pork, blood, or alcohol[403]
	• No shellfish[404]
	• Prayers are usually said before eating[405]
	• Unless ill, fast daily during day in Ramadan (Ninth month in Muslim calendar); "abstain from food, drink, sexual intercourse, evil intentions, and actions"[406]
	• Non-nutritive medications are acceptable, except orally, when fasting; nutritive solutions, (e.g., TPN) nullify fasting; if these are required, patient should not fast[407]
	• May refuse hospital food[408]
	• May use herbal remedies[409]
	• May refuse medications that contain alcohol as an ingredient[410]
	• Patient with diabetes will not take pork insulin[411]
	• May consider GI tract condition as a reflection of overall health[412]
	• Eating and elimination are very important[413]
	• May consider NOT eating (NPO) as a prelude to becoming ill[414]
Healing Environment	• Family and friends assist; there is no formal church assistance or prayer for sick[415]
	• Whenever possible, a patient's bed should be placed facing Mecca[416]
	• Purity of female is associated with family honor[417]
	• "Extreme modesty" is necessary in treating the female patient[418]
	• Female patient may wish to have notice on door "please knock" to warn them of someone planning to enter room[419]
	• Muslim clothing restrictions require a woman's body to be completely covered, including the head. Allow Muslim woman to wear own gown[420]
	• Left hand (used for washing self) is considered unclean[421]
	• Cleansing rites practiced for females after monthly period stops, postpartum, and after toileting for all Muslims[422]
	• Prays 5 times daily at specific times facing Mecca, preceded by washing "face, hands, and feet"[423]
	• Patient who cannot wash may use "dry cleansing (tayammum)" by which "he strikes his hands on a clean surface, and then brushes his palms over his hands and face"[424]
	• When Qur'an is read out loud, Muslims show respect by remaining silent, not eating or drinking; others should also be respectful during this time[425]
	• May prefer healthcare worker or provider to be same sex as patient[426]

Healing Environment (continued)	• Patient may request Imam who is "looked upon to facilitate interpretation of religious rulings at the level of individual patient;" patient's autonomy is "exercised via a conscious transfer to the chosen religious adviser"[427] • Muslim physicians or other Muslim providers on staff should be identified who will act as liaisons with Muslim patients[428] ✓ Patient may prefer to establish relationship with local Imam or Muslim leader for religious support
Pain Management	• Express pain verbally and with body language[429] • Pain may be considered a "test of faith," but Muslim faith dictates seeking relief from pain when necessary[430] • May refuse medication to relieve pain if they believe pain is spiritually helpful[431]

END OF LIFE

Advance Directives	• Faith dictates the ill obtain medical care; when treatment only prolongs dying, may refuse treatment[432] • May allow cessation of life support that has been initiated if it is determined that patient would not have agreed to life support[433]
Autopsy	• Not acceptable, except where required by law[434]
Death – Body Care	• After death, family member of like sex will prepare body in prescribed rites, including washing and rinsing of dead body[435]
Death – Special Needs	• Unless otherwise prescribed, healthcare worker may use gloves to remove lines and turn patient's head to right shoulder, close eyes and mouth, straighten body[436] • At death, patient's face should be turned toward Mecca (Saudi Arabia)[437] • Family may arrange for men to pray over patient who has died[438] • Family may grieve loudly at death, may shed tears; loud wailing, self-flagellation, rending garments, complaining, or cursing not promoted[439] • Although brain death is recognized by some Islamic scholars, end-of-life rituals are done when the body has become cold and rigor mortis is evident[440] • Allow family to stay with patient and continue rituals until signs of death have become apparent[441]
Death Process	• Family remains with dying patient, share words from Qur'an[442] • Islamic prayers should be recited as patient is dying[443] • "Brain death" is not seen as equivalent to death[444]
DNR	• May agree to DNR after discussion of terminal situation[445] • Believe discussing a terminal situation with the patient will cause death to occur earlier[446]

End-of-Life Discussion	✓ Per HIPAA, healthcare professional must obtain patient's permission to disclose health information to third parties ✓ Healthcare professional may ask patient who will make healthcare decisions for them if not themselves ✓ Health professional may discuss patient's terminal illness if applicable • When disease is terminal or there is no cure, the physician is to give a positive message to patient without lying[447] • Believes life and death are determined by God, therefore medical providers should not say anything definite to patient "about future prognosis"[448] • Recommend physician be compassionate, including the possibility of recovery "by the permission of God" thereby offering hope[449] • Muslim family immigrants may expect physician to give negative news privately to the head of the family rather than the patient[450] • American-raised Muslim may be more accepting of characteristic American disclosure in an open and frank manner[451] • The concept of futility is not widely recognized; the physician may be seen as abandoning patient or exaggerating poor prognosis[452] • Recommend the discussion be approached with help of Muslim cleric or Imam, or a Muslim physician[453]

Organ Donation	• Arab Muslim transplant may be acceptable if:[454]
	  ‣ It is only treatment that will resolve health issue
	  ‣ Success is highly probable
	  ‣ Donor or next of kin has given consent
	  ‣ Donor's death has been confirmed by Muslim doctors or living donor will be in no peril
	• Full discussion has included the transplant surgery and consequences
	• Indian Muslim: Culture does not permit transplant[455]

Withholding/Withdrawal	• Believe discussing a terminal situation with the patient will cause death to occur earlier[456] • Duties include providing "food and hydration" to the dying unless those measures would hasten death[457] • In futile care cases, withholding/ withdrawal of therapy is acceptable[458] • May allow withdrawal of life support (respirator); a minority of Islamic scholars (mostly Shi'ite) do not consider withholding and withdrawing equivalent[459] • Shi'ite do not permit withdrawal once initiated[460] • In decisions about life support, usually the father or oldest son makes a decision after consulting a Muslim scholar[461]

PERINATAL CARE

Adoption	• Not acceptable to change surname or for child to lose connections with biological parents[462]
Baptism/Birth Ceremony	• African Muslim: ceremony for naming newborn on seventh day; ritual circumcisions are performed after that[463]
Birth Process (Labor/C-Section/ Vaginal Birth)	• Husband is permitted at delivery; if husband is not present, female who is family or friend should be allowed[464] • Father or grandfather recites prayers in baby's ears after birth[465] • After birth, the placenta should be offered to parents for burial in Muslim tradition[466]
Breastfeeding	• Breastfeeding promoted; not mandatory, but sacred Scripture recommends two years for breastfeeding[467] • May give baby honey or water instead of colostrum[468] • Lack of sunlight (due to dress and veil) may result in low Vitamin D levels in lactating mother, risking deficiency of Vitamin D in baby[469]
Circumcision	• Practice male circumcision[470]
Contraception	• Birth control permitted for married; must prevent fertilization and not cause damage to reproduction capabilities[471] • Spouses agree and sometimes wife must sign consent form for contraception[472]
Family/Father Involvement	• Husband is permitted at delivery; if husband not attending, close female family or friend[473]
Fetal/End of Life	• Fetus considered tissue until day 130, when fetus is considered a "full human being"[474] • Parents will want remains[475] • Traditional washing if baby was "at least 4 months and has formed features of child;" if not, body is wrapped and buried in traditional way without washing[476]
Neonatal Illness	• During neonatal stay, if there is a lack of privacy, Muslim mother may stop breastfeeding[477]
Neonatal/ Infant End of Life	• Parents may not wish to see deceased baby, as dead are not to be seen unless necessary; photos are not usually taken[478] • Hair not to be cut, body is buried whole[479] • If newborn is expected to die shortly, father will need time to whisper into baby's ear the call to prayer[480] • Infant body should be straightened; parents generally prepare body according to specific instructions[481]

Newborn Care	• May use Kohl (contains lead) on umbilicus after discharge from hospital to encourage drying of site[482]
Prenatal Care	• Believe that blood associated with menstruation and birth makes woman "unclean"[483] • Artificial insemination acceptable between husband and wife[484] • In-vitro and artificial insemination acceptable, only if husband's sperm is used[485]
Termination of Pregnancy	• Generally not acceptable[486] ▸ Exceptions may be made in cases of great risk to mother's life and when fetus is less than 130 days

PEDIATRICS

Child/Teen Environment of Care	• Specific preparations including washing body and wrapping it; done by parent of same sex unless patient is under 12 years[487] • Ask father who should prepare body or if he would like healthcare professional to do it[488]

Jehovah's Witnesses

Note: The following information is general. Specific beliefs and practices may vary. Details on page 12.

Legend: ✓ = Suggestions for Healthcare Professionals; ▶ = Significant Details or Exceptions.

♥ CARE OF THE PATIENT	
Beliefs	• One God who created all things, named Jehovah[489] • Believe Second Coming of Christ occurred in 1914; waiting for Christ to establish millennial kingdom on earth[490] • Lord's Supper is most important; celebrated once a year[491] • No belief in immediate afterlife; don't say, "He's in a better place now"[492] • Bible is "New World Translation" in which God's name is "Jehovah"[493] • No sacraments or holy days; no birthday or holiday celebrations; members spend minimum of ten hours monthly "proselytizing"[494] • Practicing witnesses attend five meetings per week[495] • Faith healing is prohibited[496]
Blood	• Blood transfusion and blood products are prohibited[497] • May accept certain volume expanders[498] • May accept autologous transfusion that results from "closed circuit" system connected to patient's circulatory system with no storage of blood[499] • May accept some minor blood components, e.g., for hemophilia[500] • Believe that "source of soul" is in the individual's blood[501]
Diet and Nutrition	• May not eat foods which have blood added (i.e., sausages)[502] • May allow moderate use of alcohol; smoking and excesses of alcohol are forbidden[503]
Healing Environment	• Believe God is "ultimate source of all life, health, and healing"[504] • Elders, members of church may visit, pray for church member who is ill[505] • Patient likely carries Advance Medical Directive card[506]
Pain Management	• No church statement[507]
🩺 END OF LIFE	
Advance Directives	• Most members will have advance directives[508]
Autopsy	• Prefer not to have, but up to individual[509]
Death – Body Care	• No rites of faith for body of deceased[510]
Death – Special Needs	• Church members may visit with family at time of death and for some time afterward[511]

Death Process	• Believe that death is a period of total unconsciousness until resurrection occurs[512]
DNR	• Heroics to extend life are up to individual; blood, blood products are prohibited[513]
End-of-Life Discussion	• Up to individual whether to accept treatments to extend life or not[514] ✓ Per HIPAA, healthcare professional must obtain patient's permission to disclose health information to third parties ✓ Healthcare professional may ask patient who will make healthcare decisions for them if not themselves ✓ Health professional may discuss patient's terminal illness if applicable
Organ Donation	• Individual decision; consider it important to keep body with spirit[515] • May permit donation after blood removed from organ/tissue[516]
Withholding/Withdrawal	• Heroics that will prolong dying are not required[517]

👶 PERINATAL CARE

Baptism/Birth Ceremony	• No rites of faith at birth[518] • Baptism is requested when child is old enough to make decision to embrace faith[519] • Baptism is by immersion[520]
Circumcision	• Individual or family choice; not required by faith [521]
Contraception	• Birth control acceptable[522] • Sterilization not acceptable[523]
Genetic Conditions	• No church position; due to belief, church members will likely help take care of infant with anomaly and family[524]
Prenatal Care	• Artificial insemination by donor is prohibited[525] • Destroying fertilized eggs is prohibited[526]
Termination of Pregnancy	• Abortion not acceptable[527] • Life begins at conception; abortion is considered taking human life[528]

Judaism

Note: The following information is general. Specific beliefs and practices may vary. Details on page 12.

Legend: ✓ = Suggestions for Healthcare Professionals; ▶ = Significant Details or Exceptions.

❤ CARE OF THE PATIENT	

Beliefs	• Four main divisions:[529]
	  ▶ Orthodox: strictly follows traditional beliefs and practice
	  ▶ Reform: individual makes informed decisions about religious observances, however must follow ethical teachings
	  ▶ Conservative: accept Reform scholarship but maintain stricter observances of Jewish law
	  ▶ Reconstructionist: autonomy generally supersedes tradition; changes should have consensus of members
	• Three essential components in Jewish teachings irrespective of division:[530]
	  ▶ There is one God; humans were created in image of God
	  ▶ Torah: Holy book, includes teachings about God and moral duty
	  ▶ Israel: included in daily prayers, recognized as Jewish state
	• Holy Days: Sabbath is celebrated from sundown Friday to sundown Saturday[531]
	  ▶ Other holy days include Rosh Hashanah (New Year), Yom Kippur (Day of Atonement), Chanukah (Festival of Lights), and Passover
	• Believe the Messiah is still to come
	• God's laws are interpreted from Torah (the five books of Moses) and the Talmud
	• Trained and ordained Rabbi leads the congregation[532]
	• Value is placed on doing good during lifetime versus focus on afterlife[533]
	• Human body is God-given and to be treated "with respect and sanctity"[534]
	• Faith requires that one take care of health, find best care, and promote wellness[535]
	• Death is not a punishment, but a part of living[536]
	• The yarmulke or skullcap, worn by men, indicates respect for God[537]
	• May not be willing to sign forms on Sabbath or holy days[538]

Blood	• Transfusion acceptable[539]
Communication	• Judge people by actions rather than words spoken[540] • Hasidic men will not shake hands with a woman, but it should not be interpreted as rudeness[541]
Diet and Nutrition	• Laws in Torah govern what can be eaten and food preparation[542] • No pork; may practice kosher diet[543]

Diet and Nutrition (continued)	• Kosher laws are complicated and observance may differ among Jews[544] • Family may want to arrange for own food[545] • Do not serve milk and meat dishes at same meal[546] • Lactose intolerance common; many Jewish foods have high fat content[547]
Healing Environment	• Judaism includes a "commandment to visit the sick"[548] • Family and friends may visit and ask about patient's condition[549] • May not verbalize condition that is "negative to destiny" (terminal disease or condition); do not want to give "credence to morbid diagnosis"[550] • Individuals in family are expected to assist member to avoid illness and promote health[551] • May be reluctant to accept professional help for mental health problems[552] • If opposite sex patient is an Orthodox Jew, only touch while giving actual care[553] • Orthodox may request same-gender caregiver[554] • Family and friends from Temple visit; Rabbi visiting sick may pray[555] • Male patient may want to use special prayer "shawl" and yarmulke[556] • Jewish "social services" are available[557] • Many are very knowledgeable about wellness issues; may observe results of medications or treatments and adjust timing, dose, or omit depending on whether believes the medication or treatment is helping[558]
Pain Management	• Usually verbalizes pain; may be hesitant to take pain medication due to concerns about addiction[559] • Seeking relief for pain is seen as an obligation of faith[560]

END OF LIFE

DNR	• Patient has right to dignified death; deeply debated topic; family may wish to consult rabbi[561]
Advance Directives	• Considered an important form for all Jews to address; the four main divisions of Judaism have options that patients may select according to that division's interpretation of Jewish law[562] • Non-Orthodox may consider heroic measures that will only extend the "dying process" as not acceptable[563]
Organ Donation	• Transplant is acceptable and viewed as obligatory if it is to save a life[564] • View saving life as more important than keeping donor body intact; prefer direct donation[565]
Autopsy	• Discouraged traditionally unless required by law or to gain life-saving information[566] • All body parts must be buried with the body[567]

Death Process	• According to Torah, patient should be informed if he/she has serious illness[568] ▸ A controversial issue is whether to inform a patient of imminent death since some believe that the knowledge will advance death • Patient may request Rabbi be called to visit[569] • According to Jewish law, the spirit leaves the body at death; family may not want to leave body alone[570]
Death – Special Needs	• Provide quiet time when dying person recites "confessional"[571] ▸ If patient unable to recite confessional, may recite a "Sh'ma" (generally recognized as the central tenet of Judaism, comes into the liturgy as quotations from Torah) or those present may do it for patient • Respect is shown by remaining in presence of dying person; after confirmation of death, "eyes and mouth should be closed" and patient covered[572]
Death – Body Care	• Jewish community prepares body after death[573] • Orthodox: Deceased patient should not be touched by non-Jewish person[574] • Rabbi is present at time of death; unacceptable for non-Jew to handle body after death; family or member of Special Burial Society will handle body[575] • After death of patient, use gloves until Jewish member arrives to prepare body[576]
Withholding/Withdrawal	• Determined on individual basis; may consult patient's Rabbi for consistency with patient's religious beliefs[577] • Orthodox will choose heroics based on "pro-life" position; however, it is acceptable to stop when heroics are merely extending "dying process"[578]
End-of-Life Discussion	• Orthodox: all steps are taken to save life[579] • Jewish law allows heroics if treatments will likely be effective[580] • If patient is gravely ill and treatment may not be successful, heroics not required[581] ✓ Per HIPAA, healthcare professional must obtain patient's permission to disclose health information to third parties ✓ Healthcare professional may ask patient who will make healthcare decisions for them if not themselves ✓ Health professional may discuss patient's terminal illness if applicable

PERINATAL CARE

Baptism/Birth Ceremony	• Male baby is named on 8th day at the ritual circumcision[582]
Birth Process (Labor/C-Section/Vaginal Birth)	• Female family member may attend delivery and provide physical care and comfort[583] • Mother in labor may relieve pain through prayer, may accept "analgesics"[584]

Breastfeeding	• Orthodox: large families with mothers who support breastfeeding and neonatal care; one who is having breastfeeding issues may avoid letting others know due embarrassment[585] ✓ Patient may prefer provider to assess mother's technique in privacy and provide information as needed • Conservative and Reform: Community less likely to have large families and follow breastfeeding; will be open to information about breastfeeding[586]
Circumcision	• Ritual circumcision performed in front of family and group of ten adults, on eighth day[587]
Contraception	• Birth control acceptable for those not members of the Orthodox[588] • Orthodox: Contraception in male is considered contrary to "commandment to procreate"[589] • Female may use if indicated due to medical condition[590]
Family/Father Involvement	• Conservative or Reform Jew: Husband may attend birthing with wife and care for her during labor and delivery[591] • Orthodox Jew father may elect to be present at delivery but will not touch wife due to traditional beliefs[592]
Fetal/End of Life	• Until five months old, fetus is not considered capable of sustaining life on own; therefore no death rites practiced[593] • Stillborn is treated with respect; family may have member remain with body[594] • Usually parents are the only ones to view the stillborn; Orthodox may refuse to see baby or have pictures taken of deceased baby[595]
Genetic Conditions	• Within the period of 40 days after conception the fetus is considered "made of water" and abortions can be approved for fetal abnormalities[596] • Genetic conditions which may affect certain Jewish groups include: "Tay-Sachs, Canavan disease, Gaucher disease, Bloom syndrome, Dysautonomia, Fanconi anemia, Niemann-Pick disease, and cystic fibrosis"[597]
Neonatal/ Infant End of Life	• Baby would be buried as per Jewish burial rules and procedures[598] • Special rites and prayers are conducted in case of perinatal death[599] • Infant who was born alive but dies is washed according to ritual and shrouded[600] ▸ Family may have clergy perform this ceremony or, in case of the less conservative, may accept washing and shrouding by hospital nurse • Death rite is different for baby born as a live birth versus a stillborn[601] • Photos of living baby are acceptable; if less conservative parents, may be accepting of photo of deceased baby[602]
Newborn Care	• Routine newborn care except for on Sabbath when "cotton ball or paper tissue with light petroleum oil can be used to cleanse diaper area"[603]

Post-Partum Care	• May request caregiver of same sex[604] • Family helps care for new mother and baby[605] • Orthodox: May not want to be discharged on Sabbath; may ask for early discharge[606] • Discharge planning and education should be started as soon as possible[607] • Orthodox: During Sabbath there are certain taboos regarding bathing and pericare:[608] ‣ Provider may ask mother about taboos ‣ Caregiver should wear gloves after using liquid soap to wash own hands and for mother's bath • Orthodox: Until the new mother goes for prescribed ritual cleansing, husband and wife do not touch each other; husband may care for baby[609]
Prenatal Care	• Birth of child of either gender is welcome[610] • Mother is charged by faith to get prenatal care and follow wellness practices[611] • Childbirth education is acceptable[612] • In-vitro fertilization: difference of opinion on whether OK to selectively abort in cases where too many gametes or zygotes have been successfully implanted[613] • Orthodox: Female may request a female physician; if physician is male, female attendant should be allowed[614] • Orthodox: May not agree to pelvic exams during latter part of pregnancy due to possibility of bleeding • Postpartum female must have mikvah (a ritual bath) performed before resuming marital relations with husband[615]
Termination of Pregnancy	• Generally abortion is acceptable only if mother is in danger[616] • Orthodox: Within the period of 40 days after conception the fetus is considered "made of water" and abortions can be performed for fetal abnormalities[617]

Lutheran

Note: The following information is general. Specific beliefs and practices may vary. Details on page 12.

Legend: ✓ = Suggestions for Healthcare Professionals; ▶ = Significant Details or Exceptions.

[Note: Since there are more than forty Lutheran church bodies in North America alone, with mostly common beliefs, but varying doctrines and practices, the following should be viewed as general information.]

CARE OF THE PATIENT	
Beliefs	• Bible is God's Word, the foundation of faith and "standard" of practicing that faith[618] • Worship focused on rituals at altar[619] • Lutherans believe in the Father, Son, and Holy Spirit[620] • Doctrine teaches salvation through faith in Christ[621] • God administers grace through baptism and communion[622] • Sacraments are essential to the healing ministry[623] • One is born with original sin; God's grace is obtained through baptism[624] • Life is God-given[625] • Life is sacred; death is result of original sin; hope of eternal life; resurrection of the body[626] • Note: Religious observances for Christian religions may be found on the FH Diversity and Inclusion web site at *www.fhdiversityandinclusion.org*
Blood	• Transfusion and donation acceptable[627]
Diet and Nutrition	• Diet and fasting determined by individual; no specific restrictions in teachings[628]
Healing Environment	• Pastors/Ministers visit the ill, bring sacraments to them[629] • May wish to receive Holy Communion while ill[630]
Pain Management	• Very important to relieve suffering; support palliative care even when there is a risk that the medication may hasten death[631]
END OF LIFE	
Advance Directives	• Acceptable, is individual decision[632]
Autopsy	• Autopsy acceptable[633]
Death – Body Care	• Body should be treated respectfully[634]
Death – Special Needs	• Family may request to see body before removal from hospital room[635]

Death Process	• Minister will give communion in sick room; dying person becomes aware that his/her struggle is shared through the Eucharist, in congregation or sick room, through intercessory prayer, pastoral care, and lay visitation[636] • May request baptism[637]
DNR	• Treatment is not required in futile cases[638]
End-of-Life Discussion	✓ Per HIPAA, healthcare professional must obtain patient's permission to disclose health information to third parties ✓ Healthcare professional may ask patient who will make healthcare decisions for them if not themselves ✓ Health professional may discuss patient's terminal illness if applicable
Organ Donation	• Individual decision, no church standing[639]
Withholding/Withdrawal	• Does not violate teachings, but may wish to include Lutheran Pastor in discussion[640]

PERINATAL CARE

Baptism/Birth Ceremony	• Baptism is usually done by ordained Minister; in emergency can be done by any Christian[641] • Baptize infants who are presented at church by parents; baptize by pouring water over head three times[642] • Parents may want baptism for seriously ill newborn[643]
Circumcision	• Circumcision is not a religious decision, determined by individual[644]
Fetal/End of Life	• May seek baptism at birth for stillborn if a "possibility of life exists"[645]
Genetic Conditions	• No church standing on "genetic screening and counseling"[646]
Neonatal Illness	• Usually support treatment of baby unless futile[647]
Prenatal Care	• In vitro does not violate teachings, individual decision, may seek advice from Lutheran Pastor[648]
Termination of Pregnancy	• Church's position is "pro-life"[649] • In general, no teachings violated with abortion, may seek advice from Lutheran Pastor[650] • Lutheran Church Missouri Synod has a more conservative stand - abortion is not acceptable[651]

Mennonite (Anabaptists)

Note: The following information is general. Specific beliefs and practices may vary. Details on page 12.

Legend: ✓ = Suggestions for Healthcare Professionals; ▶ = Significant Details or Exceptions.

CARE OF THE PATIENT

Beliefs	• Christian group whose belief system stresses lifestyle and peace; Mennonites have missions throughout the world[652] • Church is composed of adults who freely commit to disciplined lifestyle[653] • Include "prayer and anointing with oil" as part of the healing practice[654] • Sacraments: Baptism and Holy Communion, neither of which is required for salvation[655] • Witness with their faith, words and actions; practice simplicity, look out for each other, live honestly, practice charity toward others, and work at "peace-building"[656]
Blood	• Transfusion and donation acceptable[657]
Diet and Nutrition	• No food prohibited[658]
Healing Environment	• Accept modern medicine to improve health, but understand that good health and healing are God's gift[659] • Families care for their elderly, who are well-respected and valued[660] • Makes healthcare decision based on his/her beliefs; therefore, decisions may vary from one person to another, based on individual's background and "understanding of Bible"[661]

END OF LIFE

Advance Directives	• No church position; member may have completed Advance Directives[662]
Autopsy	• Acceptable[663]
Death – Body Care	• Accept hospital practice; no last rites[664]
Death – Special Needs	• No religious rites at end of life; family of dying may desire to have family members there, for private time to pray and share memories[665, 666]
Death Process	• Death is the end of struggle, being gathered to God to await God's final victory;" dying are comforted in hope to be with God[667] • May find comfort in reading Scripture, prayers, or singing; "scriptural anointing (laying-on-of-hands) are usually welcome"[668]
DNR	• Heroics are up to individual; when making decisions, may want to consult with other members of faith family as well as biological family[669]

End-of-Life Discussion	✓ Per HIPAA, healthcare professional must obtain patient's permission to disclose health information to third parties ✓ Healthcare professional may ask patient who will make healthcare decisions for them if not themselves ✓ Health professional may discuss patient's terminal illness if applicable
Organ Donation	• Generally permit organ donation[670]
Withholding/Withdrawal	• Most would be willing to discuss "withholding/withdrawing treatment in futile situation"[671]

PERINATAL CARE

Adoption	• Adoption is acceptable[672]
Baptism/Birth Ceremony	• No religious rite at birth[673]
Birth Process (Labor/C- Section/ Vaginal Birth)	• Hospital birth is usual[674]
Circumcision	• Up to individual, not a religious issue[675]
Contraception	• Birth control acceptable[676]
Fetal/End of Life	• Parents grieve in event of fetal death[677]
Genetic Conditions	• Support counseling where genetic disease possibility is an issue[678]
Neonatal Illness	• Life is gift from God; if infant is disabled by condition, family will care for baby at home when discharged[679]
Neonatal/ Infant End of Life	• No specific religious rite at birth[680]
Prenatal Care	• In vitro: No church statement; religion would support as long as procedures support human dignity[681]
Termination of Pregnancy	• May permit therapeutic abortion[682]

Methodist, United

Note: The following information is general. Specific beliefs and practices may vary. Details on page 12.

Legend: ✓ = Suggestions for Healthcare Professionals; ▶ = Significant Details or Exceptions.

CARE OF THE PATIENT

Beliefs	• Believe in Trinity, free will, sin, the need for repentance, Scriptures, and faith in Christ as a means to salvation[683] • Observe two sacraments: Baptism and the Lord's Supper[684] • There is latitude in interpretation of doctrines among the different groups of Methodists[685] • Membership is usually granted to those 13 years and over who profess the faith[686] • Believe in afterlife with God[687] • Life after death is assured through faith[688]
Blood	• Transfusion and donation acceptable[689]
Diet and Nutrition	• No specific recommendations regarding diet[690]
Healing Environment	• May be comforted from Scripture reading, religious music; may request Holy Communion, in which case Chaplain or local Pastor should be consulted[691] • May be comforted by prayer, which can be done by healthcare professionals[692]
Pain Management	• Palliative care is acceptable[693]

END OF LIFE

Advance Directives	• Promote advance directives[694]
Autopsy	• Acceptable[695]
Death – Body Care	• No specific ceremonies for body[696]
Death – Special Needs	• Plans for funeral are made with Minister who presides over service[697] • Family may pray over deceased[698]
Death Process	• Members seek comfort and dignity for dying patient[699]
End-of-Life Discussion	✓ Per HIPAA, healthcare professional must obtain patient's permission to disclose health information to third parties ✓ Healthcare professional may ask patient who will make healthcare decisions for them if not themselves ✓ Health professional may discuss patient's terminal illness if applicable

Organ Donation	• Donation is encouraged[700]
Withholding/Withdrawal	• No religious obligation to prolong life when treatments are futile[701]

PERINATAL CARE	
Baptism/Birth Ceremony	• Practice infant and adult baptism, usually by sprinkling[702] • Parents bring infant to church for baptism[703]
Circumcision	• Up to individual family, no religious stand[704]
Contraception	• Birth control acceptable[705]
Genetic Conditions	• Support "genetic screening and counseling" [706]
Neonatal Illness	• Parents may want baptism for seriously ill newborn[707]
Neonatal/Infant End of Life	• No church statements about end-of-life care for newborn with anomalies; provide respectful care[708]
Prenatal Care	• Within a marriage, when both husband and wife agree, in-vitro fertilization is acceptable[709]
Termination of Pregnancy	• Believe in sanctity of life; however, believe that abortion may be justified in some conditions[710]

Mormon/Church of Jesus Christ of Latter-day Saints

Note: The following information is general. Specific beliefs and practices may vary. Details on page 12.

Legend: ✓ = Suggestions for Healthcare Professionals; ▶ = Significant Details or Exceptions.

CARE OF THE PATIENT

Beliefs	• Founded by Joseph Smith, who in 1820 had a vision of God the Father and God the Son. Smith was told he would re-establish the true church[711] • Book of Mormon and Bible are basis of beliefs; believe in "three persons in God (Father, Son and Holy Ghost), gift of tongues, visions, prophecy, and healing"[712] • Sacraments include "baptism, confirmation, and Lord's Supper;" ordinances include "blessing of babies, blessing of sick, consecration of oil used in blessing of sick"[713] • Believe in afterlife[714] • All will be resurrected and judgment of individuals will be based on their thoughts and actions[715] • Sabbath is Sunday; after services at the chapel, may visit with others, stay at home, or do "acts of service"[716] • Conservative with emphasis on family life[717] • Believe in anointing, prayer, laying of hands, and in God's power to heal[718] • Baptism is necessary to salvation; believe in baptism for dead with a living proxy for deceased[719] • Members enter temples, "houses of the Lord," for marriage and for necessary ordinances ("baptism and eternal marriage") for those who have died[720] • Prayer for healing by elders may be done in addition to medical care[721] • Service to others is essential; support aid programs and encourage young adults to take temporary assignments of missionary work[722]
Blood	• Transfusion acceptable[723]
Diet and Nutrition	• Promote keeping mind and body healthy, following Word of Wisdom regarding good diet[724] • Abstain from "tobacco, alcohol, coffee, tea, and illegal drugs"[725] • 24-hour fasting once a month on specified day, but ill are not required to fast[726]
Healing Environment	• May wear special "garment" of underclothing that indicates worthiness, is of special significance; patient may not wish to remove[727] • Family, friends, and church offer support; Mormon Relief Society helps members[728] • Frequently use herbal remedies[729]

END OF LIFE

Advance Directives	• No church standing; up to individual[730]
Autopsy	• Acceptable[731]
Death – Body Care	• Determined by family[732]
Death Process	• Promote dignified, peaceful death[733] • When mortal life ends, the spirit will continue; resurrection will occur in the future, with body and spirit reunited[734] • Reading Scriptures or other religious matter may provide comfort [735]
DNR	• No official stand; up to individual[736] • Heroic measures acceptable[737] • If death is "inevitable," members are not obligated to extend life through heroics[738]
End-of-Life Discussion	✓ Per HIPAA, healthcare professional must obtain patient's permission to disclose health information to third parties ✓ Healthcare professional may ask patient who will make healthcare decisions for them if not themselves ✓ Health professional may discuss patient's terminal illness if applicable
Organ Donation	• No religious position; decision on organ donation is up to individual who must decide with which choice they are most comfortable with[739]
Withholding/Withdrawal	• Acceptable to allow natural death to occur when it is inevitable[740]

PERINATAL CARE

Adoption	• Unwed Mormons frequently offer baby to be adopted; the Mormon Family Services can help find home for baby[741]
Baptism/Birth Ceremony	• Baptism by immersion > eight years[742] • Special blessing is given to babies after birth by someone in priesthood; usually in church building, but may be done in hospital or home[743] • For sick newborn, naming ceremony may take place soon after birth[744]
Birth Process (Labor/C- Section/ Vaginal Birth)	• Labor is considered natural; most will use hospital for delivery[745] • Mormon mother will keep temple garments on until delivery[746] • Father attends during labor and delivery. Other family members may also be at delivery[747]
Breastfeeding	• Prefer to breastfeed infant[748]
Circumcision	• No religious stand; up to individual family[749]

Contraception	• Birth control not acceptable unless parent ill or there is possibility of inherited anomalies[750] • Therapeutic abortions are prohibited[751]
Family/Father Involvement	• Father attends labor and delivery[752]
Fetal/End of Life	• Family considers stillbirth or miscarriage as tremendous loss; may wish to view fetus, may bury it near other relatives[753]
Genetic Conditions	• Do not usually seek prenatal testing for abnormalities; usually do not seek abortion for abnormalities[754] • May accept treatment given through use of "genetic engineering"[755]
Neonatal Illness	• Information should be given to both parents together; decisions are made together and frequently are made with prayer[756] • May choose heroics for handicapped baby[757]
Neonatal/ Infant End of Life	• Parents may request a "priesthood blessing" which offers comfort; infant in intensive care may receive more than one blessing[758] • Provide privacy for blessings[759] • Life of preemie or sick baby has religious significance; believe that infant who lives has an important mission while infant who dies was "righteous spirit who did not need the experiences of mortality" and has gone back to God[760] • For sick newborn, naming ceremony may take place soon after birth[761]
Newborn Care	• Father and family help with care for newborn[762]
Post-Partum Care	• Mother is expected to recuperate during post-partum period; family and church provide much support with care for family[763]
Prenatal Care	• Mother makes sure to appropriately take care of herself in order to do best for fetus; prenatal care is very important[764] • In vitro through use of couple's sperm and eggs is acceptable[765]
Termination of Pregnancy	• Abortion not acceptable except in case of risk to mother's life, pregnancy is from rape or incest, or the fetus has anomalies that from which it will not survive after birth[766]
PEDIATRICS	
Child/Teen Environment of Care	• Believe that those who die before the "age of eight years (age of accountability)" go straight back to God; if parent's marriage was "sealed as an eternal family unit" parents and child will be together after death[767]

Pentecostal/Assemblies of God

Note: The following information is general. Specific beliefs and practices may vary. Details on page 12.

Legend: ✓ = Suggestions for Healthcare Professionals; ▶ = Significant Details or Exceptions.

❤ CARE OF THE PATIENT	

Beliefs	• Believe in:[768]
	  ▶ Divine healing is supported by Bible and pray for sick
	  ▶ Devil is cause of disease; God gives "life and health"
	  ▶ Speaking in tongues is evidence of baptism in Holy Spirit
	  ▶ Christ's Second Coming, when he will reign for 1,000 years
	• Protestant; beliefs include Trinity[769]
	• Members acknowledge Jesus is God, salvation is through faith in Christ, Scriptures are from God, gift of tongues is evidence of baptism in Holy Spirit[770]
	• Many churches have Methodist or Baptist background; most groups following two sacraments: Baptism and the Lord's Supper[771]
	• Believe communion is healing sacrament and that one may "receive healing and strength for the body" as well as spiritual healing[772]
	• May have services for healing[773]
	• Worship on Sundays, at other times; evangelism is very important[774]
	• Practice prayer, meditation, and Scripture reading[775]
	• Dynamic in prayer, may "speak in tongues" – may be overheard "speaking in tongues" in clinical setting[776]
	• Church promotes mission work to help marginalized peoples, witnessing for the faith while serving[777]
	• After death of believer, "soul and spirit of deceased ascend to heaven and will be with Lord forever"[778]

Blood	• Transfusion and donation acceptable[779]
Diet and Nutrition	• No food prohibitions; fasting is recommended "for spiritual growth"[780]
Pain Management	• Reading of Scriptures and healing prayers may give comfort to sick[781]
🛏 END OF LIFE	
Advance Directives	• Encourage members to have advance directives[782]
Autopsy	• Individual decision[783]
Death – Body Care	• Family may be concerned about cremation but church okays it[784]

Death Process	• May ask for clergy or Chaplain to pray when patient is near death[785]
DNR	• No church policy; encourage members to pray and consult with clergy before making decision[786]
End-of-Life Discussion	• Encourage members to consult with clergy[787] ✓ Per HIPAA, healthcare professional must obtain patient's permission to disclose health information to third parties ✓ Healthcare professional may ask patient who will make healthcare decisions for them if not themselves ✓ Health professional may discuss patient's terminal illness if applicable
Organ Donation	• No church policy on organ donation; individual decision[788]
Withholding/Withdrawal	• Individual decision[789]

👤 PERINATAL CARE

Baptism/Birth Ceremony	• Dedication ceremonies take place in some churches and consist of parents presenting infant for Minister to bless[790] • Sacrament of baptism by immersion is found in most groups[791] • Do not baptize children[792]
Circumcision	• Up to individual, no church reason[793]
Contraception	• No church stand on contraception within marriage[794]
Fetal/End of Life	• Acceptable to have testing and treatment for fetus[795]
Prenatal Care	• In vitro acceptable in heterosexual couple after prayer; couple "make decisions in good conscience with guidance of Spirit of God"[796]
Termination of Pregnancy	• Abortion may be acceptable when there is risk of death to mother[797]

Presbyterian

Note: The following information is general. Specific beliefs and practices may vary. Details on page 12.

Legend: ✓ = Suggestions for Healthcare Professionals; ▶ = Significant Details or Exceptions.

[Note: Since there are more than a dozen Presbyterian denominations in North America alone, with mostly common beliefs, but varying doctrines and practices, the following should be viewed as general information.]

♥ CARE OF THE PATIENT	
Beliefs	• Relationship between God and man requires no clerical intermediary, but depends on a personal relationship with God[798] • Sacraments are: Baptism and Holy Communion[799] • Baptism is not necessary for salvation[800] • Believe in divine healing through faith and prayer[801] • Believe in triune God: Father, Son, and Holy Spirit[802] • Members practice meditation, prayer, and reading Scripture[803] • Communal worship is important, usually on Sundays[804] • Consider mission work important, working for social justice, stewardship of time, talent, resources, and planet[805]
Blood	• Transfusion and donation acceptable[806]
Diet and Nutrition	• No restrictions[807]
Healing Environment	• Pray for patient when member is ill; church should be notified so that members can pray for patient[808] • Patient may be comforted by Scripture readings and healing prayers[809] • Special trained laypersons from church often support those who are ill, through prayer and helping in the home[810] • Members try to obtain the best medical care possible[811]
🩸 END OF LIFE	
Advance Directives	• Church supports advance directives[812]
Autopsy	• Acceptable[813]
Death – Body Care	• Body is to be handled with dignity and respect; no other specific care recommended[814]
Death – Special Needs	• Family may request to see deceased before removal from hospital room[815] • Family may ask for prayers to be offered for the deceased which can be done by Chaplain, church clergy, family, friends and healthcare personnel[816]

Death Process	• Patient or family may request baptism or Lord's Supper[817] • At death, faithful will be with God[818] • Death is a natural part of life, soul goes to "heaven" at death, to be with God[819]
End-of-Life Discussion	✓ Per HIPAA, healthcare professional must obtain patient's permission to disclose health information to third parties ✓ Healthcare professional may ask patient who will make healthcare decisions for them if not themselves ✓ Health professional may discuss patient's terminal illness if applicable
Organ Donation	• Donation is encouraged; promote signing donor cards[820]
Withholding/Withdrawal	• No religious position in futile cases; up to individuals[821] • Patient has right to die with dignity and be provided with adequate pain management[822]

PERINATAL CARE

Baptism/Birth Ceremony	• Parents may want a seriously ill newborn baptized[823] • Baptism usually done by Minister by pouring or sprinkling water on child's head in front of church members who are asked to assist parents in raising the child as a Christian[824]
Circumcision	• No religious stand[825]
Contraception	• Contraception up to individual[826]
Fetal/End of Life	• At death, fetus should be handled with respect; provide parents with comfort[827]
Genetic Conditions	• Church supports genetic counseling[828]
Prenatal Care	• No opposition to in vitro; up to individuals[829]
Termination of Pregnancy	• Presbyterian views and practices on this issue differ widely[830]

Roman Catholic

Note: The following information is general. Specific beliefs and practices may vary. Details on page 12.

Legend: ✓ = Suggestions for Healthcare Professionals; ▶ = Significant Details or Exceptions.

❤ CARE OF THE PATIENT	
Beliefs	• Roman Catholic faith and doctrines are founded on Christ and Bible[831] • Roman Catholic worship is primarily focused on Mass and receiving Eucharist[832] • Christ is present in host and wine of Eucharist[833] • Observe Sundays and seven special days as holy days where members worship at Mass; may attend Mass daily[834] • Sins after baptism are forgiven through sacrament of reconciliation[835] • Sacrament of sick is administered by "Priest, deacon, or lay minister" to patient who is ill[836] • God is the source of life, health, and healing[837] • Many groups in parishes visit ill members[838]
Blood	• Transfusion acceptable[839]
Diet and Nutrition	• Avoid excesses in food[840] • Fast and abstinence Ash Wednesday, Fridays in Lent, and Good Friday[841] • Fasting not required when ill[842]
Healing Environment	• Reading Scriptures or other devotions may provide comfort[843] • May receive comfort from healing prayers, which may be offered by healthcare professionals[844] • May keep religious items such as rosary, medals, or scapula on person or nearby[845]
Pain Management	• May use prayer to seek relief from pain[846] • Support alleviation of "pain and suffering;" do not support pain relief methods that place patient in "state of unconsciousness, unless those methods are essential for relief"[847]

🛏 END OF LIFE	
Advance Directives	• No restrictions on advance directives[848] • Encourages patient to provide documents on healthcare wishes and update, as needed[849] • Surrogate should follow "Catholic moral principles and patient's wishes"[850]
Autopsy	• Acceptable; body is to be treated with respect[851]

Death Process	• Pain management for dying is very important to maintain comfort and dignity[852]
	• At death the soul leaves the body to enter into eternal life[853]
	• Family may request baptism, sacrament of sick or other sacraments[854]
DNR	• Heroic measures are not prescribed[855]
	• Not duty-bound to continue heroics if they will only extend dying process[856]
	• Duty to preserve life; may reject life-prolonging measures that do not offer reasonable benefit[857]
End-of-Life Discussion	✓ Per HIPAA, healthcare professional must obtain patient's permission to disclose health information to third parties
	✓ Healthcare professional may ask patient who will make healthcare decisions for them if not themselves
	✓ Health professional may discuss patient's terminal illness if applicable
Organ Donation	• Transplant is acceptable, seen as sacrifice for brotherly love[858]
	• Donation of body is acceptable[859]
Withholding/Withdrawal	• Withholding/withdrawing heroics is acceptable when it is artificially extending life in a futile case[860]
	• Personal choice is valued except in physician-assisted suicide, which is not allowed[861]
	• Not duty-bound to continue heroics if they will only extend dying process[862]

PERINATAL CARE

Baptism/Birth Ceremony	• Baptism through pouring or immersion is required for infant and adult[863]
Circumcision	• Circumcision is determined by individual, not a religious requirement[864]
Contraception	• Church prohibits birth control other than natural methods[865]
	• Abortion and sterilization are not acceptable[866]
Fetal/End of Life	• Baptism is necessary[867]
Genetic Conditions	• Church supports dignity of all humans including those of handicapped newborns; heroics or treatment would be determined by benefits weighed against burden to infant[868]
Neonatal/ Infant End of Life	• Parents may want baptism for seriously ill newborn[869]
	• See "Genetic Conditions"
Termination of Pregnancy	• Abortion not acceptable[870]

Sikhism

Note: The following information is general. Specific beliefs and practices may vary. Details on page 12.

Legend: ✓ = Suggestions for Healthcare Professionals; ▶ = Significant Details or Exceptions.

❤ CARE OF THE PATIENT	
Beliefs	• Sikh is seen as a Hindu reformation; founder combined features of Hindu and Islam[871]
	• Founder was a Guru; nine Sikh gurus followed, each adding significantly to the development of Sikhism[872]
	• Believe in:[873]
	▶ One God
	▶ Member relates to God directly, no intermediary
	▶ Self-directed worship
	▶ Equality among all people
	▶ Reincarnation many times before achieving oneness with God
	• After baptism, a Sikh wears the five religious symbols - the "five Ks" of dress:[874]
	▶ Kesh (uncut hair)
	▶ Kangha (wooden comb)
	▶ Kara (iron wrist band)
	▶ Kirpan (short sword)
	▶ Kach (short trousers/breeches)
	• Some members "take Amrit" (like confirmation), then follow the rules below:[875]
	▶ Go to "temple" every day
	▶ Follow specific diet
	▶ Have "special prayers"
	▶ Practice the "five Ks" of dress
	• Salvation is freedom from the birth-rebirth cycle, achieving oneness with God[876]
	• Karma (deeds performed in each life) "determines how a soul is reborn during reincarnation"[877]
	• Believe all people and religions are equal[878]
	• Follow "rules of conduct, which include living a life of honesty, truth, restraint, family-oriented, and piety"[879]
	• May consider illness as "will of God," but believe that they should seek treatment to return to healthy state[880]
Blood	• Transfusion and donation acceptable[881]

Communication	• Touching person of opposite sex is not acceptable; most will fold hands and greet person verbally[882] • Limit unnecessary touching and respect personal space of patient[883] • Oldest adult male traditionally is spokesperson[884] ✓ Per HIPAA healthcare professional to obtain patient's permission
Diet and Nutrition	• Many are vegetarians; those who eat meat would not consume beef[885] • Most do not use tobacco, alcohol, or consume foods that contain alcohol products[886, 887] • May refuse to eat food with which they are unfamiliar[888] ✓ Patient may need healthcare professional to describe ingredients; may help encourage eating[889]

Healing Environment	• Five K symbols should not be removed without permission and only after washing hands; removal of the turban or pants (which symbolize sexual morality) for a procedure may embarrass individual[890, 891]
	• Sikh's head hair is sanctified, should be covered[892]
	• Do not cut hair or beard[893]
	• If necessary to remove hair:[894]
	  ▶ Get patient and/or family permission first for either gender patient
	  ▶ Surgical patient may be willing to use paper cap during surgery
	  ▶ Removed turban should be treated respectfully, given to family
	• Book of prayers is to be touched only with washed hands[895]
	• May have "holy water, called Amrit" which is sugar and water for drinking; this water is special and should be handled with respect and not be thrown out[896]
	• Most prefer to be treated by same gender[897]
	• Prefer running water (shower) for bathing; hygiene is very important[898, 899]
	• Water should be provided in area for toileting[900]
	• Provide separate container with water[901]
	• Traditionally, sons take care of parents[902]

END OF LIFE

Advance Directives	• Encouraged to complete directives[903]
Autopsy	• Acceptable, however some may refuse in belief that the deceased "suffered enough"[904]
Death – Body Care	• Face should be "peaceful" and clean, "eyes and mouth closed"[905] • Family may want to wash the body, then "a white cotton shroud" is placed on the body, while also maintaining the five Ks[906] • Body may be washed with fresh yogurt to eliminate bacteria[907]

Death – Body Care (continued)	• Non-Sikhs are allowed to care for the deceased, but should remember to leave the five Ks and not cut hair on head or face[908] • Touching deceased's feet is respectful; family, friends and healthcare professionals may touch feet[909]
Death – Special Needs	• Maintain the five Ks[910] • Sikh's head hair is sanctified and should be kept covered[911] • At death, hair and/or beard should not be cut. Body should be buried whole[912]
Death Process	• Comfort may be derived from reciting passages of holy book or having someone else read[913] • Patient may prefer privacy[914] • Some patients may wish to sip holy water, or have it sprinkled around them[915] • Patient may show increased attachment to the five Ks[916] • Many family and friends will visit[917] • Most are stoic about death[918] • Weeping and wailing loudly is discouraged[919]
DNR	• No restrictions on heroics[920]
End-of-Life Discussion	✓ Per HIPAA, healthcare professional must obtain patient's permission to disclose health information to third parties ✓ Healthcare professional may ask patient who will make healthcare decisions for them if not themselves ✓ Health professional may discuss patient's terminal illness if applicable
Organ Donation	• Acceptable[922]
Withholding/Withdrawal	• Do not encourage heroics in futile situation[923]

PERINATAL CARE

Baptism/Birth Ceremony	• Baptism occurs in temple, after reaching the age of responsibility[924] • Naming ceremony on 40th day; the name Singh (lion) is added to son's name, the name Kaur (princess) added to daughter's name[925]
Birth Process (Labor/C-Section/ Vaginal Birth)	• Family may say prayers for neonate and mother; mother may meditate during labor; baptized mother will wear five Ks[926] • Baptized mother may wear Kachha (breeches) on one leg during birth; shaving private area may be acceptable, if necessary[927] • Traditionally new mother rests; may need encouragement to ambulate[928] • May place the Kara (bracelet) on infant's right wrist[929]
Breastfeeding	• Encouraged as the best food for baby[930]

Circumcision	• Not a part of faith; up to individuals[931]
Contraception	• Acceptable within marriage[932, 933]
Fetal/End of Life	• Body of stillborn or late miscarriage, as well as infant who died, should be given to parents for funeral rites[934]
Neonatal Illness	• Traditionally, mother and child together for first 40 days[935]
Prenatal Care	• Encourage large families[936, 937] • Believes ensoulment occurs at conception[938] • In vitro is permitted within a marriage[939] • Traditionally prefer male children[940] • May be iron deficient due to vegetarian diet[941]
Termination of Pregnancy	• Not acceptable except in case where health of mother is in danger[942] • Most consider egg and sperm donation unacceptable[943]

Unitarian

Note: The following information is general. Specific beliefs and practices may vary. Details on page 12.

Legend: ✓ = Suggestions for Healthcare Professionals; ▶ = Significant Details or Exceptions.

CARE OF THE PATIENT

Beliefs	• Believe in:[944]
	  ▶ Worth and dignity of each person
	  ▶ Justice and equality
	• Common values are stated in the Principles and Purposes, however members do not have to follow for membership[945]
	• Celebrate Christian, Jewish, and pagan holidays[946]
	• "Lord's Supper" is administered by some churches[947]
	• Faith healing is not part of their belief system[948]
	• Church does not follow a creed[949]
	• Local congregations are "self-governing;" a congregation may give certain powers to elected trustees[950]
	• Each congregation may differ in beliefs and worship, from formal church liturgy to group or lecture style[951]
	• Promote the goal "of world community with peace, liberty, and justice for all"[952]
	• Unitarian focus is on this life, not on afterlife[953]

Blood	• Transfusion acceptable[954]
Diet and Nutrition	• All food types acceptable[955]
Healing Environment	• Patient may want Minister of congregation to be notified and to make visit[956] ✓Patient may prefer healthcare professional to ask about helpful religious practices[957] • Most want to be informed about treatment and be a partner in their healthcare[958]

END OF LIFE

Advance Directives	• Acceptable, encourages use[959]
Autopsy	• Acceptable[960] • Frequently donate body for medical education[961]
Death – Body Care	• No specific or special actions promoted[962] • Treat body "with respect and dignity"[963]

Death – Special Needs	• Family may request time with the deceased "to say final goodbyes"[964]
Death Process	• Individual has right to "die with dignity" rather than try to delay death[965]
DNR	• Individual right and decision; support non-heroics for terminal patient[966]
End-of-Life Discussion	• Most members hope for a "natural" death[967] ✓ Per HIPAA, healthcare professional must obtain patient's permission to disclose health information to third parties ✓ Healthcare professional may ask patient who will make healthcare decisions for them if not themselves ✓ Health professional may discuss patient's terminal illness if applicable
Organ Donation	• Permitted[968] • Individual decision; helping others fits in with "ethical living and justice-seeking" values[969]
Withholding/Withdrawal	• Quality of life and human dignity is important ; may not wish to prolong life when quality of life is unacceptable[970]

PERINATAL CARE

Baptism/Birth Ceremony	• May perform baptism of infant as symbol of dedication[971]
Circumcision	• Permissible[972]
Contraception	• Birth control acceptable[973]
Fetal/End of Life	• When fetus dies, parents may request a "naming or blessing ceremony"[974]
Prenatal Care	• In vitro is supported[975]
Termination of Pregnancy	• Most are "pro-choice" and abortion is acceptable[976]

Cultures

I N A CULTURAL GROUP, INDIVIDUALS HOLD A "COMMON SET OF CHARACTERISTICS NOT shared by others, typically including common ancestry, language and religion, a sense of historical continuity, and interactions with persons in the same group."[977] Culture is learned; it is acquired through life's experience and passed on from one generation to the next. It encompasses beliefs about life and death, life values, and traditional activities including how to treat illnesses. The table below outlines the percentage of Americans who self-identify with a particular culture.[979, 980] Understanding how different cultures view healthcare helps you to tailor questions and treatment plans to the patient's needs. Although you cannot become an expert in the norms and traditions of every culture, being sensitive to general differences can strengthen your relationship with your patients.[981]

Cultural Identity	% In the United States
White, Non-Hispanic	65.6%
Black, Non-Hispanic	12.8%
American Indian and Alaska Native	1.0%
Asian or Pacific Islander	4.5%
Hispanic or Latino	15.4%

"American" is used to broadly define people living in the United States. The United States has an Anglo majority that is politically and economically dominant. One of the defining characteristics of the country as a nation is its legacy of slavery and the persistence of economic and social inequalities based on race.[982]

African American

African Americans (also referred to as Black Americans or Afro-Americans) are citizens or residents of the United States who have origins in any of the black populations of Africa. In the United States, the terms are generally used for Americans with at least partial Sub-Saharan African ancestry.[983]

Most African Americans are the direct descendants of captive Africans who survived the slavery era within the boundaries of the present United States, although some are—or are descended from—immigrants from African, Caribbean, Central American, or South American nations.[984]

African American history starts in the 17th century with indentured servitude in the American colonies and progresses to the election of an African American as the 44th President of the United States – Barack Obama. Between those landmarks there were many other events and issues, both resolved and ongoing, that were faced by African Americans. Some of these were: slavery, reconstruction, development of the African-American community, participation in the great military conflicts of the United States, racial segregation, and the Civil Rights Movement.[985]

Black Americans make up the third largest racial minority in the United States and form the third largest racial group, after Hispanics, in the United States.[986]

Arab

An Arab is a resident of Arab cultural and linguistic heritage and/or identity, who traces ancestry to any of the various waves of immigrants of the countries comprising the Arab World.[987]

Countries of origin include Morocco, Algeria, Tunisia, Libya, and Egypt in North Africa, and Lebanon, Syria, Palestine (Gaza Strip and West Bank, plus Arab Israelis within what is Israel), Jordan, Iraq, Saudi Arabia, Yemen, Oman, United Arab Emirates, Qatar, Bahrain, and Kuwait in West Asia. Sudan and other countries where Arabic is an official language as a consequence of their membership in the Arab League, but where it is not the majority spoken vernacular, are not included.[988]

This cultural group is comprised of highly diverse groups with differing ancestral origins, religious backgrounds and historic identities. Assyrians, Circassians, Kurds, and Berbers may also identify themselves as "Arab Americans." The ties that bind are a shared heritage by virtue of common linguistic, cultural, and political traditions.[989] "Middle Eastern and North African American" may be more appropriate cultural terms.

Asian

The culture of Asia is comprised of the cultural heritage of many nationalities, societies, and ethnic groups in the region, traditionally called a continent from a Western-centric perspective, of Asia. The region or "continent" is more commonly divided into more natural geographic and cultural sub regions, including Central Asia, East Asia, South Asia (the "Indian subcontinent"), North Asia, West Asia, and Southeast Asia. Geographically, Asia is not a distinct continent; culturally, there has been little unity or common history for many of the cultures and peoples of Asia.[990]

Asian art, music, and cuisine, as well as literature, are important parts of Asian culture. Eastern philosophy and religion also play major roles, with Hinduism, Taoism, Confucianism, Buddhism, Christianity and Islam all playing major roles. One of the most complex parts of Asian culture is the relationship between traditional cultures and the Western world.[991]

Asian Americans are Americans of Asian descent. In popular American consciousness, the term generally refers to persons with ancestry from the Sinosphere (see: Orientals), which includes Chinese, Filipinos, Korean, Japanese and Vietnamese Americans, though in definition they encompass any minority group whose national origin is from the Asian continent.[992] Asian American is the accepted term for most formal purposes, such as government and academic research, although it is often shortened to Asian in common usage.[993]

Gypsy (Romani)

The Romani or gypsy people are an ethnic group living mostly in Europe, who trace their origins to medieval India. Known mostly as being travelers, Romani are widely dispersed, with their largest concentrated populations in Europe, with more recent populations in the Americas.[994] Their Romani language is divided into several dialects, which add up to an estimated number of speakers larger than two million.[995] The Romanian cultural presence can be seen in classical music, newspapers, church, cultural organizations and groups, such as the Romanian-American Congress or the Round Table Society NFP. Religion, predominantly within the Romanian Orthodox Church, is an important trace of the Romanian presence in the United States, with churches in almost all bigger cities throughout the country. American children of Romanian origin often learn to speak both the Romanian and English languages fluently. Romanian cuisine is also praised very often in the United States. One of the best known foods of Romanian origin is Pastrami.[996]

Latino

Hispanic is a term that originally denoted a relationship to the ancient Hispania (geographically coinciding with the Iberian Peninsula). During the modern era, it took on a more limited meaning, relating to the contemporary nation of Spain.[997]

Still more recently, primarily in the United States, the term has also (or alternatively) been used to denote the culture and people of countries formerly ruled by Spain, usually with a majority of the population speaking the Spanish language. These include Mexico, the majority of the Central and South American countries, and most of the Greater Antilles.

Hispanic and Latino Americans are Americans with origins in the Hispanic countries of Latin America or in Spain. The group encompasses distinct sub-groups by national origin and race, with ancestries from all continents represented. Some members of the community prefer Hispanic and others Latino, the latter being more common in the western United States and the former in the eastern.[998]

Hispanics and Latinos constitute 15.4 percent of the total U.S. population, or 46.9 million people, forming the second largest ethnic group, after non-Hispanic White Americans (a group which is also composed of dozens of sub-groups). Again, Hispanic and Latino Americans are the largest *ethnic* minority in the United States.[999]

Native American

Native Americans in the United States are the indigenous peoples from North America now encompassed by the continental United States, including parts of Alaska and the island state of Hawaii. They comprise a large number of distinct tribes, states, and ethnic groups, many of which survive as intact political communities. The terminology used to refer to Native Americans is controversial: according to a 1995 US Census Bureau set of home interviews, most of the respondents with an expressed preference refer to themselves as American Indians or Indians.[1000]

Native Americans today have a unique relationship with the United States of America because they can be found as members of nations, tribes, or bands of Native Americans who have sovereignty or independence from the government of the United States.[1001]

Pakistani

Pakistan has many ethnic and linguistic groups and the unifying factor is Islam. Over 97 percent of Pakistanis are Muslims. The ethnic groups in Pakistan are: Punjabis (44.15%), Pashtuns (15.42%), Sindhis (14.1%), Seraikis (10.53%), Muhajirs (7.57%), Balochis (3.57%) and others (4.66%).[1002]

About 98 percent of languages spoken in Pakistan are Indo-Iranian (sub-branches: 75% Indo-Aryan and 20% pure Iranian), a branch of Indo-European family of languages. Most languages of Pakistan are written in the Perso-Arabic script, with significant vocabulary derived from Arabic and Persian. Punjabi (Shahmukhi), Seraiki, Sindhi, Pashto, Urdu, Balochi, Kashmiri (Koshur), etc., are the general languages spoken within Pakistan. The majority of Pakistanis belong to various Indo-Aryan-speaking ethnic groups, while a large minority is made up of various people from and those from Dardic language groups. In addition, small groups' language isolates such as Burusho and Brahui-speaking peoples also live in the country. The major ethnic groups of Pakistan in numerical size include: Punjabis, Pashtuns, Sindhis, Seraikis, Muhajirs, Balochis, Hindkowans, Chitralis and other smaller groups.[1003] Pakistani Americans are currently classified as Asian Americans or Other Americans by the United States Census Bureau.

West Indian

The term West Indian is used to describe populations of the Caribbean. It is estimated to have been around 750,000 immediately before European contact, although lower and higher figures are given. From 1500 to 1800 the population rose as slaves arrived from West Africa such as the Ashanti, Kongo, Igbo, Akan, Fon and Yoruba as well as military prisoners and captured slaves from Ireland. People from Asia, Great Britain, Italy, France, Spain, the Netherlands, Portugal and Denmark also immigrated to the West Indians, creating industry and the cultural, mixed-race melting pot that continue to exist today. The total regional population was estimated at 37.5 million by 2000.[1004]

The 20 Cultures in this section are:

- American: African-American
- American: European-American
- American: Native American/American Indian
- Asian: Chinese
- Asian: East Indian
- Asian: Filipino
- Asian: Japanese
- Asian: Korean
- Asian: Pakistani
- Asian: Vietnamese
- Gypsy (Romani)
- Latino: Brazilian
- Latino: Colombian
- Latino: Cuban
- Latino: Dominican
- Latino: Mexican
- Latino: Puerto Rican
- Middle Eastern: Arab
- West Indian: Haitian
- West Indian: Jamaican

American: African-American

Note: The following information is general. Specific beliefs and practices may vary. Details on page 12.

Legend: ✓ = Suggestions for Healthcare Professionals; ▶ = Significant Details or Exceptions.

♥ CARE OF THE PATIENT	
Beliefs	• Many follow Protestant, Catholic, or Islamic faiths[1005] • May believe in "life after death"[1006] • May practice "laying of hands" as believe some have healing powers[1007] • May practice folk medicine in addition to traditional beliefs in health, illness; may have close ties with church[1008] • May believe that illness is a punishment from God, due to some dissonance in his/her life or "bad spirits"[1009, 1010] • Frequently use prayer to as a remedy for illness; believe that when illness occurs, one is not in accord with nature[1011] • May consult healers who use herbs or roots (depending on region)[1012] • Female may wear copper or silver bracelet to protect herself[1013] ✓ Patient may prefer healthcare professional to ask for permission before removing an item • Family may include extended family[1014]
Blood	• Donation may be acceptable, if donating for family[1015]
Communication	• Value close personal space[1016] • Nonverbal cues interpreted as interest may not mean the patient is listening or understanding; clarify terminology used by provider and by patient[1017] • Depending on region, may use eye contact when talking, but not while listening; may look the other way[1018] • Verify that patient is listening[1019] • Patient may see timing of medications/appointments as flexible[1020] • Greet patient formally (e.g. with Mr./Mrs. and Surname)[1021] • May be loud and animated in discussion and use body language[1022]
Diet and Nutrition	• Diet is usually "high fat and salt" with little fruit or vegetables[1023] • Consider green leafy vegetables important for health and "bowel function"[1024] • May be lactose intolerant[1025]
Healing Environment	• Family very supportive during crisis[1026] • Many families are matriarchal where women are looked to for treatment decisions and promoting wellness. As seriousness of event increases, more in family are consulted for input, and decisions regarding treatment may be delayed[1027]

Healing Environment (continued)	• May take pharmaceuticals "PRN" instead of routine as prescribed[1028] • Various internal and external preparations are used to treat illness and to maintain wellness[1029]
Pain Management	• May believe pain is an indication of illness; take medication only if in pain[1030] • Some avoid taking pain medication in concern about "addiction"[1031] • May be willing to take medicine or "non-pharmacological methods" for relief[1032] • May not ask for pain medicine in the desire to be "perfect" patient; may believe that pain is "God's will"[1033]

END OF LIFE

Advance Directives	• May have concerns that planning would hasten death[1034] • Family may make decisions for patient; unlikely patient will make advance directives[1035]
Autopsy	• Acceptable if necessary[1036]
Death – Body Care	• Usually leave body care to professionals[1037]
Death – Special Needs	• Family's method of coping at time of patient's death will vary according to "education and socioeconomic background of bereaved;" many will receive support from church members, friends, and others outside of family[1038]
Death Process	• May believe that death is but a passage from this life with evil to another life; therefore, funeral may be a celebration of deceased's life[1039] • Family may want to be present when patient dies[1040] • Patient may want to die in hospital[1041] ✓ Healthcare professional may provide information and offer options regarding beliefs about hospice, heroics, and terminal care
DNR	• Believe only God knows length of life; God can heal, so the focus is on getting well[1042] • Value life; generally support heroic measures until the death of patient[1043] • May be concerned that DNR would result in poorer care[1044]
End-of-Life Discussion	• May wish condition be disclosed to spokesperson who will then reveal condition to patient; however, some believe condition is "between patient and God"[1045] ✓ Per HIPAA, healthcare professional must obtain patient's permission to disclose health information to third parties ✓ Healthcare professional may ask patient who will make healthcare decisions for them if not themselves ✓ Health professional may discuss patient's terminal illness if applicable

Organ Donation	• May permit in case of close family[1046] • Depending on religious beliefs, may believe body of deceased should be "whole" for afterlife[1047]
Withholding/Withdrawal	• May not support withdrawal[1048] • May discuss with patient[1049]

PERINATAL CARE

Baptism/Birth Ceremony	• Depending on the region, selecting the newborn's name may be significant; there may be a "naming ceremony"[1050]
Birth Process (Labor /C- Section/ Vaginal Birth)	• Appreciative for pain relief, but may use non-pharmacological methods like music, massage[1051] • Prefer female caregiver, but it is more important that healthcare professional be capable and caring than be female[1052] • During labor may be "loud and verbally expressive"[1053]
Breastfeeding	• Breastfeeding depends on education of mother; education about "benefits of breastfeeding" encourages most mothers to do so[1054]
Circumcision	• Acceptable[1055]
Contraception	• Acceptable[1056] • Specific methods used may be determined by knowledge level about methods, privacy when used, and desire to avoid discussions about sexuality[1057] • Oral contraception most used method[1058]
Family/Father Involvement	• Father may or may not be present at birth[1059] • In some groups, nuclear and extended family are at the birth[1060]
Fetal/End of Life	• Mother may or may not grieve when there is loss early in pregnancy[1061]
Genetic Conditions	• May believe condition is "God's will" or punishment for parents' activities[1062] • May refuse testing before birth due to belief that outcome is in God's hands; may be concerned that amniocentesis will cause a miscarriage[1063]
Neonatal Illness	• Mother may believe that her activities during pregnancy are cause for neonatal/fetal condition[1064]
Neonatal/ Infant End of Life	• Mortality rates are higher than rest of US population; newborn frequently weighs less at birth[1065] • Other factors that contribute to mortality rates include differences in "housing, exposure to environmental pollutants, low wages, inequities in employment, limited access to public facilities," and time between pregnancies[1066]

Neonatal/ Infant End of Life (continued)	• Loss of baby is a catastrophic, especially since new baby is a sign of hope; bereavement is "intense"[1067] • Family may have "viewing" with interment for neonate; may have an elaborate funeral; family eats together afterward[1068]
Newborn Care	• Baby may be "swaddled" to protect the baby from "air" or to prevent respiratory illnesses[1069] • May use band or coin on umbilicus to prevent "protrusion"[1070]
Post-Partum Care	• Traditionally mother will be supported to rest and avoid "cold air"[1071] • Time to clear out "impurities;" may take traditional remedies like teas, castor oil, and douching (after menstruation begins)[1072]
Prenatal Care	• See pregnancy as a "natural condition," usually celebrated[1073] • Prenatal care varies depending on education of mother; preference for natural delivery[1074] • At risk for small infant and infant mortality[1075] • May have "cravings;" mother may believe this is due to fetus' needs[1076] • If mother is lactose intolerant, vitamin supplements and calcium should be considered[1077] • May hold various beliefs and taboos related to activities that may harm fetus[1078] ✓ Healthcare professional may ask patient about specific beliefs or fears
Termination of Pregnancy	• Abortion not acceptable; children are "gifts from God"[1079]

PEDIATRICS

Child/Teen Environment of Care	• With death of child, there may be an elaborate funeral; family eats together afterward[1080]

American: European-American

Note: The following information is general. Specific beliefs and practices may vary. Details on page 12.

Legend: ✓ = Suggestions for Healthcare Professionals; ▶ = Significant Details or Exceptions.

♥ CARE OF THE PATIENT

Beliefs	• Many practice a Judeo-Christian faith; however, many other faiths practiced[1081] ✓ Patient may prefer to have a Chaplain or church leader visit German: Many follow the Lutheran, Jewish, or Roman Catholic faiths[1082] Irish: Many are Protestant or Roman Catholic[1083] Italian:[1084] 　▶ Many are Roman Catholic 　▶ Older Roman Catholic patients are especially influenced by faith • Depending on faith practice, may have religious statues, or other religious symbols[1085] 　▶ Religious items should not be removed from patient or patient's room, if necessary ask for permission • May believe that health comes from God[1086] • Homosexuality may or may not be acceptable[1087] ✓ Patient may prefer healthcare professional avoid discussion with family about patient's same gender sexual orientation
Blood	• Transfusion and donation acceptable[1088] ✓ Healthcare professional may ask patient to verify position on blood; Jehovah's Witnesses, as a matter of faith, do not accept blood or blood products
Communication	• Depending on the geographical area, speech may be fast or slow[1089] • Generally, European Americans' conversations may be louder than many other groups[1090, 1091] 　▶ Germans: Voice is not loud; communication is "precise, explicit and direct" 　▶ Irish: "Ordinary conversation is controlled and relaxed; loud voice may be considered hostile" 　▶ Italians: Within the family, discussions may appear to be heated with more than one person talking at the same time • Most maintain direct eye contact during discussion[1092]

Communication (continued)	• Those of same gender do not generally touch unless belong to same family or are good friends[1093, 1094]
	  ▸ German: Acceptable to touch when necessary for care; explain reason for touch in patient's private areas before touching
	  ▸ Irish: Generally do not touch during conversation with family
	  ▸ Italians: Generally very tactile with family
	• Touch patient on arm or shoulder after getting patient's permission[1095]
	• Handshakes are acceptable when being introduced or meeting[1096]
	• Greetings:[1097]
	  ▸ Use patient's title (e.g., Mr., Mrs.) and family name unless patient requests otherwise
	  ▸ Usually willing to give own personal information

Diet and Nutrition	• Usual foods eaten in the United States are high fat and low fiber[1098]
	• Meal times usually depend on cultural practices, geographical area, and day of the week (e.g., Sunday main meal may be mid-day, while main meal during the week may be at night)[1099]
	✓ Healthcare professional may ask patient about mealtimes and main meals; timing of medication may need to be adjusted according to when patient usually eats
	• German:[1100]
	  ▸ Three meals daily
	  ▸ Foods typically high in fat and starches with light meal at night
	• Irish:[1101]
	  ▸ Three meals daily
	  ▸ Meals generally include bread, "meat, potatoes, and vegetables"
	  ▸ If Roman Catholic, may abstain from meat Fridays during Lent and eat fish instead
	• Italian:[1102]
	  ▸ Elders and less acculturated may still eat main meal at noon, with a light meal late in day; may fast during religious holidays, especially during the Lenten season
	  ▸ Diet traditionally has "complex carbohydrates, little meat and protein"; "staples are pasta, cheese, vegetables, bread, fruit and dessert"

Healing Environment	• Many use alternative therapies along with medical treatments[1103] • May use "folk healers and magic-religious healers"[1104] ✓ Healthcare professional may ask patient about any foods, traditional treatments, over-the-counter medications or other practices used to maintain health or treat illness • German: Persons helping in making decisions about healthcare health care depends on generation and religion; spokesperson role may be assumed by father or other[1105]

Healing Environment (continued)	• Irish: May be male or female leader of family who makes healthcare decisions; in acculturated family, "adult child may be spokesperson"[1106] • Italian: Due to respect for elders, making decisions about healthcare may include elders and those who are deemed important to family; "spokesperson may be the eldest male or family member who is educated"[1107]

Pain Management	• Many believe that patients should receive comfort measures[1108]
	 • Assess patient for pain; provide appropriate measures[1109]
	  ▸ Germans: May not report pain unless asked; accept most routes for medication
	  ▸ Irish: May consider pain as a part of life and must be tolerated; may view person who admits pain as weak
	  ▸ Italian: May not admit pain to family in order not to cause them distress or worry; may be afraid of pain and believe it is "unnatural"
	 ✓Healthcare professional should assess patient for pain and discuss benefits of pain medication on healing process

⊞ END OF LIFE

Advance Directives	• May have advance directives or be willing to initiate one[1110]
Autopsy	• German: May be acceptable, depending on religion, especially when needed for legal or medical reasons[1111] • Irish: Acceptable "when it is necessary"[1112] • Italian: Autopsy may not be acceptable, body is "sacred"[1113]

Death – Body Care	• Rites for care of body:[1114]
	 ✓Healthcare professional may ask family if there are any special rites
	  ▸ German: Care of body may depend on religious practice
	  ▸ Irish: Care of body is done with "respect and modesty"
	  ▸ Italian: Family who were not present at death may want to view body before it is removed from room; may prefer to have mortuary do body care and preparation

Death – Special Needs	• May be subdued in expressing grief[1115] • German: Special needs may depend on patient's faith[1116] • Irish: Numbers of family present may require additional space and privacy; post preparation of body, family females may "keen, a wailing lamentation" and then wake, "a celebration of life," begins[1117] • Italian: May not seek support from the hospital staff but from family members and religious leader[1118]
Death Process	• Many follow practice of having someone remain with dying[1119] • Many are agreeable to hospice care[1120]

Death Process (continued)	✓ Healthcare professional may ask patient's understanding of hospice and expectations regarding heroics • German: Immediate family should be advised of impending death; depending on religion, may have certain prayers or rites for patient[1121] • Irish and Italian: Family may want to be notified of "impending death" so that they can be present to support patient; when death is close, family may want Priest to be called[1122] ✓ Per HIPAA healthcare professional to obtain patient's permission
End-of-Life Discussion	• German: For terminal illness, healthcare professional should tell patient and family together[1123] • Irish: If patient wishes to tell anyone, will usually disclose information to close family; usually stoic and may not wish to discuss illness or status[1124] • Italians: Family may expect to be told of terminal illness before patient; once patient has been told, may not discuss further to avoid distressing patient[1125] ✓ Per HIPAA, healthcare professional must obtain patient's permission to disclose health information to third parties ✓ Healthcare professional may ask patient who will make healthcare decisions for them if not themselves ✓ Health professional may discuss patient's terminal illness if applicable
Organ Donation	• Most are accepting of transplantation or donating organs[1126] • Healthcare professional may ask patient to verify his/her position on transplantation

 PERINATAL CARE

Birth Process (Labor /C-Section/ Vaginal Birth)	• Ask patient if there are any ethnic beliefs or practices for birth and incorporate any that are not harmful[1127] • German: Amish and German Baptist may prefer home birth; Cesarean section is prohibited for Amish and may result in "excommunication from community"[1128] • Irish: May avoid any vocalization of pain during labor and delivery; very modest; will usually follow physician's recommendation for vaginal or Cesarean birth[1129] • Italian: Most delivery vaginally; may be loud during labor pain and will accept medication to relieve pain[1130]
Breastfeeding	• Encouraged and acceptable to most mothers[1131] • Mother may believe that she should only eat bland diet to "avoid upsetting baby"[1132] • German: generally promote breastfeeding until age 1-2 yrs and encourage mothers to eat and drink foods that will promote milk[1133]

Breastfeeding (continued)	• Irish: promote breastfeeding, however breastfeeding may be done for a short time[1134] • Italian: breastfeeding may be practiced[1135]
Circumcision	• German: Usually do not practice[1136] • Irish: Usually practice circumcision[1137] • Italian: Practice is common is US[1138]
Contraception	• Many accept most contraception methods[1139] • German: depending on religion, may or may not practice contraception[1140] • Irish: depending on religion, may or may not practice contraception[1141] • Italian: contraception is up to couple[1142]
Family/Father Involvement	• Many fathers participate in childbirth classes with the mother and in the delivery room[1143] ✓Father may prefer to participate in birthing activities • German: Father may or may not want to be present[1144] • Irish: Usually mother prefers labor and delivery with, may want father to participate in birth[1145] • Italian: depending on acculturation and generation, may want father to participate in birth[1146]
Genetic Conditions	• May be attributed to an unfortunate event during pregnancy or God's punishment for some activity of the parents[1147] • German: May believe condition is hereditary; German Amish do not accept prenatal testing since they do not accept abortion[1148] • Irish and Italian: May believe condition is God's will[1149]
Neonatal Illness	• May be attributed to an unfortunate event during pregnancy or God's punishment for some activity of the parents[1150] • Irish: Issues should be discussed in privacy with mother and father of infant; parents may blame themselves[1151] ✓Healthcare professional may want to use "neutral language" to discuss neonatal illness to try to avoid parents assuming blame for illness
Newborn Care	• May have cultural beliefs about certain activities[1152] • May believe that baby should have an "abdominal band" or "metal object over the umbilicus" to keep it flat[1153] • German: Immediate family members, including father, may help care for baby[1154] • Irish: Family may or may not help with baby[1151] ✓New parents with no family help may need information on baby care • Italian: Female family members help in care and give information to new mother[1155]

Post-Partum Care	• German: Grandmother may stay with new parents for extended time to help; "Amish and German Baptist communities" may help with support[1156] • Irish: May have no help from extended family[1157] • Italian: Mother's female relatives may help for a few weeks[1158]
Prenatal Care	• Most mothers seek prenatal care and participate in activities such as healthy eating and resting[1159] • May have cultural beliefs about not participating in certain activities during pregnancy (e.g., birthmarks caused by certain foods or actions)[1160] ✓ Patient may prefer healthcare professional to incorporate ethnic beliefs or practices for prenatal care
Termination of Pregnancy	• Abortion is "controversial"[1161] ▸ May be acceptable ▸ Depends on patient's religious beliefs

American: Native American/American Indian

Note: The following information is general. Specific beliefs and practices may vary. Details on page 12.

Legend: ✓ = Suggestions for Healthcare Professionals; ▶ = Significant Details or Exceptions.

 CARE OF THE PATIENT

Beliefs	
	• Beliefs, magic, folklore, disease treatment and herbal medicine differ among Native American groups[1162]
	• Spiritual leader learns traditional knowledge with traditional teachings, rituals and ceremony through apprenticeship which continues throughout life[1163]
	• Most groups believe in a higher power who has created all; individual communicates with this power (God) without intermediary[1164]
	• All of God's creation is interconnected and interrelated[1165]
	• Believe all of life has a natural cycle, all of life is sacred and to be treated with respect; there are four aspects to beings and all four need to be addressed to provide the best healthcare: "physical, spiritual, emotional, and mental"[1166]
	• Indian Priest often synonymous with medicine man/woman, the person who establishes etiology as well as remedy for illness[1167]
	• Among approximately 500 different tribes, each has own culture regarding treatment of illness[1168]
	• Traditional Indian medicine focuses on holistic, behaviors to achieve harmony (wellness)[1169]
	• Healing process moves individual from illness (negative) to harmony and health; thinking positive is important to the process[1170]
	• May seek medical doctor for specific conditions and traditional healers for others; may see traditional healer and Western doctor for the same illness, but each is seen for a "different aspect" of the condition[1171]
	• Good health results from having balance of "mind, body, heart/ emotion and spirit; since physicians usually pay more attention to the physical, folk healers help to bring the "other elements into balance"[1172]
	• Very family oriented[1173]
	• Care of elders accepted as part of life responsibility[1174]
	• Navajo:[1175]
	▶ Culture blends religion and healing practices, which are part of daily life
	▶ Blessing way - healing rites to remove illness through various "stories, songs, rituals, prayers, symbols and sand paintings"
	• Family participate in ceremonies related to beginning and end of life and at time of illness[1176]
	• In case of amputation, patient/family may desire to bury the limb[1177]

Blood	• May be acceptable[1178] • Up to individual[1179]
Communication	• Frequent use of silence and non-verbal communication; consider it rude for person they don't know to talk loudly to them, write notes during conversation or to interrupt[1180, 1181] • Physical space is very important; some Navajo patients may not adapt easily to hospital environment[1182] • "Excessive eye contact" considered an insult[1183] • Handshakes should be "lightly and quickly"; hard handshakes are considered ill manners[1184] • Patient may be careful in communication to avoid making anyone feel inferior or to lose credibility; value truth; silence may indicate thoughtful evaluation of the discussion[1185] • May use metaphors to describe condition and avoid speaking about self[1186] • May refer to relatives by "familial term" as a sign of respect; however, the relationship may be traditional or spiritual rather than biological[1187]
Diet and Nutrition	• Usually follow tribal food practices[1188] • Diet depends on food availability and cost of foods[1189] • May be lactose intolerant[1190] • Diet is primarily "carbohydrates and fats"[1191] • For healthcare teaching, use term "nutrition (seen as positive) versus diet (seen as negative or deprivation)"[1192]

Healing Environment	• May avoid discussions about illness or bodily functions[1193]
	• Family provides support during health crisis[1194]
	• Patient may desire native healer to address spiritual health[1195]
	• Patient may prefer to be treated by someone of same gender[1196]
	• If patient is wearing a medicine bag:[1197]
	  ▸ Make every effort to have it remain in place
	  ▸ If necessary to remove medicine bag, give to family or place where patient can see it
	  ▸ Replace as soon as possible
	• May be unacceptable to cut patient's hair[1198]
	✓ Patient may prefer to discuss how to dispose of shaved or cut hair
	• Navajo: Extended family as well as immediate family is very important; family provides support; expect extended family to be present[1199]

Pain Management	• May believe that illness is atonement for a past or future infraction[1200] • "Value of tolerance without complaint;" not likely to express pain, however might indicate not feeling well[1201] ✓ Healthcare professional may offer pain medication if warranted

END OF LIFE

Advance Directives	• May be unwilling to sign informed consent or other documents[1202] ✓ Healthcare professional may ask the patient or family about their wishes
Autopsy	• May not be acceptable[1203]
Death – Body Care	• Do not move body until checking with family; family may wish to pray, conduct ritual before the body is moved[1204] • Refrain from touching body if possible since some believe that the spirit remains with the body for some time after death[1205] • Family may want to cut "a lock of hair from the deceased to be used as part of a year-long 'soul keeping' ceremony"[1206]
Death – Special Needs	• Do not use name of deceased[1207] ✓ Whenever possible healthcare professionals should not say name of patient who has died; use relationship, (e.g., "your sister") ✓ Healthcare professional may want to ask family what do with personal effects of deceased • Navajo: Family participate in ceremonies for birth, death, and illness[1208]
Death Process	• May avoid touching dying patient or discussion of death[1209] • Maintain positive outlook in patient's presence[1210] • Overt signs of grief may be expressed once patient has died[1211]
DNR	• May not wish to discuss DNR if there is poor prognosis in belief that it may bring death forward[1212] ✓ Patient may prefer to discuss health directives or terminal condition
End-of-Life Discussion	• Prefer that this issue be discussed with family rather than patient[1213] • Family prefer to be told to provide time for all to get together[1214] ✓ Per HIPAA, healthcare professional must obtain patient's permission to disclose health information to third parties ✓ Healthcare professional may ask patient who will make healthcare decisions for them if not themselves ✓ Health professional may discuss patient's terminal illness if applicable
Organ Donation	• May not be acceptable[1215]
Withholding/Withdrawal	• Up to individual; concept of "medically futile" is not a part of beliefs[1216]

PERINATAL CARE

Baptism/Birth Ceremony	• Great Basin Tribes: Naming ceremony done when family decides[1217] • At "naming ceremony" baby becomes "full member of community;" if baby dies before "naming ceremony" (at one month or later) it is not a full part of the tribe and will have no funeral[1218]

Birth Process (Labor/C- Section/ Vaginal Birth)	• Crow: May use sweat baths each week during pregnancy, which is believed to make labor easier; find delivery in hospital acceptable[1219] • Crow: Mother may have taken Peyote during labor[1220] ✓ Patient may prefer to use traditional remedies ✓ Healthcare professional may inquire about which remedies may have been taken • Great Basin Tribes: Usually only females attend mother in labor and delivery[1221] • May use herbs or meditation during labor[1222] • Birth is a "sacred and holy event"[1223] • Some tribes practice religious rites at birth[1224]
Breastfeeding	• Crow: Breastfeeding is less popular now[1225] • Great Basin Tribes: Support breastfeeding[1226] • Generally breastfeeding or bottle acceptable[1227]
Circumcision	• Up to individual[1228]
Contraception	• Crow: Traditionally used breastfeeding for contraception; may be open to other methods[1229] • Great Basin Tribes: Younger generation find oral contraceptives acceptable; implants or intrauterine devices are unacceptable[1230] • Female may not be willing to discuss with male provider[1231]
Family/Father Involvement	• Crow: Customarily do not attend labor or delivery; younger may remain for labor and rarely for delivery[1232] • Father's involvement or role depends on tribal custom[1233]
Fetal/End of Life	• Great Basin Tribes: Funeral and ceremonies same as for adult or child; 1 year of mourning[1234]
Neonatal/ Infant End of Life	• Great Basin Tribes: Funeral and ceremonies same as for adult or child; 1 year of mourning[1235] • If newborn is not expected to survive, family may desire to have ritual that would have been done at home post discharge[1236] • At "naming ceremony" baby becomes "full member of community;" if baby dies before "naming ceremony" (at one month or later) it is not a full part of the tribe and will have no funeral[1237]
Newborn Care	• Crow: Umbilical cord will be saved when it dries up and falls off, placed in decorative wear to protect health of child[1238] • Crow: Will name baby at 4 days; grandmother teaches how to care for baby[1239] • Great Basin Tribes: Swaddle babies, usually for first month; save umbilical cord[1240] • Newborn is highly valued among Indians

Newborn Care (continued)	• Great Basin Tribes: May not bathe baby for 1 month; may have a naming ceremony for the baby[1241] • Baby may have dark spots ("Mongolian") on low back[1242] • Parents and extended family provide care[1243] • Navajo mother uses touch to promote mother/newborn bonding[1244]
Post-Partum Care	• Crow: Grandmother teaches new mother how to care for baby[1245] • Great Basin Tribes: Mother, new baby remain home for 30 days[1246] • Tribal customs vary from exercise to bed rest[1247]
Prenatal Care	• Crow Tribe: Pregnancy is seen as a natural event and prenatal care is not seen as essential; may seek care later in pregnancy than typical US culture[1248] • Crow: Does not get baby items ready for birth in case baby dies during pregnancy[1249] • Great Basin Tribes: may not discuss pregnancy or get care in first three months due to belief this may affect pregnancy[1250] • Great Basin Tribes: May follow traditional taboos on certain foods during pregnancy; may avoid certain activities in belief that those would cause bad thoughts and be bad for the fetus[1251] • Other tribes: May be accepting of prenatal care[1252] • Customs may include not touching hair during pregnancy[1253]
Termination of Pregnancy	• Abortion is not forbidden or supported; up to individual[1254]

Asian: Chinese

Note: The following information is general. Specific beliefs and practices may vary. Details on page 12.

Legend: ✓ = Suggestions for Healthcare Professionals; ▶ = Significant Details or Exceptions.

♥ CARE OF THE PATIENT	
Beliefs	• Generally practice one of the following four: "Taoism, Buddhism, Islam or Christianity"; may follow Chinese medicine, herbalists and other alternative therapies prior to seeking Western medicine or use concurrently with the Western treatments[1255] • Family unit is greater than one person in it; elders are important and consulted when making decisions[1256] • Believe in Yin/Yang balance in all aspects of life; through balance can reach "optimal health"[1257] • May believe disease develops when yin and yang are not in balance[1258] • Treat whole patient; traditional medicine includes "cupping, acupuncture and herbal medicine"[1259] • Wellness promoted; believe physical and spiritual harmony provide for good health[1260] • May refuse to take medications when does not feel ill[1261]

Blood	• Believe that blood is not replenished by body; therefore, may not be willing to donate or have blood test done[1262]
	  ▶ Donations may not be acceptable
	  ▶ May not want to have blood tests performed

Communication	• Silence and nonverbal expression used in communication; patient tries to maintain harmony[1263] ✓ Patient may prefer healthcare professional avoid physical contact during conversation unless conducting an exam or administering services ✓ Patient may prefer healthcare professional to explain why contact is necessary • Not comfortable or accepting of touch from those they do not know[1264] • Family honor and loyalty are important[1265] • Greetings:[1266] ✓ Greet patient by Mr./Mrs. with last name to show respect • Maintain eye contact with elder, avoid with others[1267] • May respond to a question with nod or shake for answer[1268] ✓ Healthcare professional should clarify patient's response, use appropriate eye contact, touch • Older Chinese may be illiterate; discuss and ask questions to determine patient's understanding[1269]

Communication (continued)	• Greet patient by Mr./Mrs. with last name to show respect[1270]
Diet and Nutrition	• Traditional diet is becoming higher in fat and sugar; new mother may follow customary strict diet[1271] • Practitioner of Taoism, following the theory of balance, will eat and drink in moderation[1272] • May follow Yin/Yang and eat only certain foods when ill (e.g., post-op or after delivery may eat only Yang foods such as chicken, beef, fried foods)[1273] • Generally meals include rice and noodles with little meat; vegetables are eaten with meat for balance[1274]
Healing Environment	• Chinese are very modest and may not give out personal information[1275] • When discussing serious condition, family may want to be part of discussion[1276] ✓ Patient may prefer healthcare professional to include oldest male or eldest son in healthcare discussion ✓ Per HIPAA healthcare professional to obtain patient's permission • May practice coin rubbing to "draw out" illness[1277] • Family may want to protect patient from knowing if prognosis is poor; family is seen as decision maker, rather than the patient[1278] • Family takes care of patient[1279] • Provide female patient with female nurse[1280] • May refuse surgery in belief that body must remain whole[1281] • Word for "4" is associated with death; therefore, it has a negative connotation. Patient may not want to stay in a room with "4" or with "7" which reminds one that spirits come back seven days after death[1282, 1283] • May follow Feng Shui practice that includes placement of furniture to promote flow of "positive energy;" Feng Shui dictates that bed should preferably face south and be sideways to door[1284] • Offensive to receive paper with name or lettering in red ink, for example, a prescription; this is due to the fact that at "death or anniversary of death," the person's name is documented in red[1285]
Pain Management	• May refuse pain medication or intervention the first time it is offered due to social custom of refusing something the first time it is offered[1286] • May use acupuncture for pain[1287] • May be pleasant and quiet, concealing emotion or pain[1288, 1289] ✓ Patient may use body language and non-verbal indications to show pain

END OF LIFE

Autopsy	• May be acceptable[1290] • In belief that body integrity is important, may not permit autopsy[1291]

Death – Body Care	• Family may wish to wash the deceased[1292]
Death – Special Needs	• Family may bring in "special amulets and cloths from home to place on the body"[1293]
Death Process	• If patient is terminal or dying, family usually calmly accepts death[1294] • Family may take patient who is dying to hospital in belief that "dying at home will bring bad luck; others prefer to die at home so spirit of the dead has a place to rest[1295, 1296] • For the Taoist, death is the balance for life and is not feared; believe that the "soul" is with the deceased until burial[1297] • Oldest son arranges for funeral[1298]
DNR	• Quality of life is more important than duration; may not agree to life support measures[1299] • May refuse to discuss DNR as many believe discussion about death will "cast a death curse" and will hasten patient's death[1300] • For young patient, may want heroics in spite of inevitability of death[1301]
End-of-Life Discussion	✓ Per HIPAA, healthcare professional must obtain patient's permission to disclose health information to third parties ✓ Healthcare professional may ask patient who will make healthcare decisions for them if not themselves • Health professional may discuss patient's terminal illness if applicable
Organ Donation	• May be acceptable[1302] • According to Confucian and traditional medicine: Body integrity is important, therefore generally refuse organ donation; Taoist accepts organ donation[1303]
Withholding/Withdrawal	• Quality of life is more important than prolonging it; family may request heroics be stopped if burden of costs is issue[1304] • For young patient, may want heroics in spite of inevitability of death[1305]

👶 PERINATAL CARE

Birth Process (Labor/C-Section/ Vaginal Birth)	• May prefer normal delivery to Cesarean section[1306] • Mother may want to remain clothed for labor and delivery; may follow custom of not bathing for 1-4 weeks after birth[1307, 1308] • For a Cesarean section, mother may want to select "auspicious" time for delivery[1309] • After delivery, the Taoist mother may make an offering in thanksgiving[1310]
Breastfeeding	• Promote breastfeeding; cow and goat milk unacceptable[1311] • May choose bottle feeding if returning to work soon[1312]
Circumcision	• Acceptable[1313]

Contraception	• Acceptable[1314]
	• Methods used are similar to US culture[1315]
Family/Father Involvement	• May believe that the laboring mother must eat well to provide stamina for labor[1316]
	✓ Health professional may need to explain to mother that nausea and vomiting may occur at end of labor and a full stomach may be a problem
	• Fathers generally do not attend labor or delivery; couple who has been in the US for some time may expect father to provide support for labor[1317]
	• Usually female family member will attend birth[1318]
Fetal/End of Life	• May believe stillborn or aborted fetus is not part of family; no grieving takes place for lost fetus[1319]
Neonatal/ Infant End of Life	• For young patient, may want heroics in spite of inevitability of death[1320]
	• Do not have usual funeral rites for those who die under 18 years old; family will "minimize" any reference to death; do not discuss in public[1321]
Newborn Care	• Most babies have "Mongolian spots (dark bluish spots over the lower back and buttocks)"[1322]
Post-Partum Care	• May follow practice of wrapping up and keeping doors and windows closed to protect from draft ("wind"); believe that in postpartum condition mother's "pores" are open[1323]
	• May refuse bath since water is considered "cold" no matter what the temperature; eat only "hot" foods to maintain balance[1324]
	✓ Mother may avoid eating certain foods on tray; ask which foods she may eat
	• May follow practice of rest for a month to recuperate from birth; usually the maternal grandmother will care for new mother and baby[1325]
	• Mother may be with infant only for breastfeeding during the first month of baby's life[1326]
Prenatal Care	• May see pregnancy as a "natural" state[1327]
	• Asking questions related to sex are "taboo" and should be asked "tactfully and indirectly"[1328]
	• May be concerned that Yin foods should be eliminated from diet as pregnancy is seen as Yin condition and Yang is needed for balance[1329]
	• Many need vitamin, calcium, mineral and iron supplements during pregnancy as well as postpartum; may be lactose intolerant[1330]
	✓ Mother may benefit from nutrition consult and nutrition education
	✓ Mother may stop supplements without notifying physician if she experiences unpleasant gastrointestinal effects
Termination of Pregnancy	• May be acceptable[1331]

PEDIATRICS

Child/Teen Environment of Care	• Keep evil spirits from hurting the child by having child wear an amulet that has "an idol or Chinese character painted in red or black ink and written on a strip of yellow paper"[1332]
	✓ Patient may prefer healthcare professional to receive permission before removing amulet
	• For young patient, may want heroics in spite of inevitability of death[1333]
	• Do not have usual funeral rites for those who die under 18 years old; family will "minimize" any reference to death; do not discuss in public[1334]

Asian: East Indian

Note: The following information is general. Specific beliefs and practices may vary. Details on page 12.

Legend: ✓ = Suggestions for Healthcare Professionals; ▶ = Significant Details or Exceptions.

♥ CARE OF THE PATIENT	
Beliefs	• May follow Hindu, Sikh or Islam faiths[1335] • May practice traditional or religious healing along with western medicine[1336] • May believe that illness is an imbalance in body (body accumulates toxins) or may believe that illness is due to actions in previous lives[1337] • May use hot/cold foods to balance hot/cold conditions (e.g., balance "hot" pregnancy with "cold" fruits and vegetables[1338]
Blood	• May have concerns that blood loss makes the patient weaker; may be willing to receive blood from close family[1339]
Communication	• Most speak softly; loud tone considered rude, or representative of anger in speaker[1340] • May avoid discussion of condition or treatment; most, especially older people, do not discuss private matters about sex or sexual organs[1341] • Eye contact with elderly or superior may be considered disrespectful; do not maintain eye contact with individuals who are strangers or of opposite sex[1342] • Value personal space[1343] ✓ Patient may prefer healthcare professional to explain assessment or procedures that require close contact • Pointing with finger is an unacceptable gesture; offer food, medicine or other items with right hand only[1344] • Greeting:[1345] ▶ Address formally with title for respect
Diet and Nutrition	• May be vegetarian[1346] • Diet includes foods cooked in "oil and ghee (clarified butter)"[1347] • May use hot/cold foods to balance hot/cold conditions (e.g., balance "hot" pregnancy with "cold" fruits and vegetables[1348] • May observe fasting[1349] • Many eat with right hand only; wash hands prior to and after meals[1350]
Healing Environment	• Usually a close family member stays with the patient and may wish to help with care[1351] • May desire serious condition be discussed with spokesperson; spokesperson then discloses information to patient if deems it appropriate[1352]

Healing Environment (continued)	• Male family (father, husband or oldest son) is spokesperson or maker of decisions[1353, 1354] • May want close family to attend discussion for consent; used to verbal agreement[1355] ✓ Per HIPAA healthcare professional obtain patient's permission • "Silence" may indicate agreement or wish not to oppose healthcare professionals recommendations; rely on health professionals to make decision that is best for the patient[1356] • Most follow washing protocol after elimination, using left hand for toileting[1357, 1358] ▸ Provide water container near toilet or bedpan and a way to wash hands after toileting • Body language expresses feelings; may not express feelings otherwise, depending on acculturation[1359] • Patient rests and family members take over activities[1360] • Depending on religion, may not cut hair[1361] • Most prefer "daily shower"; however, someone who is ill may elect for a bath in bed[1362] • Due to modesty, female may wish to wear own gown in hospital; do not consider hospital gown modest[1363] • Do not support vaginal exams for pre-marriage or virginal female[1364]
Pain Management	• May use traditional remedies; narcotics are acceptable, but may prefer analgesic injections[1365]

END OF LIFE

Advance Directives	• Hindu: Encourage advance directives be prepared[1366] • Muslim: If treatment only prolongs dying, may refuse treatment[1367] • Sikh: Encouraged to complete directives[1368]
Autopsy	• Not acceptable unless necessary[1369]
Death – Body Care	• Family may want body washed and dressed; close family wash body if Hindu or Sikh[1370]
Death – Special Needs	• Important to allow patient's family at bedside at death; family may grieve openly[1371] • May wish for Priest or Pastor, if Christian[1372]
Death Process	• Attitude is reflection of faith[1373] • Desire for healthcare professional to advise family first if patient terminal or death is near; they will decide when or if to tell patient[1374] ✓ Per HIPAA healthcare professional obtain patient's permission • Many family members may visit patient before death[1375] • May wish to die at home; family will do faith rites when patient dies[1376]

DNR	• Hindu: Up to individual; Artificially prolonging life viewed as interfering with karma[1377]
	• Muslim: May agree to DNR after discussion of terminal situation[1378]
	• Muslim: May consent to stopping heroics if it is determined that patient would not have agreed[1379]
	• Sikh: No restrictions "on resuscitation attempts"[1380]
End-of-Life Discussion	• May desire serious condition be discussed with spokesperson; spokesperson then discloses information to patient if deems it appropriate[1381]
	• Male family (father or oldest son) is spokesperson or maker of decisions; spokesperson may be husband or father[1382, 1383]
	✓ Per HIPAA, healthcare professional must obtain patient's permission to disclose health information to third parties
	✓ Healthcare professional may ask patient who will make healthcare decisions for them if not themselves
	✓ Health professional may discuss patient's terminal illness if applicable
Organ Donation	• May refuse due to faith[1384]
Withholding/Withdrawal	• Hindu: Do not encourage prolonging death[1385]
	• Muslim: Duties include providing "food and hydration" to the dying unless those measures would hasten death[1386]
	• Sikh: Do not encourage heroics in futile situation[1387]

PERINATAL CARE

Adoption	• Depends on faith; Muslim do not condone due to change in surname. Need for child to keep connections with biological parents/ family[1388]
Baptism/Birth ceremony	• Depends on faith[1389]
Birth Process (Labor /C- Section/ Vaginal Birth)	• May want to walk; may not want pain medication in belief that this will lengthen time to delivery[1390]
	• Vocal expressions during labor are OK; may not want to know sex of baby until "placenta delivered" because female birth may stress mother and interfere with delivery of placenta (preference for boy child)[1391]
	• Female family are in delivery room to provide support[1392]
Breastfeeding	• Supported and encouraged for a minimum of six months; may breast feed until baby is two or three years old[1393]
Circumcision	• Acceptable for males[1394]
Contraception	• May be acceptable[1395]
	• Depending on acculturation, may have little knowledge of conception and contraception, irrespective of educational level[1396]

Contraception (continued)	• Acceptable to use birth control; oral and intrauterine devices most prevalent types used[1397]
Family/Father Involvement	• Father does not usually attend delivery[1398]
Fetal/End of Life	• Muslim: Fetus is considered "full human being" after 130 days[1399]
Genetic Conditions	• May believe that actions of mother before birth caused condition or that actions in former lifetime caused[1400]
Neonatal Illness	• May refuse heroics if parents do not perceive child will be "normal"[1410] • Usually any problems with baby should be addressed with mother first; if serious, father or mother-in-law notified first[1401] ✓ Per HIPAA healthcare professional obtain patient's permission
Newborn Care	• Female relatives assist mother for 2-6 months post delivery[1402] • Daily baths with gentle massage; keep baby warm and with mother[1403]
Post-Partum Care	• Traditionally mother and baby will be at home for first 40 days; mother rests and is given certain foods and herbs to restore energy[1404] • Depending on faith, may take bath weekly or may take special bath with traditional medicinal value daily for first 10 days[1405]
Prenatal Care	• Avoids "pepper and papaya" during pregnancy due to belief that those will result in delivery prematurely; pregnancy is "hot" and cold foods are encouraged[1406, 1407]
Termination of Pregnancy	• Not generally supported; may be based on health of mother, religious or economic concerns[1408]

PEDIATRICS

Child/Teen Environment of Care	• Family does not discuss puberty or sex[1409] • May refuse heroics if parents do not perceive child will recover to previous state[1410]

Asian: Filipino

Note: The following information is general. Specific beliefs and practices may vary. Details on page 12.

Legend: ✓ = Suggestions for Healthcare Professionals; ▶ = Significant Details or Exceptions.

CARE OF THE PATIENT

Beliefs	• Majority follow Roman Catholic faith. Some believe that illness is beyond their control[1411]
	• Therapies include home remedies; may use a combination of traditional remedies and professional[1412]
	• Promote wellness; consult healthcare professional for acute illness; mental illness carries a "stigma"[1413]
	• Believe in "evil eye"[1414]
	• Family is important vs. individual[1415]
	• May believe illness is caused by imbalance or some misdeed of person[1416]
	• Patient may believe condition/illness is preordained and is "will of God;" may be non-compliant with medications or treatment[1417]
Blood	• May not be acceptable[1418]
	• May be more concerned about blood donation causing "imbalance" than being recipient of transfusion[1419]
Communication	• Eye contact is minimal[1420]
	• Avoid offending others; concerned about "losing face" and may avoid verbalization of personal position or feelings particularly when in group[1421]
	• Conversation[1422]
	✓ Patient may prefer healthcare professional to have a social conversation before beginning serious discussions or interventions
	• Respect healthcare worker; whatever discussed is serious[1423]
	• Patient may remain silent or give an affirmative answer rather than disagree[1424]
	✓ Healthcare professional may want to verify that patient understands
Diet and Nutrition	• May follow "hot/cold" beliefs regarding properties of food[1425]
	• Ethnic food includes "rice, fish, and vegetables"; diet has high sodium content (for example, soy sauce)[1426]
	• May be lactose intolerant[1427]
	• May refuse food at first offering[1428]
Healing Environment	• Son/daughter may stay with parent; may want to give hands-on care [1429]
	• Personal cleanliness is very important[1430]

Pain Management	• Frequently do not complain of pain[1431] • Patient may endure pain in the belief that pain is the will of God[1432] ✓Healthcare professional may ask patient if he/she has pain and offer medication

END OF LIFE

Advance Directives	• May be unwilling to plan care due to taboo in "planning for one's death"[1433]
Autopsy	• May not be acceptable unless necessary for medical reasons[1434]
Death – Body Care	• Family members may want to prepare the body by washing[1435]
Death – Special Needs	• Family members may want to "say goodbye" before the body is removed to the morgue[1436]
Death Process	• Patient may have attitude of acceptance to illness/death as God's will; may be important to notify Priest to visit patient prior to death[1437] • Family will want be at the bedside of dying patient and to pray for the soul immediately after death[1438] • Overt bereavement displays may occur after patient dies[1439]
DNR	• May refuse DNR; family decides[1440]
End-of-Life Discussion	• Family may want to shield patient if prognosis is poor in the belief that it will burden patient and increase suffering[1441, 1442] ✓Per HIPAA, healthcare professional must obtain patient's permission to disclose health information to third parties ✓Healthcare professional may ask patient who will make healthcare decisions for them if not themselves ✓Health professional may discuss patient's terminal illness if applicable
Organ Donation	• Organ donation may be refused[1443]
Withholding/Withdrawal	• Support heroics for religious reasons; may believe it is morally wrong to omit life-sustaining measures[1444]

PERINATAL CARE

Birth Process (Labor/C- Section/Vaginal Birth)	• Daily bath is important except immediately after birth; may or may not be traditional in following custom of refusing bath for 10 days after birth[1445] • New mother may keep covered with blankets and clothing no matter the temperature; breastfeeding practiced[1446]
Breastfeeding	• Promote breastfeeding and drinking hot soups to encourage "milk production"[1447]
Circumcision	• Male circumcision is acceptable[1448]

Contraception	• Acceptable[1449] • Practice rhythm method[1450]
Family/Father Involvement	• Father traditionally not present at birth[1451] • Some may prefer female relative at birth[1452]
Genetic Conditions	• Birth of handicapped child may be seen as a gift from God to help family become better people, a curse, or a result of mother not taking care of herself while pregnant[1453]
Neonatal Illness	• May believe that illness is from "evil eye"[1454] • Any problems with infant should be discussed with father and family before discussion with mother; recommend that physician disclose issue to new mother afterward[1455] ✓ Per HIPAA healthcare professional obtain appropriate permission
Newborn Care	• Babies frequently have dark spots (called "Mongolian spots") on lower back or buttocks[1456] • May cover navel of baby to prevent "air from entering" baby's body through cord and thereby causing illness[1457]
Post-Partum Care	• Mother is with newborn round the clock, but care is shared with family[1458] • Personal cleanliness is important and mothers may take "sponge bath" more than once a day[1459]
Prenatal Care	• Will seek care during pregnancy unless cost is an issue; family encourages rest and good food[1460] • May avoid certain foods and vitamins in belief that foods will affect appearance of baby[1461] • If physician is male, may be "embarrassed" with pelvic exam[1462]
Termination of Pregnancy	• Abortion is not acceptable[1463]

Asian: Japanese

Note: The following information is general. Specific beliefs and practices may vary. Details on page 12.

Legend: ✓ = Suggestions for Healthcare Professionals; ▶ = Significant Details or Exceptions.

♥ CARE OF THE PATIENT	
Beliefs	• Practice various religions, however cultural values originate from "Zen, Buddhist, Confucius, and Shinto" teachings. Some believe imbalance causes illness and that treatment should be aimed at restoring balance[1464] • For a favorable outcome, may seek input of Priests before making decisions; social rank and use of titles important; expect healthcare professional to know what is best for patient[1465] • Some may depend on the healthcare professional to make decisions for them rather than select from options presented[1466]
Blood	• Transfusion acceptable[1467]
Communication	• Touch used with infants; less physical contact with adults[1468] • Acceptable to shake hands, other touch, eye contact is disrespectful[1469] • May agree for politeness, but not follow directions for care[1470] • Formal, reserved behavior with little physical contact between adults[1471] ✓ Patient may prefer healthcare professional to limit touch
Diet and Nutrition	• Rice is a staple; diet is low fat but high in sodium (soy sauce)[1472] • Diet may include many fried foods and high caloric foods[1473] • May avoid milk products due to lactose intolerance, which is found frequently in culture[1474] • Eat uncooked fish[1475]
Healing Environment	• Word for "4" is associated with death; therefore, it has a negative connotation. Patient may not want to stay in a room with "4" or with "7" which reminds one that spirits come back seven days after death[1476] • Respect physician, those in charge; patient may consult family for medical decisions[1477] • Culture values group decision and harmony as more important than individual choice[1478] • Bath is important, but may be omitted when patient is sick; family gives "personal care"[1479] • Patient/family may take assistance from family members but not outsiders or social service[1480]

Healing Environment (continued)	• Family:[1481]
	▸ Is important; eldest son usually is responsible to care for parents
	▸ Some family members remain at bedside of elderly family member in hospital
	▸ Is patriarchal; father makes family decisions
	✓ Healthcare professional should approach patient before procedures to ask whether patient wants physician to discuss results with patient or family
	✓ Per HIPAA healthcare professional obtain appropriate permission
Pain Management	• Culture which often does not verbalize pain; healthcare professional may administer less than adequate pain medication due to this[1482]
	• Patient may expect healthcare professional to pick up on non-verbal cues as to pain[1483]
	• May refuse, in belief that medicine will be addictive[1484]

⬛ END OF LIFE

Advance Directives	• Culture dictates protection of elderly from knowledge of terminal situation; may be difficult to obtain advance directives[1485]
	• The more accustomed the patient is to Western life, the more likely the patient will be open to discussion of advance directives[1486]
Autopsy	• May be acceptable[1487]
	• Believe that body should remain whole; the more accustomed to Western life, the more likely to agree to autopsy[1488]
	• Shinto: Autopsy permitted[1489]
Death – Body Care	• Body should be clean and dressed for viewing[1490]
Death – Special Needs	• Family may want to stay with dying patient[1491]
	• Shinto Japanese: Family remains with body until buried or cremated[1492]
Death Process	• No public expression of grief; may mask grief during discussion about death of someone close[1493]
DNR	• May be willing to consider DNR if is accustomed to and familiar with Western medicine practice[1494]
	• Value physician's input, may decide on basis of discussion with physician; may find it difficult to stop heroics once initiated[1495]
	• Values group family decision making[1496]
End-of-Life Discussion	• Hopes for a "peaceful death;" patient and family may not want to discuss terminal situation so that patient does not worry about it[1497]
	• Prefer that prognosis be discussed with family, not patient[1498]
	✓ Per HIPAA, healthcare professional must obtain patient's permission to disclose health information to third parties

End-of-Life Discussion (continued)	✓Healthcare professional may ask patient who will make healthcare decisions for them if not themselves ✓Health professional may discuss patient's terminal illness if applicable
Organ Donation	• Generally donation and transplant not acceptable[1499] • Believes that body should remain whole; the younger generations, more accustomed to Western life, are more likely to agree[1500] • Hindu, Buddhist: Organ donation/transplant up to individual • Shinto: Generally refuse organ donation[1501]
Withholding/Withdrawal	• May be difficult to get agreement to stop heroics, once initiated[1502] • Those more accustomed to Western medicine practice may accept withdrawal[1503]

👤 PERINATAL CARE

Baptism/Birth Ceremony	• Depends on spiritual beliefs, religion[1504]
Birth Process (Labor/C-Section/Vaginal Birth)	• May wear amulet from Shinto shrine to provide for good birthing; usually worn around neck during pregnancy[1505] • Endures labor without analgesic; believes that bearing pain makes better mother[1506] • May not show pain or ask for relief; expect healthcare professional to recognize the need for relief and provide a remedy[1507]
Breastfeeding	• No colostrum to newborn[1508] • Usually breastfeed[1509] • Traditionally babies are weighed pre- and post-breastfeeding; feedings are supplemented if determined that baby did not get enough milk[1510] ✓Healthcare professional may want to educate patient on the importance of colostrum and how demand increases the quantity of milk produced
Circumcision	• Acceptable, up to individual[1511]
Family/Father Involvement	• Father and maternal grandmother likely to attend delivery[1512] • Father frequently takes passive role, does not coach mother[1513]
Fetal/End of Life	• No funeral rites for stillborn or miscarriage[1514]
Genetic Conditions	• Family may believe this is "punishment" for prior behavior in family[1515]
Neonatal Illness	• Father is to be consulted before mother, so that father can attend mother when illness is discussed with mother[1516] • Parents may want "aggressive" treatment[1517]
Newborn Care	• Mother takes care of baby; father who has been exposed to US practice may participate in child care[1518]

Newborn Care (continued)	• Traditionally baby is "named on seventh day with ceremonial writing of name"[1519]
Post-Partum Care	• Postdelivery rest; mother may refuse bath/shampoo for seven days post-delivery[1520]
	• Mother may plan to move in with grandparents who will care for her and baby for two to three months[1521, 1522]
	• End of postpartum period celebrated on day 100 with ceremony[1523]
Prenatal Care	• Mother seeks prenatal care[1524]
	• Japanese are passive; may not ask for help, but expect to provide help without being asked[1525]
	• In Japan, use of ultrasound is frequent during pregnancy; may expect US physician to order during most visits[1526]
	• Taboos on certain foods believed to affect fetus[1527]
	• During pregnancy woman is to keep from getting "chilled" as this may harm the mother or fetus; wear socks to keep feet warm and may not use air conditioner[1528]
	• Promote rest during pregnancy[1529]
	• Traditionally, pregnancy is "woman's fulfillment" and pregnant patient is "pampered"[1530]
Termination of Pregnancy	• Abortion may be acceptable[1531]
	• May seek abortion if testing reveals abnormalities[1532]

Asian: Korean

Note: The following information is general. Specific beliefs and practices may vary. Details on page 12.

Legend: ✓ = Suggestions for Healthcare Professionals; ▶ = Significant Details or Exceptions.

	CARE OF THE PATIENT
Beliefs	• May follow belief system of Tao, Confucius, Buddha, or Christianity; may practice a mix of traditional and Christian religion[1533]
	• Promote wellness, care of own body[1534]
	• Use therapies including acupuncture and traditional treatments; herbs are frequently used[1535]
	• May believe that illness is because of actions that he/she had taken, bad luck, or "imbalance of hot and cold"[1536]
	• Family-oriented society, family input on decision-making but male makes final decision[1537]
	✓ Per HIPAA healthcare professional obtain appropriate permission
Blood	• May not be acceptable[1538]
	• Loss of blood takes away strength and allows "soul to leave the body" through loss; receiving blood, therefore, may provide entry for another's spirits[1539]
Communication	• Touching is considered impolite unless person is good friend of same gender; family does hands-on care of patient[1540]
	• Respectful to avoid eye contact and physical touch with those outside of family or friends; family oriented; family is involved in giving care to hospitalized family member[1541]
Diet and Nutrition	• Breakfast is the main meal of day; when first offered food or drink, social custom dictates refusal[1542, 1543]
	• Rice and Chinese cabbage are staples; lactose intolerance seen frequently[1544]
Healing Environment	• May seek Western medical care; respect physicians and nurses[1545]
	• May agree (or nod to imply agreement) for the sake of harmony and saving face, but be noncompliant with instructions[1546]
	• Word for "4" is associated with death and therefore has a negative connotation. Patient may not want to stay in a room with "4" or with "7"[1547]
	• Offensive to receive paper with name or lettering in red ink, for example, a prescription; this is due to the fact that at death or death anniversary, the person's name is documented in red[1548]
	• "Coin rubbing" is practiced on children and older adults; red marks may look like abuse[1549]

Pain Management	<ul><li>May be concerned about addictions; prefer pain medication by mouth or IV rather than IM[1550]</li><li>May not express pain[1551]</li><li>Assess for non-verbal indications of pain[1552]</li></ul>

🜀 END OF LIFE

Advance Directives	<ul><li>Culture dictates protection of elderly from knowledge of terminal situation; it may be difficult to obtain advance directives[1553]</li><li>Decision maker for family reviews documents for patient before patient can sign[1554]</li></ul>
Autopsy	<ul><li>May not be acceptable except for instances where cause of death is unknown[1555]</li></ul>
Death – Body Care	<ul><li>Family may wish to bathe body after death[1556]</li></ul>
Death – Special Needs	<ul><li>Family may wish to have time with deceased before removal from room[1557]</li><li>Traditionally at death of Korean, name is written in red ink[1558]</li></ul>
Death Process	<ul><li>Death is transition to another life; at death of patient family may be emotional and loud[1559]</li><li>Family may wish to take elder back to home country before death[1560]</li><li>May not consider "brain death" as equivalent to death[1561]</li></ul>
DNR	<ul><li>May not be in favor of prolonging life; death and dying fairly well accepted[1562]</li></ul>
End-of-Life Discussion	<ul><li>Among older Koreans, more patriarchal; in younger generations, more family involved in decisions, although male may make final determination[1563]</li><li>May wish family leader to be informed first and that person will let patient know prognosis[1564]</li></ul> ✓ Per HIPAA, healthcare professional must obtain patient's permission to disclose health information to third parties ✓ Healthcare professional may ask patient who will make healthcare decisions for them if not themselves ✓ Health professional may discuss patient's terminal illness if applicable
Organ Donation	<ul><li>Generally transfusion and donation not acceptable[1565]</li><li>Based on Confucianism may refuse donation/organ transplantation in belief that donor body must not be disfigured[1566]</li></ul>
Withholding/Withdrawal	<ul><li>Patriarchal culture where male determines life-support decision; families may wish to return patient to native country before patient dies[1567]</li><li>May consider removing life support as contrary to God's will and disrespectful to elder[1568]</li><li>May not be in favor of prolonging life; death and dying fairly well accepted[1569]</li></ul>

PERINATAL CARE

Birth Process (Labor/C-Section/ Vaginal Birth)	• May not want medication in order to have a natural birth[1570] • May want to "walk, squat, or crawl;" encouraged to withstand pain[1571] • Rest is very important for mother after the birth[1572] • After birth, mother traditionally drinks special soup to encourage milk production[1573]
Breastfeeding	• Breastfeeding promoted[1574] • May use home remedies to promote milk[1575] • Some initiate breastfeeding at birth, others on third day; some Koreans accustomed to US practices may give bottle feedings instead of breastfeeding[1576]
Circumcision	• May refuse circumcision[1577]
Contraception	• Generally withdrawal or douching are methods of contraception[1578]
Family/Father Involvement	• Father does not attend delivery[1579] • Father may not actively participate in newborn's care[1580]
Fetal/End of Life	• No rites practiced for stillborn birth; consider that baby as not having been born and may wish for hospital disposal[1581]
Genetic Conditions	• Discuss any problems with father before talking to mother due to fact that mother may believe that she caused problem[1582]
Neonatal Illness	• May prefer for condition be discussed with father and he will let the mother know[1583]
Newborn Care	• Infant remains in home for at least a month, not taken out in public[1584] • Baby is picked up when cries; may sleep with mother[1585]
Post-Partum Care	• Mother takes care of baby, rest is encouraged; family will help with other duties of mother[1586] • Time of rest varies and may be from 7 days to 90[1587] • Mother keeps warm and newborn is swaddled[1588] • Certain foods are given to new mother ("seaweed soup and steamed rice"); anything consumed must be warm[1589]
Prenatal Care	• May not seek prenatal care until fifth month[1590] • Typical Korean prenatal visits include no physical exam; mother may not be aware of typical US OB exam that may include a Pap smear[1591] ✓ Healthcare professional may want to discuss exam to be done with sensitivity to modesty needs • Prefer provider of same sex[1592]

Prenatal Care (continued)	• Information about personal issues like breast exams and bowel habits would not be divulged until patient is comfortable in relationship with provider[1593] • Certain foods are prohibited during pregnancy[1594] • May be lactose intolerant and consequently do not consume milk products[1595] • Family supports pregnant woman in maintaining a positive, calm attitude for a good pregnancy[1596] • Mother may believe infant at birth should be small; may wear binder and work very hard in belief that these will help her deliver a small baby[1597]
Termination of Pregnancy	• Abortion is acceptable[1598]

 PEDIATRICS

Child/Teen Environment of Care	• Family may practice folk therapies that mark skin (e.g., moxibustion, cupping)[1599] • Marks may appear to be abuse[1600] ✓ Healthcare professional may want to carefully question patient and family to determine whether these were made by folk therapies

Asian: Pakistani

Note: The following information is general. Specific beliefs and practices may vary. Details on page 12.

Legend: ✓ = Suggestions for Healthcare Professionals; ▶ = Significant Details or Exceptions.

CARE OF THE PATIENT

Beliefs	
	• Religious beliefs are mostly Muslim[1601]
	▶ Practice Islam
	▶ Majority belong to Sunni and Shi'ite (Shi'ah) sects
	▶ There are also many Hindus, Parsis, and Christians
	▶ Sunni Muslims follow the practice and teachings of the Prophet Mohammed
	▶ Shi'ite Muslims seek religious guidance from religious leaders called Imams
	• Religious practices include a belief in the five pillars:[1602]
	▶ One God (Allah) and his prophet, Mohammed (Shahada)
	▶ Prayer five times a day after ritual ablution, at home or in congregation at a mosque
	▶ Fasting during the month of Ramadan (ninth month of the Muslim calendar)
	▶ Giving alms tax (zakaat)
	▶ Pilgrimage to Mecca at least once in a lifetime
	• Sabbath prayers on Friday afternoon are important[1603]
	• Islam influences all parts of life – birth, marriage, family, politics, economics, and social relationships[1604]
	• May seek help of traditional healers, herbalists (hakim), as well as modern medicine; promote wellness[1605]
	• Belief in spiritual healing, i.e., reciting verses of the Koran eliminates illness or eases suffering[1606]
	• Spiritual leader (pir), prays for sick and gives him/her a packet of verses (taawiz) to wear[1607]
	• Family members provide spiritual care by praying in groups or reading passages from the Koran to the patient[1608]
	• Religious holidays based on the lunar calendar[1609]
	▶ During religious holidays give charity to the poor, widows, and orphans
	▶ Practices include group prayer and visiting with family, relatives, and neighbors
	• Some immigrant families celebrate Easter, Thanksgiving, and Christmas[1610]

Blood	• Blood transfusion is acceptable[1611] • Patients may prefer to receive blood from same religion[1612]

Communication	• English is the official language of Pakistan[1613]
	• National language is Urdu[1614]
	• Pakistanis speak other languages, i.e., Punjabi, Sindhi, Pashto, Gujarati, Kashmiri, and Baluchi[1615]
	• Greet verbally with gestures[1616]
	  ▸ Inappropriate gestures include pointing a finger during conversation; use facial expression instead of hand gestures
	• Uncommon to address older persons by first or last name[1617]
	  ▸ Greet patient formally with Mr. or Mrs. and last name
	  ▸ Members of the same peer group will address each other and those younger by first name
	  ▸ Older persons should be treated politely, with respect
	• Muslims greet by placing the palm of the right hand to their forehead, bow slightly and say, "Asallam Wallaiqum," which means "peace and prosperity"[1618]
	• Commands can be given to younger persons, but older persons expect to be treated with respect[1619]
	• Tone of voice is very important for showing respect[1620]
	  ▸ Soft tone indicates respect
	  ▸ Loudness and giving commands, and emotional outbursts can be interpreted as disrespect
	• Silence is shown as approval. A nod or smile, or silence acknowledges understanding[1621]
	  ▸ Patient is unlikely to indicate he/she does not understand; will sign due to respect for provider
	  ▸ May direct questions to family members
	• Usually direct with healthcare professionals[1622]
	  ▸ Older persons may speak with stories rather than answering questions directly
	  ▸ For issues of consent, may prefer that a close family member be present
	  ▸ Tend to rely on health professionals to make treatment decisions
	• Father, husband, or older brother may make a decision of consent for a female patient[1623]
	• For interpreters, prefer close family member who is older or in the same age group and gender[1624]

Diet and Nutrition	• Typically eat two to three meals a day. Preferring a big meal in middle of day and a smaller meal at supper. May prefer supper late in the evening.[1625] • Sometimes prefer snacks with evening tea[1626] • Prepare lavish meals for guests[1627]

Diet and Nutrition (continued)	• May prefer using clay cookware, which is considered to be healthy[1628]
	• Avoid distractions, such as watching television, reading, or excessive talking, while eating[1629]
	• Food that cannot be eaten together[1630]
	▸ Fish and dairy, red meat and dairy, or sour fruit and dairy all believed to produce toxins in the body
	• Hot or cold may refer to content instead of temperature, i.e., eat cold food during hot weather and hot food during cold weather[1631]
	▸ Hot foods include meat and fish, eggs, honey, most oils, nuts and seeds, most herbs, and spices
	▸ Cold foods include milk, butter, cheese, yogurt, most vegetables and fruits, and some grains and legumes, such as wheat, rice, barley, and lentils
	• Most meals include rice or flat baked wheat bread (chapati) eaten with meat, vegetable, or lentil curry[1632]
	▸ Breakfast typically includes cereals, bread, eggs, tea, and milk
	▸ Lunch and dinner is typically rice or chapati with another dish
	• Sweet dishes not typically part of the diet[1633]
	▸ Typically entertain guests with cookies or salty snacks
	• Common beverages include water, buttermilk (lasi), or mango shakes, believed to relieve indigestion[1634]
	▸ Hot tea with milk is taken over coffee
	• If Muslim, pork and alcohol strictly prohibited. Only eats fish with scales and fins (no shellfish)[1635]
	• Muslims fast from sunrise to sunset during the month of Ramadan[1636]
	▸ Young children, people who are traveling or ill, and women who are breastfeeding, menstruating, or pregnant are exempt
	• Recommend fasting for fever, gastrointestinal (GI) problems, cold, or arthritic pain[1637]
	• During acute illness, may prefer bland, liquid, or easily digested foods[1638]
Healing Environment	• Usually prompt in seeking care for symptoms that cause discomfort[1639]
	• Patients prefer clinician of same gender[1640]
	• Men shake hands and hug each other but women usually do not[1641]
	• May view direct eye contact as rude or disrespectful. Muslim men and women will lower their gaze in the presence of the opposite sex[1642]
	• Avoid touching those of the opposite gender if they are not married or blood relatives[1643]
	▸ Traditionally, unmarried men and women maintain two to three foot distance from each other or will socialize in separate areas of a room
	• Considered obscene to step on or touch someone with a foot. If this happens, apologize immediately to avoid giving offense[1644]

Healing Environment (continued)	• Privacy is important when discussing personal matters[1645]
	  ▸ Family matters are not discussed in public or with non-family members
	  ▸ Not time-conscious except for medical appointments and work
	• Men prefer to wear loose pants[1646]
	• Women prefer not to wear hospital gowns that reveal body parts, preferring to cover head and chest and wear clothing that reaches below the knee[1647]
	✓ Healthcare professional should refrain from asking women to remove clothing unless there is a clear medical need
	  ▸ Menstruating women will take a full bath and wash hair at the end of their period, before praying
	  ▸ Patients who have undergone surgery or have respiratory tract infection prefer bedside bath
	• Patients prefer private toilets but will accept urinals, bedpans, or bedside commodes[1648]
	• Must purify themselves (washing hands, face, feet) before praying[1649]
	• Taawiz must only be removed by healthcare professional after patient or family member gives permission. May be tied to patient's gown[1650]
	• Close family members prefer to stay with patient to assist with daily care[1651]
	  ▸ Mother, wife, daughter, or other female member of family for sick family members instead of another female non-family member
	  ▸ Other family members may bring fruit or home-cooked meals during hospital stay
	• Chronically ill patients prefer to do their own self-care (i.e., diabetic blood testing, dietary control, and monitoring of blood pressure)[1652]
	• Pakistanis prefer to be hospitalized only if they are seriously ill[1653]

Pain Management	• Usually try traditional remedies such as "certain leaves and herbs" before Western medicine; believe natural substances cure many ailments. May take herbal medicines concurrently with other medicine. Keep over-the-counter medicine imported from Pakistan as first aid home remedies[1654] • Fear addiction to medications; may stop taking medicines as soon as pain or other symptoms are gone[1655]

END OF LIFE

Autopsy	• Usually will refuse, unless required. Muslims request that if an autopsy is performed, the organs be returned to the body afterward[1656]
Death – Body Care	• After someone dies, the arms and legs are straightened and the eyes closed, toes fastened together with bandage and body covered with a sheet[1657] • For deceased adults, the body is ritually washed by another Muslim of same gender, prior to burial, then wrapped in a white cotton shroud and placed in the coffin[1658]

Death – Body Care (continued)	• Do not believe in embalming[1659] • Body buried as soon as possible after death[1660]
Death – Special Needs	• Acceptable for family to express grief and mourn openly by crying [1661]Mourn for three days and then hold a memorial gathering (within a week of death and then a month later)[1662] • Family may call spiritual leader to give patient holy water to drink to purify the body before dying[1663]
Death Process	• When death is near, immediate family is told and called to stay by bedside to witness loved one's passing and offer special prayers to ease suffering[1664] • May call religious leader to offer special prayers[1665] • Death is accepted as a natural part of the journey to the afterlife[1666] • Family may initially allow patient to be placed on life support, but will not allow as a long-term solution[1667]
End-of-Life Discussion	• If patient is "terminal, significant other(s) are to be told first" and they will decide when to tell patient[1668] ✓ Per HIPAA, healthcare professional must obtain patient's permission to disclose health information to third parties ✓ Healthcare professional may ask patient who will make healthcare decisions for them if not themselves ✓ Health professional may discuss patient's terminal illness if applicable
Organ Donation	• Organ transplants are acceptable[1669] • Muslims usually resist organ donation because Islam forbids it[1670]

PERINATAL CARE

Baptism/Birth Ceremony	• Party may be held to celebrate birth[1671] • Muslim family may perform Aqiqah ceremony where the newborn's head is shaved and one or two goats are sacrificed[1672]
Birth Process (Labor/C-Section/ Vaginal Birth)	• Prefer hospital deliveries in the US[1673] • Encourage women to walk during labor[1674] • Advise light meals[1675] • Female family members support woman in labor[1676] • Usually refuse pain medications because they may delay delivery[1677] • Woman in labor usually assumes passive role and follows direction of healthcare professional or family members[1678] • Encouraged to suppress expression of pain, but some moaning, grunting, and screaming may be acceptable[1679] • Preferred vaginal delivery but Cesarean is acceptable, if necessary[1680] • Do not reveal sex of baby until placenta is out[1681] • Show baby to mother first, then the father, then other family[1682]

Birth Process (Labor/C-Section/ Vaginal Birth)(continued)	• In Muslim families, father or grandfather recites the Muslim calls to prayer to ensure infant hears these words first as an invitation to follow God[1683]
Breastfeeding	• Lactation is encouraged for at least six months and can breastfeed for as long as two to three years[1684] • Working mothers can combine with bottled formula[1685] • Lactating mothers encouraged to eat carbohydrates and fats for sufficient milk supply[1686]
Circumcision	• Male circumcision is an Islamic ritual that should be performed before age seven[1687]
Contraception	• Sex before marriage not acceptable, a woman may be disowned by her family[1688] • Birth control is acceptable for married couples[1689]
Family/Father Involvement	• Father may take childbirth education[1690] • Father usually not present at delivery; however, more educated men prefer to stay with wife to offer emotional support[1691] • May participate in care of infant[1692]
Genetic Conditions	• Believed that genetic defects occur when pregnant woman picks up sharp objects (scissors, knives, and needles) during a lunar or solar eclipse[1693] • Believe that when a child is born with genetic or congenital defects that the mother was exposed to chemicals or toxins during pregnancy[1694]
Neonatal Illness	• Prefer to have news given to mother first. If illness is serious may tell father or mother-in-law first[1695] ✓ Healthcare professional to obtain appropriate permission from patient per HIPAA ✓ Per HIPAA healthcare professional to obtain patient's permission • Expect a physician, rather than a nurse, to inform of diagnosis[1696] • Generally will accept a nurse's opinion about managing ongoing health problems[1697]
Newborn Care	• Mother, maternal grandmother, or older women in family hold and comfort infant[1698] • Older women in the family typically assist with baby for six weeks to three months post delivery[1699] • Common to give baby massages with oil after a bath and swaddle the baby[1700]
Post-Partum Care	• Believe mother should stay warm after birth[1701] • Mother eats special foods with meals to restore energy[1702] • Mother may only bathe once a week, taking partial baths and washing perineal area with warm water each time she uses the toilet[1703] • Mother is often given back massages with warm oil[1704]

Prenatal Care	• Modest and private; do not generally discuss sexual matters or anatomy; prefer same sex caregiver[1705]
	✓ Pregnancy viewed as healthy state
	• In first trimester avoid "hot" foods, i.e., meat, eggs, nuts, herbs, spices - which are believed to cause miscarriage[1706]
	• Usually seek prenatal care, mother and mother-in-law or elder female family member often offer advice[1707]
	✓ Healthcare professional should educate patient as to signs and symptoms for which she should go to medical doctor
	• Expectant mother avoids emotional stress and shock and performs usual tasks, avoiding heavy lifting[1708]
	• Therapeutic abortion acceptable if mother's life is in danger, but Islam forbid abortion by choice[1709]
	• A fetus is considered a person 120 days after conception[1710]

 PEDIATRICS

Child/Teen Environment of Care	• Mother will stay and care for children in hospital[1711]
	• Men typically make healthcare decisions for young girls[1712]
	• Children rarely make independent decisions[1713]

Asian: Vietnamese

Note: The following information is general. Specific beliefs and practices may vary. Details on page 12.

Legend: ✓ = Suggestions for Healthcare Professionals; ▶ = Significant Details or Exceptions.

♥ CARE OF THE PATIENT	
Beliefs	• May follow belief system of Buddha, Confucius, or Tao or may practice a blend of the three[1714] • Therapies used include herbals, coin rubbing, and acupuncture[1715] • May believe illness is caused by imbalance of hot and cold[1716] • Consider respect and harmony as most important; eye contact is disrespectful when addressing someone older or of higher social standing[1717] • Believe that Western meds are stronger; may take reduced dosage due to this belief, and smaller stature of Vietnamese[1718] ✓ Healthcare professional may want to explain that dosage is based on patient's weight • Believe that "perspiration removes body toxins;" may believe decrease of perspiration in US and stress is cause of illness[1719] • May consider routine visit by Chaplain a signal that the patient is critical[1720] ✓ If visits are regularly scheduled and not initiated by the patient, healthcare professional may want to explain the purpose of a Chaplain visit beforehand
Blood	• May not be acceptable[1721] • Loss of blood takes away strength and allows "soul to leave the body" through loss; receiving blood, therefore, may provide entry for another's spirits[1722] • May believe that loss of blood is permanent and results in weakness[1723]
Communication	• Unacceptable to touch patient's head, unless necessary; may believe the soul resides in head, will lose soul if head is touched[1724] • Touch only when necessary; explain necessity to patient first; afterward, touch opposite side of head to keep soul from escaping[1725] • Palm up is offensive in communication[1726] • Eye contact is disrespectful when addressing someone of higher social standing or older[1727] • May smile rather than express emotions, concerns, or complaints[1728] • With people who are not family, usually desire more personal space[1729]
Diet and Nutrition	• Traditionally low fat/sugar, high carbohydrate diet mainly of rice with leafy vegetables[1730]

Diet and Nutrition (continued)	• Those more accustomed to US lifestyle take in more calories and are sedentary, leading to overweight[1731] • Do not usually take drinks with ice[1732] • May be lactose intolerant[1733] • Encourage prenatal salty diet with little fruit or vegetables[1734]
Healing Environment	• Greeting:[1735] ▸ Address patient formally with Mr. or Mrs. and last name • Believe that ill health is from not having yin-yang in balance; imbalance may have various sources, including "spirit taking over body"[1736] • Consider Western pharmaceuticals as "hot," affecting balance in body; may lower dose when feel imbalance[1737] • Herbs or teas in traditional medicine are believed to "cool" the body and may be taken to balance "hot" Western medicines[1738] • May nod or indicate agreement to show respect and avoid conflict[1739] ✓ Healthcare professional should verify patient's understanding • Usually do not offer medical information; accompanying family may provide information[1740] • Very modest; only touch between waist and knees when absolutely required for treatments, test, care[1741] • If plan of care or treatment for female patient includes examination of torso or pelvic area, arrange for same sex provider[1742] ✓ Patient may prefer for health care professional to carefully explain necessity and process for exam, and remain with patient during exam • Family, including extended, support patient; family does hands-on care for patient[1743] • Traditionally the husband/father makes decisions; wife may not agree, but will allow husband to decide in order to maintain peaceful relations[1744] • May believe that soul can leave body through invasive procedures, resulting in poor health or death[1745] • Does not count age from actual birth date; birthday is celebrated on New Year's Day (Tet)[1746]
Pain Management	• Patient unlikely to express pain; the individual may consider pain to be his/her fate[1747] ✓ Patient may use non-verbal cues to indicate pain • May have concerns about addiction; may be "stoic"[1748]

 END OF LIFE

Autopsy	• Autopsy acceptable, but may be difficult to obtain unless family understands reason for autopsy[1749]

Death – Body Care	• Family helps prepare body of deceased and places coin in mouth as aid to spirit[1750]
Death – Special Needs	• Family may request time with deceased before removal of body[1751]
Death Process	• May want family to receive news of terminal state rather than telling patient, so that patient is not worried[1752] ✓ Per HIPAA healthcare professional obtain patient's permission • In preparation for patient's death, family/friends help dying patient remember the good he/she did in lifetime[1753] • May prefer to die at home; one who dies away from home "becomes a wandering soul with no place to rest"[1754] • Overt expression of emotions is considered a weakness, except for the widow at the burial of her spouse[1755]
DNR	• Usually avoid extending the dying process, but it may be difficult to get consent for DNR[1756]
End-of-Life Discussion	• Eldest male (husband or oldest son) is usually "spokesperson" for family and makes decision; female will likely defer to male in decisions to maintain harmony[1757] ✓ Per HIPAA, healthcare professional must obtain patient's permission to disclose health information to third parties ✓ Healthcare professional may ask patient who will make healthcare decisions for them if not themselves ✓ Health professional may discuss patient's terminal illness if applicable
Organ Donation	• Organ donation not acceptable[1758] • Buddhists believe that removal of organs may result in lack of that part in next life[1759]
Withholding/Withdrawal	• May consider delay in removing life support to a "more auspicious date"[1760] • Family member may wish to consult with religious leader for advice before withdrawal of heroics[1761]

 PERINATAL CARE

Birth Process (Labor/C-Section/ Vaginal Birth)	• Prefer to ambulate during labor[1762]
	• Deliver in "squatting" position[1763]
	• Attended by close female member of family[1764]
	• Following delivery:[1765]
	  ▸ Mother seeks to restore balance of hot/cold by intake of warm drinks
	  ▸ Showers are prohibited; provide "sponge" baths instead
	  ▸ Mother may appear to ignore newborn as a measure to protect the newborn from the "evil eye"

Breastfeeding	• Promote breastfeeding, but do not feed baby colostrum[1766]
Circumcision	• Usually do not perform circumcision[1767]
Contraception	• Acceptable, unless Roman Catholic[1768]
Family/Father Involvement	• Female family will keep father away from delivery, but he should be accessible. Father who is more accustomed to US practice may take childbirth prep classes and attend to laboring mother[1769]
Genetic Conditions	• May believe this is retribution for actions of family[1770] • See "Neonatal Illness"
Neonatal Illness	• Prefer that the information be given to father who then decides who will disclose the information to mother; prefer physician presence when information is disclosed to mother[1771] ✓ Per HIPAA healthcare professional obtain patient's permission
Newborn Care	• Mother takes care of baby, but female relatives help for the first few months[1772]
Post-Partum Care	• Mother will eat more "hot" foods to "replace and strengthen her blood"[1773]
Prenatal Care	• Intimate touch allowed only in private; may not agree to pelvic exam[1774] • During pregnancy, mother is to avoid "strenuous activity" and avoid "sexual activity"[1775]
Termination of Pregnancy	• Not acceptable[1776] • Contradicts belief that soul enters at conception[1777]

Gypsy (Romani)

Note: The following information is general. Specific beliefs and practices may vary. Details on page 12.

Legend: ✓ = Suggestions for Healthcare Professionals; ▶ = Significant Details or Exceptions.

CARE OF THE PATIENT

Beliefs	• Faith practice based on Roman Catholic, Pentecostal belief systems; may use statues of saints[1778]
	• Believe illness is self-inflicted; if returned to "state of purity and conforming to correct social behavior," the illness will resolve[1779]
	• Respect for elders; elder has role in making decisions regarding patient treatment[1780]
	• Family and clan loyalty is the most important value[1781]
	• Close-knit culture that views others as impure; do not leave patient alone; many of clan will stay at same time with patient[1782]
	• Believe in supernatural and may use "herbs, charms, sing, curse, or spit on floor" to ward off death; may take herbs, wear charms, and red items to repel "evil spirits"[1783]
	• Family members may request Priest to visit patient; herbal medicines may be brought to the patient by gypsy spiritualist[1784]
	• Primarily seek care in acute situations[1785]
	• Believe good luck has been lost by those who become ill[1786]
Diet and Nutrition	• Diet high in fat content and highly seasoned[1787]
	• Culture has specific practices for food preparation[1788]
	• Believe eating certain foods will promote good health; believe health and luck go together[1789]
	• The heavier person is seen as healthy[1790]
	• Some adults may fast on Fridays[1791]
	• May bring in food in disposable containers to avoid items considered contaminated (used by non-Gypsies)[1792]
	✓ Staff may provide disposable food containers and utensils
Healing Environment	• View hospital as source of disease and isolation; hospitals are seen as "unclean"[1793]
	• May request pills by color, share with family[1794]
	• Gypsies generally do not follow preventive care measures and may be non-compliant with follow-up care, especially when it requires changes in lifestyle[1795, 1796]
	▶ Explain need to take full course of medications; may be non-compliant once patient begins to feel better
	• Body secretions from top half of body are not thought to be unclean; Roma believe sputum to be curative[1797]

Healing Environment (continued)	• Consider top half of body clean and must be separate from bottom half which is considered unclean[1798]
	✓ Patient may prefer healthcare professional and staff to wash hands before touching patient
	✓ Patient may prefer healthcare professional to use separate bath soap/linens for top half and bottom half of patient's body
	• Family members may request Priest to visit patient; herbal medicines may be brought to the patient by gypsy spiritualist[1799]
	• Patient assessment and care should be done by same sex person as patient[1800]
	• Patient/family distinguish between Gypsy illness and non-Gypsy; patient will use gypsy cures or go to the "drabami" (Gypsy women who are knowledgeable about medicines) for Gypsy illness, use physicians to cure other[1801]
	• Patient may be unable to read or write; discuss information requiring signature, establish knowledge base of patient regarding disease[1802]
	▸ Consider using videos, pictures, or other education materials to instruct
	▸ Consider lifestyle when discussing post-discharge care, as patient may be migratory
	• Custom of members of clan is to support ill through physical presence[1803]
	✓ To avoid multiple requests for information, healthcare professional may request a contact who will share information with family
	✓ Per HIPAA healthcare professional obtain patient's permission
	✓ Healthcare professional may consider placing patient in a bed which allows unrestricted visits to minimize disturbance to other patients or the giving of care; for example, provide room closest to unit entrance
Pain Management	• Expressive about pain; prefer "oral or IV" pain medication but no rectal meds[1804]

 END OF LIFE

Autopsy	• Generally not acceptable[1805]
Death – Special Needs	• Final words of dying are "very significant" and family will want to hear what the patient says; "feelings of person at moment of death indicate to relatives what will happen in the next year"[1806]
	• May light a candle by window when death is near, to "light the way" for the soul; family do not verbalize deceased's name in concern that deceased may "haunt" them[1807]
	✓ Family may prefer for healthcare professional to avoid using deceased's name when talking with them

Death Process	• Large numbers of clan arrive at hospital and camp out when Gypsy is dying; overt expressions of grief;[1808] some may believe that at death of "King" or "Queen" of gypsies, the soul of the deceased goes to the closest person present; others may ask to have dying patient moved outside or window opened to allow soul to be freed at death[1809]
End-of-Life Discussion	• Patient and family avoid discussion of matters pertaining to death[1810] ✓ Per HIPAA, healthcare professional must obtain patient's permission to disclose health information to third parties ✓ Healthcare professional may ask patient who will make healthcare decisions for them if not themselves ✓ Health professional may discuss patient's terminal illness if applicable
Organ Donation	• Generally not acceptable[1811] • Believes that after death the soul "retraces its steps" for the first year, body must remain together[1812]

👤 PERINATAL CARE

Breastfeeding	• Breastfeeding practiced[1813] • Mother may eliminate some foods from her diet to avoid colic in baby[1814]
Circumcision	• Male circumcision acceptable, but not usually done[1815]
Family/Father Involvement	• Father not present at delivery[1816]
Genetic Conditions	• Usually accepting of conditions, take care of child at home[1817]
Neonatal/ Infant End of Life	• Death of infant is bad luck; parents may have grandparents or hospital authorities take care of burial[1818]
Newborn Care	• New baby kept from visitors, cared for only by mother[1819] • Traditionally clean baby's navel and place ashes on it for protection[1820] • If newborn fusses, becomes ill when visitor in, believe visitor gave baby evil eye[1821]
Post-Partum Care	• Very sensitive to and embarrassed with discussions/examinations/ treatments of lower body and lower body excretions[1822] • Mothers are unclean for nine days post birth and may not "cook, or touch men"[1823]

Prenatal Care	
	• No prenatal care due to non-acceptance of vaginal exams[1824]
	• Pregnancy and birth considered "impure;" patient may prefer to be in hospital for birth to keep home "clean"[1825]
	• During birth family "tie and untie knots" in belief this keeps umbilical cord from tangling[1826]
	• Newborn's name is not verbalized; no photography; covered with father's clothing to designate who is father[1827]
	• Anything the mother touches after birth is thrown away since she is "unclean"[1828]

Latino: Brazilian

Note: The following information is general. Specific beliefs and practices may vary. Details on page 12.

Legend: ✓ = Suggestions for Healthcare Professionals; ▶ = Significant Details or Exceptions.

CARE OF THE PATIENT

Beliefs	• Most Brazilians are non-practicing Roman Catholics; however, there are other increasing religions such as Evangelical and other Protestant[1829]
	
	• Other religions include "Mormons, Jews, Muslims, Buddhists," and Umbanda; the rationale for many religions is due to Brazil's constitution, which guarantees freedom of religion[1830]
	
	• "Roman Catholics folk practices focus on saints, promises, and pilgrimages"[1831]
	
	• "Syncretism" is frequently seen where individuals follow "beliefs and practices" from more than one religion[1832]
	
	• Many believe in miraculous events, which they consider the result of intercession of saints[1833]
	  ▶ Many believe in "religious/spiritual healing;"
	  ▶ May seek Roman Catholic Priests during emergencies
	
	• Spiritists, practice laying on of hands, and folk healers give herbal remedies and offer "prayer and blessings"[1834]
	
	• Believe that sickness is caused by "fate" or God; may also believe patient is ill because of environmental changes[1835]
	
	• May believe that "suppression of strong negative emotions" results in "ataque" or "susto" and can be the source of mental problems[1836]

Blood	• Blood transfusions acceptable[1837]
Communication	• Portuguese literacy; variations in level of literacy of the English language and most do not speak Spanish[1838] • Physical greetings are with a hug, except in "business situations;" then women may hug, but men usually do not do so[1839] • Greetings: "Handshakes are appropriate when strangers are introduced or in formal situations for both greetings and goodbyes;" a kiss on each cheek is for a "family member, friend, or acquaintance"[1840] • Brazilians may use the title "Doutor/Doutora" (doctor) when addressing someone of "higher status;" they are more likely to address their co-workers using "Senhor/Senora" in addition to their first name[1841] • Speech volume is high and may talk over someone; interruptions are frequent and acceptable[1842] • Brazilians are often detailed-oriented when providing information but are courteous[1843] • Brazilians consider it rude to say no to a healthcare professional[1844]

Communication (continued)	• Written consent is not routine in Brazil; explanation in US consent forms of "possible complications and risks," may cause anxiety and worry for patients[1845]
	• Questions: "Patients and family members may be reluctant to question medical professionals about treatment options or to request second opinion"[1846]
	• Brazilians give direct eye contact when communicating; exception is lower class people avoiding direct eye contact with superior, to show respect[1847]
	• Brazilians do not observe personal space; if one moves to provide more space, Brazilian may be offended[1848]
	• Culture is highly tactile; touch is associated "with friendship and concern rather than intimacy"[1849]
	• May not arrive on time when it comes to personal and social occasions, but are usually prompt for business occasions[1850, 1851]
	▸ May need to emphasize time constraints for appointments and importance of meeting-assigned time parameters
	• Gestures are a normal part of conversations; however, the "American sign for OK (with thumb and forefinger)" is considered vulgar by Brazilians; to convey everything is good, use the "thumbs up"[1852]
	• Brazilians value privacy in their home and family matters, but within the family, little is considered private information[1853]
	• Decision-making role is often the duty of the parents or spouse[1854]
	• Males are the head of household of traditional families[1855]
Diet and Nutrition	• Brazilians eat three meals a day, with breakfast as the smallest meal; the main meal is at noon, with a lighter meal in the evening[1856]
	• Typical breakfast "consists of coffee with hot milk, French bread, and butter"[1857]
	• Main meal "consists of rice, beans, meat, and a vegetable or salad"[1858]
	• Evening meal may be "similar to lunch or a light meal, e.g., soup, hot milk and coffee, with bread or cake"[1859]
	• To increase appetite, one should take vitamins[1860]
	• Cooking food includes seasoning; Brazilians usually do not add seasoning once food is served[1861]
	• Beverages or water are taken without ice; may take soda with meals and "drink strong black coffee with sugar (cafezinho) after meals, also during mid-morning and/or mid-afternoon"[1862]
	• May believe certain food combinations can lead to illness or make illness worse; for example, may avoid cold items when one has respiratory problems; combinations such as milk and specific fruits are believed to be potential causes of illness[1863]
	• Roman Catholic Brazilians often eat fish on Fridays, during Lent season[1864]

Diet and Nutrition (continued)	• In cases of "liver dysfunction" (mal do figado), bland diets, and avoidance of fatty and spicy foods[1865] • Ill persons are usually given herbal teas and soups such as "chicken soup and rice soup"[1866]
Healing Environment	• Women may prefer/request for female caregivers due to modesty concerns[1867] • Physical appearance is important for both sexes; hygiene is highly practiced (bathing, shampooing)[1868] • Prefer to bathe prior to meal; may believe that post-meal activity affects digestion process[1869] • Brazilians often use "periwash" after urinating or passing a bowel movement[1870] • Patient values self-care; if unable to do self-care, may ask family member to help[1871] • May believe in spiritual clothing/amulets – "crucifix, rosaries, religious medallions, and figas (amulet in figure of clenched fist – used to ward off evil)"; "colored ribbons tied around wrists or ankles as part of petition to Virgin Mary, which are not removed"[1872] • Women are primary caregivers of the family; others (family or caregivers) are expected to give attention and care to ill person[1873] • Many Brazilians are hesitant to go through screening; they do not want the test to reveal illness/condition or deal with "bad news"[1874] • Homosexuals are included in family activities, but gender status may not be formally disclosed[1875]
Pain Management	• Both sexes have "low threshold for pain," with males tolerating less than females[1876] • Vocalization of pain may include "moaning, crying, or screaming"[1877] • May use home remedies; some follow prescriptions and treatments ordered[1878] • It is common for friends and family to share medications[1879] • Many Brazilians often prefer intramuscular or intravenous medications; may relate infusions to how sick the patient is[1880] • May use a variety of treatments such as "homeopathy, acupuncture, medicinal herbs, and spiritual healing" along with traditional medicines[1881] • May postpone medical care in US if they think doctor will "only prescribe Tylenol;" may rely on medications obtained from Brazil where many antibiotics and other drugs are available without prescription[1882]

END OF LIFE

Autopsy	• Autopsy may not be acceptable.[1883]

Death – Body Care	• After death, family may kiss or touch deceased and choose clothing to dress deceased; no rituals are practiced; family may desire interment in Brazil[1884]
Death – Special Needs	• Family may desire prolonged visitation with deceased before body is removed to morgue[1885] ✓ Health care professional may need to explain hospital and funeral services in US
Death Process	• Unforeseen death may be perceived as "fate, or God's will;" maintain religious beliefs "about life after death"[1886] • Patient may prefer to stay at the hospital with acute illness, otherwise may prefer to stay at home[1887] • May not desire hospice care due to belief that denying the patient "therapeutic measures" means giving up on possibility of recovery if death is certain:[1888] ✓ Healthcare professional may want to advise family as soon as possible to allow time for family to say good-bye ✓ Healthcare professional may offer to call priest, religious leader, or chaplain
DNR	• May not be open to DNR since family want to maintain hope for recovery[1889]
End-of-Life Discussion	• Those Cubans who have recently immigrated or who are less accustomed to Western medical practices may want the information about serious or terminal illness shared first with the spouse, eldest child, or spokesperson; those who have spent more time in US and are accustomed to Western medical practices generally want to know about their condition[1890] • Family may want to protect patient from knowledge about terminal status[1891] ✓ Per HIPAA, healthcare professional must obtain patient's permission to disclose health information to third parties ✓ Healthcare professional may ask patient who will make healthcare decisions for them if not themselves ✓ Health professional may discuss patient's terminal illness if applicable
Organ Donation	• May not be acceptable; donation not routine[1892] • More acceptable among "the youngest, the higher educated," and those belonging to families of higher economic status[1893]
Withholding/Withdrawal	• Generally will want all efforts made to extend life or to give palliative care[1894]

PERINATAL CARE

Baptism/Birth Ceremony	• Roman Catholics baptize infant after discharge from hospital[1895] • Parents may want baptism for a seriously ill newborn[1896]
Birth Process (Labor /C- Section/ Vaginal Birth)	• During labor mother may scream - has low threshold for pain[1897] • May choose Cesarean section for convenience, fear of problems with birth; may not accept normal birth after having had Cesarean[1898] • Episiotomy is favored to "restore tight vaginal opening to afford male partner sexual pleasure"[1899]
Breastfeeding	• Many women prefer to feed with "powdered dry milk" with the assumption that this will help them regain their pre-pregnancy shape sooner[1900]
Circumcision	• Males and females not typically circumcised[1901]
Contraception	• May be acceptable[1902] • Although the Roman Catholic church prohibits contraception except for the rhythm method and abstinence, most "married or partnered women" use other measures to prevent pregnancy[1903] • Many request tubal ligation in conjunction with Cesarean section; tubal ligation in Brazil requires consent of the husband in "women older than 25 who have at least two living children;" consent of male in Brazil is not necessary for other methods used to prevent pregnancy[1904]
Family/Father Involvement	• Father does not usually attend labor or delivery[1905, 1906]
Genetic Conditions	• Genetic defects caused by "God's will" or incidents during pregnancy; may also believe this is "associated with defective sperm, sometimes associated with excessive alcohol use"[1907]
Neonatal Illness	• Believe that exposure to fresh air may make infants/children ill[1908] • If child is sick:[1909] ✓ Healthcare professional should inform mother and father ✓ If mother is single, healthcare professional should tell her with family members or friends present
Neonatal/ Infant End of Life	• Infant death is attended with little sadness as the infant is considered "pure and is regarded as an angel"[1910] • Parents may want baptism for a seriously ill newborn[1911]
Newborn Care	• In the first 40 days, newborn is kept inside home except for visits to doctor; when outside, baby is completely covered[1912]
Post-Partum Care	• New mother is expected to refrain from strenuous activity and remain at home for 40 days after delivery; she is expected to rest with family members providing help[1913]

Prenatal Care	• Pregnancy is considered a special time; family tries to meet "desires or cravings (deseos)" of pregnant woman[1914] • May ask for ultrasound test to determine baby's gender[1915] • Prenatal care is practiced and desired, as well as childbirth preparation classes; may not access if no insurance coverage for costs[1916] • Discouraged from strenuous work and swimming during pregnancy; "taboos warn against sexual relations during pregnancy"[1917]
Termination of Pregnancy	• Abortion not acceptable[1918] • Brazilian law prohibits abortion with punishment for both the person undergoing the procedure and the one performing it[1919] • Traditional remedies in the form of teas may be taken to bring on a late menstrual period, which may result in a "natural abortion"[1920]

Latino: Colombian

Note: The following information is general. Specific beliefs and practices may vary. Details on page 12.

Legend: ✓ = Suggestions for Healthcare Professionals; ▶ = Significant Details or Exceptions.

❤ CARE OF THE PATIENT	
Beliefs	• The predominant religion is Roman Catholic, at greater than 90 percent[1921]
	• Illness is caused by patient's bad behavior, as a punishment or God's will[1922]
	• Mental illness is caused by an overwhelming situation; it disgraces family[1923]
	• Feelings of happiness and good are associated with good health as well as being able to maintain usual "role in life"[1924]
	• Extended family very influential; elder or oldest sister/brother acts as spokesperson[1925]
	• Males are decision-makers while females are caregivers to either sex patient[1926]
	• Colombians are respectful of elders; family members are caregivers when elders are ill[1927]
	• Admitting a patient to a facility for institutionalization is a last resort when there is no caregiver, but is regarded as desertion[1928]
	• Homosexuality is not acceptable[1929]
Blood	• Transfusions are acceptable, if necessary[1930]
Communication	• Spanish is the "national language;" generally literacy level determined by socioeconomic class[1931]
	• May be "very affectionate and friendly"[1932]
	• Colombians use direct eye contact with family and friends; may avoid direct eye contact with elders, "authority figures" and healthcare professionals (e.g., doctors, nurses)[1933]
	• May be emotional and loud; often hands are in motion while talking[1934]
	✓ Patient may prefer for healthcare professional to provide comfort by holding his/her hand or touching patient's shoulder while relaying "bad news."
	• For greeting, use formal title, Mr., Mrs., Miss, followed by person's last name[1935]
	• Men shake hands with both sexes, women "clasp each other's wrists," or greet with cheek to cheek for family and friends[1936]
	• Planning is usually for short-term; may be flexible about time and late for appointments[1937]
	✓ Healthcare professional may emphasize need to be on time for appointments

Communication (continued)	• Modest; will permit sharing private information if needed for care[1938]
	• In disclosing serious illness, family may ask the healthcare professional to deliver the information with them present or choose to tell patient themselves; may not wish to tell the patient how sick he/she is, especially if "the patient is a child or elderly parent"[1939]
	✓ Per HIPAA healthcare professional obtain patient's permission
	✓ In the event of serious illness, patient may prefer healthcare professional to consult with a close family member as to how to properly communicate news
	• Written consent is not routine in Colombia; healthcare professional may need to explain that "most procedures in US require written and signed consent from patient"[1940]
	▸ Explain this process slowly, requesting input from patient often to verify understanding and provide time for patient's questions
	▸ Patient may be "embarrassed" to ask questions, may need some prompting to ask
Diet and Nutrition	• Typically have three meals per day with lunch the largest; major meal in the US is usually at night[1941]
	• Breakfast is "coffee or chocolate and bread; lunch usually includes soup"[1942]
	• Lunch and dinner "staples are rice and potatoes; vegetables are scarce in diet"[1943]
	• Fruit juice taken with meals, usually watered down[1944]
	• May follow food beliefs influenced by religion (e.g., Roman Catholic will eat only fish rather than meat on Fridays during Lent)[1945]
	• Prefer stock from meat to chicken soup when ill[1946]
	• If Colombians have a cold, fever, or respiratory infection, they avoid cold or iced drinks; instead they "drink hot herbal tea (chamomile, mint, flaxseed, thyme, or rosemary)" or a hot beverage consisting of "diluted unrefined sugar cane paste, possibly with lime (agua de panela)"[1947]
	• During menstruation, women do not consume foods considered acidic[1948]
Healing Environment	• Room may contain images of the Virgin or Crucifix; family may wish to surround image(s) with candles, if allowed; religious family members may pray or say rosary if patient is very ill[1949]
	• When Colombians cannot access medical care, may use a "traditional healer (curandero) who uses special herb mixtures, prayers, or massage"[1950]
	• Patients may not seek care until very sick and some seek Western medicine along with traditional methods; family members usually care for them[1951]
	▸ May need to explain need for patient to walk and to participate in self-care as part of recovery process
	• Very modest, especially with caregiver of opposite sex[1952]
	▸ For toileting with bedpan or urinal, provide privacy

Healing Environment (continued)	✓ Patient may prefer to use a gown, robe, and hospital pants so that his/her body is not unnecessarily exposed[1953] • If healthcare professional is female, male patient may be distressed by examination or intervention needed in private areas[1954] • Roman Catholic Colombians often carry special clothing or amulets such as "medallions (escapularios), rosary beads, and religious figures and pictures"[1955] ✓ Patient may prefer healthcare professional to not remove these items without cause or permission ✓ If removal necessary, give to family
Pain Management	• Women in pain are more vocal and emotional; men are usually stoic[1956] • Oral or IV medications are preferable to intramuscular or rectal[1957] • May have concerns about addiction to pain medicine, which results in not following directions for taking pain medication[1958] • May apply "ice/heat to control pain, massage to control muscular pain"[1959] • May have access to medications from Colombia, which are sold over the counter[1960] ✓ Healthcare professional may ask patient if he/she is taking any medications not prescribed

🩺 END OF LIFE

Autopsy	• Acceptable if necessary to identify cause of death[1961] ✓ Per HIPAA healthcare professional obtain patient's permission ✓ After patient dies, healthcare professional may ask family spokesperson whether this is acceptable
Death – Body Care	• Family members may want to view deceased before the body leaves the room[1962] • Family may wish clean and dress the body; no special rituals[1963] • In Colombia, interment is usually within one to one and one-half days[1964] ✓ Healthcare professional may need to inform family that interment in US is generally at least three days after death
Death – Special Needs	• May have religious items near patient[1965]
Death Process	• Patient may prefer to stay at the hospital in cases of acute illness; however, in chronic or terminal cases may prefer to spend last days at home[1966] • May accept hospice care if understand that this does not mean forsaking care for patient[1967] • Roman Catholics believe that "one should be at peace and without sin at time of death"[1968]

Death Process (continued)	✓ With appropriate HIPAA permission, healthcare professional may inform head of family (spokesperson), away from patient room so that the family can be advised
	• Patient or family may request "sacrament of sick" for patient[1969]
	✓ Patient may prefer healthcare professional to call Priest or religious leader when to visit patient for confession, communion, or to receive sacrament
	• Priest at bedside is very important if patient is gravely ill[1970]
End-of-Life Discussion	• Prefer that healthcare professional inform spokesperson about impending death, away from patient's room[1971]
	✓ Per HIPAA, healthcare professional must obtain patient's permission to disclose health information to third parties
	✓ Healthcare professional may ask patient who will make healthcare decisions for them if not themselves
	✓ Health professional may discuss patient's terminal illness if applicable
Organ Donation	• May be acceptable[1972]

 PERINATAL CARE

Baptism/Birth ceremony	• Roman Catholics baptize, usually at church[1973]
Birth Process (Labor /C-Section/ Vaginal Birth)	• May take small amounts of liquids, but not solids, during labor[1974]
	• Relatives not usually present during labor and delivery; maternal grandmother may provide support[1975]
	• Anesthesia not customary, but may be accepted[1976]
	• Laboring mother may exhibit stoicism, passivity, and/or become loud[1977]
	• Cesarean section is more likely to be requested by those of upper class status; during periods of extreme pain, mother may ask for Cesarean section[1978]
Breastfeeding	• Usually breastfeed, especially those of "low to middle" socioeconomic levels[1979]
Circumcision	• Male circumcision acceptable, usually performed at birth; female circumcision unacceptable[1980]
Family/Father Involvement	• Acceptable for married couples; following Roman Catholicism does not appear to affect decision to use/ not use contraception; generally use condoms, especially in younger couples[1981]
	• May deny pregnancy and use traditional "menstrual inducing techniques" early in pregnancy[1982]
	• Recent immigrants who are educated are more likely to practice rhythm method[1983]

Genetic Conditions	• If problems are present with baby, discuss with father first, or close relative to ascertain best way to tell mother; physician should disclose news to mother[1984]
	• Genetic defect may be attributed to parents' actions[1985]
Neonatal Illness	• Parents may want baptism for seriously ill newborn[1986]
Newborn Care	• During the first 40 days, baby generally not taken out in public except for visits to doctor[1987]
	• May give newborn "sugar water;" baby is shielded by "hats, mittens, and booties" from "drafts" which are believed harmful, irrespective of temperature[1988]
	• Baby's bracelets to ward off the evil eye are a common sight[1989]
Post-Partum Care	• Baby's maternal grandmother and aunt may care for newborn and mother; newborn's father may also participate[1990]
	• May limit types of foods consumed and activities during the traditional "quarantine" period of 40 days postpartum[1991]
	• May place "cotton in their ears to avoid air entering their system"[1992]
	• Shower is customary on second day postpartum; female relative may provide perineal care[1993]
	• Mother given a high protein diet, usually chicken, for first month[1994]
Prenatal Care	• Seek prenatal care if financially possible, unless recent immigrant from rural Colombia; when "childbirth" instruction is possible, parents generally participate[1995]
	• Mother is expected to rest, consume plenty of nourishing food, especially protein-rich foods[1996]
Termination of Pregnancy	• By law, abortions are illegal[1997]
	• In Roman Catholic faith it is considered "a sin;" however, abortions do occur and are more acceptable in "urban" families[1998]
	• May deny pregnancy and use traditional "menstrual inducing techniques" early in pregnancy[1999]

Latino: Cuban

Note: The following information is general. Specific beliefs and practices may vary. Details on page 12.

Legend: ✓ = Suggestions for Healthcare Professionals; ▶ = Significant Details or Exceptions.

❤ CARE OF THE PATIENT	
Beliefs	• Majority of population (85%) are Roman Catholic; rest follow African Cuban Santeria, Protestant or Jewish spiritual beliefs[2000] • In order to promote a sense of well-being and support, a visit from the patient's local religious leader may help[2001] • "Santeria" or "Regla de Ocha" is a blend of African tribal and Roman Catholic beliefs; "Santeria is viewed as a link to past and is used to cope with physical and emotional problems"[2002] ✓ Patient may prefer healthcare professional to offer privacy when patients and/or families want to conduct religious prayer or rites, as long as sanitation and safety regulations are observed • May be reluctant to accept treatment for illness or condition that cannot be "seen" or does not have symptoms[2003] • May assume illness is result of nervousness, stress, or germs, evil spells, or Voodoo[2004] • May worship specific saint; reciting rosary and praying is familiar practice[2005] • May use amulets to protect from supernatural evil[2006] ▶ To reduce anxiety, allow patient to continue wearing amulet, religious articles, if at all possible • In order to maintain good health, it is important to avoid bad news, extremes, or stress[2007] • Patient with a mental illness is a stigma; family may not admit to illness or accept treatment[2008] • May suffer "anxiety and depression" from leaving Cuba, family, friends, and having little contact from family remaining in Cuba[2009] • Cubans primarily seek Western medicine when ill; however, may also utilize spiritual healers as last resort[2010]
Blood	• Transfusions allowed[2011]
Communication	• Cubans primarily speak Spanish, often rapidly[2012, 2013] • Many communicate in "Spanglish, a mixture of Spanish and English;" those with higher education are more likely to use English as choice of spoken language in the home[2014] ✓ Patients who are less familiar with English may need assistance with filling out required forms • Cubans often use two surnames - the mother and father's family names; at marriage a woman adds her husband's surname[2015]

Communication (continued)	✓ Healthcare professional may need to verify the patient's legal name
	✓ Patient may prefer healthcare professional to use a formal greeting, especially the elderly, with Senor (Mr.), Senora (Mrs.), or Senorita (Miss), unless patient desires a different address
	• Prefer relationships that are non-confrontational, "smooth," and show respect for others; value "intimate interpersonal relationships over impersonal" business relationships[2016]
	• Cubans are often late for appointments; focus is on current issues[2017]
	✓ Healthcare professional may want to stress the importance and necessity of arriving on time for scheduled visits
	• Support and care is provided by nuclear and extended family, including godparents[2018]
	• Cuban homes often include several generations; all are involved in decision-making process[2019]
	▸ Home care often provided by the extended family
	✓ Per HIPAA healthcare professional obtain patient's permission
	✓ Patient may prefer for healthcare professional to communicate directly with the decision maker for family
	✓ For invasive procedures, patient may prefer healthcare professional to obtain verbal consent from family as well as closest relative
	• Touching and close contact is acceptable with family and friends; frequently use hand gestures when speaking[2020]
	• Anticipate direct eye contact; lack of eye contact indicates dishonesty or disrespect[2021]
	• Formal greeting for strangers; family greet with hug and kiss on cheek, handshake customary between men[2022]
	• Cubans articulate loudly, may seem unfriendly; commands or requests may seem demanding[2023]
	• Privacy is enormously imperative, only those permitted by patient or approved spokesperson are privy to personal health information; often patient or family will prefer information be withheld from patient[2024]
	• Believe that patient should not be given negative information; this would be additional burden for patient[2025]
	• Family may discuss health issues with eldest in family before agreeing to procedure or plan; if patient is terminal, family may expect healthcare professional to discuss it with patient's spouse or oldest child[2026]
	✓ With appropriate HIPAA permission, allow family to determine whether or not to tell patient
Diet and Nutrition	• Traditional Cuban diet may be high in fat, cholesterol, sugar, and fried foods; rice and beans are usually served, but very few vegetables[2027, 2028]
	• Traditional staples include "root crops like yucca, yams, malanga, and boniato" as well as "plantains and grains"[2029]
	• Dishes are often cooked with "sofrito (olive oil, garlic, tomato sauce, vinegar, wine, lime juice) and spices;" frequently meat is marinated in citrus juice[2030]

Diet and Nutrition (continued)	✓ Healthcare professional may inquire about usual cooking and traditional food eaten; calorie-laden flavorings may be added • May be intolerant of milk products[2031] • Routinely have "almuerzo," the main meal, at noon and "comida as late as 10-11 PM"[2032, 2033] ✓ Healthcare professional may inquire about meal times to adjust medication doses appropriately • Cubans consider being heavy as "positive, healthy, and sexually appealing"[2034] ✓ Healthcare professional may prefer to advise patients, if needed, about the health risks linked with obesity and partner with them with a qualified professional; i.e., a nutrition/dietician • Believe in consuming "fresh foods, soups, and broths when ill," but light meals[2035] • Beverages often consist of cold fluids; taboo to consume certain foods with certain drinks; "many foods used as home remedies"[2036]
Healing Environment	• Family present at hospital around the clock, especially in relation to a gravely ill patient[2037] • Both sexes are "very modest;" prefer bathing daily[2038] • May assume that washing hair worsens illness and results in chills/drafts; nail care for women is essential[2039] • Toileting in bathroom is preferred over bedpan; "regularity is priority," with peri-care (soap and water) afterward[2040] • Clothing or bed may have religious medallions attached to it[2041] • Patient may be totally passive in receiving care; self-care not considered norm[2042] • May not be proactive in obtaining healthcare assistance; may request help only when critical[2043] • Family often the chief source for health counsel; elder women supply conventional home remedies such as teas or mixtures to alleviate mild to moderate symptoms or to try to cure usual illnesses[2044] • Definition of health means non-existence of pain[2045] ✓ Healthcare professional may provide teaching about "preventive measures and health promotion activities" ✓ Healthcare professional may also teach the extended family, as this will increase likelihood that the patient will follow instructions[2046] • Regard plump, rose-colored cheeks as a sign of good health; thin seen as sign of poor health[2047] • Decision maker and family protector is generally the "most educated, respected, or eldest family member, usually male;" women are usually passive but supportive, providing care for family[2048] • Family oriented with love and respect for parents and elders; provide care for them at home[2049, 2050]

Healing Environment (continued)	• Doctors are held in high esteem and patients usually will follow doctor's recommendation[2051]
	• Many use conventional "medicinal plants in the form of teas, potions, salves, or poultices;" some share others' prescriptions[2052]
	✓ Healthcare professional may inquire about traditional remedies used. This will determine if any item may be contraindicated or harmful to patient treatment. Safe remedies should be continued if possible
	✓ Determine what over-the-counter (OTC) or prescriptive drugs the patient may be taking
	✓ Healthcare professional may need to instruct patient on dangers of OTC or using medication prescribed for others
	• Homosexuality is not acceptable; often do not disclose gender identity[2053]
Pain Management	• Female appears to have higher tolerance to pain than male; Cubans do not want to be addicted to pain medication and stop as soon as possible[2054]
	• Culturally suitable to articulate feelings of pain; threshold for pain in male is usually lower than female[2055]
	• Believe intramuscular medication has better effect[2056]
	• Usually patient is passive. Family females will provide care as well as manage symptoms[2057]

END OF LIFE

Autopsy	• May not be acceptable[2058]
Death – Body Care	• No specific rites or dress[2059]
Death – Special Needs	• May request lighted candles which are believed to illuminate the spirit's way to the next life[2060]
	✓ Healthcare professional may ask whether electric candles are permitted and acceptable to family
Death Process	• Family may desire to be with deceased patient overnight[2061]
	• Support of the extended family at death is vital[2062]
	• Loud crying occurs during grieving, along with other physical expressions of sorrow[2063]
	• At death of patient, men may be stoic, as death is often seen as a part of life[2064]
	▸ Stoicism does not imply lack of feelings for patient at end of life
	• Many family members and friends usually congregate around dying person[2065]
	• Roman Catholics believe prayers said for the dying provide a "peaceful passage" from this life to the next; "rosary beads, crucifixes, or estampitas (little statues of saints)" are placed in the patient's room[2066]

Death Process (continued)	• Death rites for those believers of Santeria may consist of "animal sacrifice, chants, ceremonial gestures"[2067] ✓ Patient may prefer healthcare professional to call a local religious leader ✓ If possible, healthcare professional should provide space for family members to congregate near the dying patient
DNR	• To Cubans DNR means one has abandoned hope of recovery; this practice is not acceptable[2068] • Generally will want all efforts made to extend life or give palliative care[2069]
End-of-Life Discussion	• Depending on acculturation, patient may wish to know of terminal condition[2070] • Family may not wish to inform patient of impending death, family will stay near until death occurs[2071] • Hospital death preferred, due to desire for hospital medical care[2072] ✓ Per HIPAA, healthcare professional must obtain patient's permission to disclose health information to third parties ✓ Healthcare professional may ask patient who will make healthcare decisions for them if not themselves ✓ Health professional may discuss patient's terminal illness if applicable
Organ Donation	• May not be acceptable[2073]
Withholding/Withdrawal	• Believe in heroics and necessary treatments to prolong life or provide palliative care[2074]

👪 PERINATAL CARE

Baptism/Birth Ceremony	• Majority are Roman Catholic, whose practice includes baptism[2075] • Cubans desire babies, children who are chubby[2076]
Birth Process (Labor /C-Section/ Vaginal Birth)	• Woman's mother may be present, husbands may or may not attend during labor process and delivery; desire to have medical doctor for delivery[2077] • Laboring woman will have an inactive role generally; vocalizations of pain are loud[2078] • Prefer to deliver in the hospital as believe that "infant and maternal mortality" is lower with hospital birth[2079]
Breastfeeding	• Traditionally, breastfeeding is strongly encouraged; mother may elect to bottle feed when given formula choices in US[2080] • Breastfeeding is practiced[2081] • Believe that breastfeeding is better than bottle, but breastfeeding may lead to breast "deformity"[2082] • Baby transitions to solid foods and bottle at an early age; bottle weaning often transpires at about 4 months due to the belief that "a fat child is a healthy child"[2083]

Circumcision	• Male circumcision is not norm in Cuba; no female circumcision[2084]
Contraception	• May be open to use of birth control, unless religious[2085] • Recent immigrant may be accustomed to oral contraceptives; condom use is not usual as males believe condoms interfere with sensation during intercourse[2086]
Family/Father involvement	• Traditionally, father is not present; mother who is more aware of US practice may be open to father's involvement in birth[2087] • Fathers attend labor/delivery, usually as observer rather than coach[2088]
Fetal/End of Life	• Usually parents will name stillborn[2089] • Mother may believe that condition is "punishment for her sins"[2090]
Genetic Conditions	• Problems with baby should be communicated with father and then maternal grandmother, but not directly with the mother[2091] ✓ Per HIPAA healthcare professional obtain patient's permission
Neonatal Illness	• If baby needs neonatal intensive care unit, mother will usually be at baby's crib and provide care[2092] • Mother may believe that condition is "punishment" for her sins or that she saw a child with that condition during pregnancy; some will accept condition as part of God's plan[2093]
Neonatal/Infant End of Life	• Family will expect terminal infant to receive last rites[2094] • Parents may want baptism for seriously ill newborn[2095] • Death of baby affects extended family who support parents; may accept death with attitude that baby's death was God's will[2096]
Newborn Care	• Mother may expect to have baby with her from birth on, unless baby has medical condition; Cubans customarily have rooming-in[2097] • Traditionally will use binder over umbilicus to prevent it from sticking out and to "keep the intestines from falling out"[2098] ✓ If mother is using binder, healthcare professional may remind her to keep it sufficiently loose for drying and use cotton to avoid infection • May believe blindness and deafness is caused by "cutting the infant's hair or nails in first 3 months"[2099] ✓ Healthcare professional should obtain permission prior to cutting baby's hair or nails
Post-Partum Care	• Female family members will care for "mother, infant, and housework" during the 40 days post birth designated for postpartum care; mother's role is to breastfeed and care for the baby[2100] • Avoid sexual relations during 40 days post birth; may wear girdle to help return to pre-pregnancy condition[2101] • Believe mother may contract infection during postpartum period if she walks, is exposed to cold, or does not cover feet[2102]

Post-Partum Care (continued)	• Woman's mother and sister usually care for new mother and infant for 41 days; typically do not leave home during this period[2103]
	• Believe postpartum mother should not hear "bad news" or have stress as either may affect mother or baby negatively[2104]
Prenatal Care	• Seek care during pregnancy, unless cost is issue[2105]
	• Parents very receptive to attendance at childbirth classes[2106]
	• Women usually follow the provider's directions, don't question[2107]
	• Recent immigrant may have "calcium deficiency and be undernourished due to limited supplies of calcium, calcium-rich foods, and protein" in Cuba; may also have micronutrient deficiencies[2108]
	• Cuban women have a high incidence of high blood pressure developing during pregnancy; malnutrition is seen frequently[2109]
	• Pregnancy is considered a normal event; both future grandmothers provide support and information during prenatal period as well as after the birth; immigrant may have limited or no support system[2110]
	• Grandmother's role is important in making decisions about pregnancy and baby, but more fathers are getting involved[2111]
	• Rest for mother is supported; no arduous activities[2112]
	• Keep loud noises and people with abnormalities away from pregnant women; may believe that these will affect the fetus[2113]
Termination of Pregnancy	• More accepted among recently arrived Cubans[2114]

Latino: Dominican

Note: The following information is general. Specific beliefs and practices may vary. Details on page 12.

Legend: ✓ = Suggestions for Healthcare Professionals; ▶ = Significant Details or Exceptions.

♥ CARE OF THE PATIENT	
Beliefs	• High percentage of Roman Catholics (95%); other gods and practices have also been introduced by African heritage[2115]
	• Common practice is to have small shrines around the house with saints and likeness of Virgin Mary; heritage combines the following spiritual aspects:[2116]
	▶ Christianity
	▶ Spiritism (espiritismo or promoting spiritual wellness through moral behavior)
	▶ Santeria (merging Roman Catholic saints and African gods)
	▶ Witches (brujos)
	▶ Healers (curanderos)
	• In spiritism, a medium acts as intermediary to receive information on how to make the petitioners' soul pure through his/her moral behavior[2117]
	• Santeria common practices "include worshipping African gods (orishas)" that are related to certain saints in Roman Catholic faith[2118]
	• May petition God for help with illness and offer religious activities in exchange for God's assistance[2119]
	• Dominicans believe in link between spirituality and illness[2120]
	• Illness often seen as "punishment, a lesson to be learned or God's will;" first step may be to pray for God's healing[2121]
	• Mental illness as a stigma, a "punishment for moral" sins or the result of a "spell or curse;" care is provided by family at home and family usually agreeable to psychotherapy and psychotropic medications[2122]
	• Gays and Lesbians most likely do not disclose their gender orientation; Dominicans do not recognize homosexuality or transsexuals[2123]
	• Dominican's most basic and "powerful social unit" is the nuclear and extended family[2124]
Blood	• Transfusion acceptable[2125]
Communication	• Castellano (Castilian) Spanish is the language spoken; may have learned English in Dominican school[2126]
	• Dominicans are polite and greet others with respect; address older women by "Senora" or "Dona" and last name, men by "Senor" or "Don" and last name[2127]
	• Greet all members in a group upon arrival with a "social kiss on each cheek;" handshake acceptable for newcomer of either sex[2128]

Communication (continued)	• Tone of voice can be loud and emphatic[2129]
	• Prefer non-confrontational conversation, although tend to be blunt; if they do not agree, they will indicate so[2130]
	• Recent arrival to US or someone who is not sure regarding English pronunciation may use family member to interpret; patient usually prefers interpreter of same gender[2131]
	• Dominicans do not tell patient about terminal situation; want news to be given to family member who is closest relative; frequently family decides it is best not to disclose news to patient[2132]
	✓ Healthcare professional to obtain permission from patient per HIPAA
	• Based on resources, education and status, families can react differently to serious illness; patient or family distribute patient information to family members in certain prescribed order[2133]
	• Dominicans anticipate that health care professionals will be "sensitive and compassionate"[2134]
	• May be leery of signing consents unless they trust the professional who explains it[2135]
	✓ Patient may prefer to establish trusting relationship with healthcare professional before consent to treat or provide services is given
	• Typically reluctant to take part in research; concerned there will be no help if something goes wrong, and concerned about being used as "guinea pigs"[2136]
	• Direct eye contact is used; generally less personal space is acceptable unless with person of opposite gender; do not want closeness to be misconstrued in sexual way[2137]
	• Extremely animate and emotional when speaking, using hands and body language; improper gestures similar to US culture[2138]
	• May not share feelings with strangers, although may share with family and friends[2139]
	• Communicate "private information" with healthcare professional if pertinent to healthcare; however, sexual information is not usually shared[2140]
	• May "touch one another on the arms and shoulders; pinch on cheek is OK, especially with children"[2141]
	✓ Patient may prefer healthcare professional to obtain permission before touching the patient
	• Dominicans have a flexible orientation to time; may be late for appointments[2142]
	• Head of family in a traditional household is often dominant male, typically the family spokesperson[2143]
Diet and Nutrition	• Traditional meal pattern is three meals a day, with lunchtime as the largest meal[2144]
	• A typical breakfast often consists of "white farmer's cheese (queso blanco), eggs, and salami, all fried"[2145]

Diet and Nutrition (continued)	✓ In place of bread, sometimes mashed green plantains may be served
	• A typical dinner is "eggs, salami, plantains, and homemade soup"[2146]
	• Staples are "beans, rice, meat, and salad;" many favorite foods are fried[2147]
	• Espresso is consumed at all meals; occasionally hot chocolate is also provided[2148]
	• May use herbal teas to treat illness; may drink ethnic beverages that are fortified with vitamins[2149]
	• Families gather at meals, sharing news; it is considered rude to have the television or radio on at meal times[2150]
	• May follow hot/cold balance of disease: "Hot" medications or "hot" foods are taken for "cold" illnesses and cold foods are omitted for "cold" illness[2151]
	• During Holy Week or other religious holidays, may fast or refrain from eating meat products[2152]
Healing Environment	• Unacceptable for caregivers to be of opposite gender, especially for physical care[2153]
	• Prefer daily baths; for skin care Dominicans often use many natural products, applied on skin until dry and then rinsed off[2154]
	• Ill patients may refrain from bathing due to beliefs about balance in hot/cold theory; may believe getting cold increases "humoral imbalance" when have fever[2155]
	• After toileting, Dominicans choose to wash (rather than use just toilet paper); also prefer perineal care[2156]
	▸ If bedpan or commode is required, ensure privacy to protect modesty
	• Dominican culture is "a mixture of Spanish, Taino, Indian, and African slave influences that consist of protective and healing traditions;" persons who have made a religious promise often wear white clothing with colored sash[2157]
	• Many embellish their attire with assorted "charms, amulets, and healing pouches;" a black onyx charm on a baby wards off evil eye; necklaces with pendants of saints are worn; statues of saints are placed at patient's bedside[2158]
	• May affix bags of herbal mixtures to clothing for "protection and healing;" if necessary to remove special amulets or medals, patient/family usually agree[2159]
	✓ Patient may prefer for healthcare professional to give protection/healing remedies to a family member, should they need to be removed
	• Patients usually do self-care; if patient is unable, family members will provide care[2160]
	• Sick are often inactive, permit family members to care for them[2161]
	• Family members generally remain with patient 24 hours a day - at least one member remains with the patient, if possible[2162]

Healing Environment (continued)	• Expectation is that all family members and close friends will visit; visitors offer comfort and are supportive to patient and family[2163]
Pain Management	• Improper for individuals to admit or seem weak; men especially do not express "pain or discomfort and are expected" to put up with it[2164] • May not seek medical care until symptoms prevent normal function[2165] • May refuse "narcotics" even after a discussion about the importance of narcotics to care; concerned about dependency[2166] • Non-prescription methods of pain management are OK[2167] • May intermix traditional remedies such as herbs, ointments, and teas with Western medicine[2168] • Most allow others to do their care in acute or chronic illness[2169]

END OF LIFE

Autopsy	• Autopsy is unacceptable unless required[2170] ✓ Healthcare professional may inquire with spouse, mother, or the individual who was closest to the deceased
Death – Body Care	• Body of deceased is taken to funeral home for preparation[2171]
Death – Special Needs	• Most family members come to the bedside if patient passes at hospital; customary to burn candles near the body of deceased[2172] • Family comes together at the wake or funeral; most will travel to Dominican Republic if interment services will be held there[2173]
Death Process	• In religious families, family may call clergy[2174] • Family prefer to be advised of patient's imminent death; may not tell patient[2175]
End-of-Life Discussion	• Prefer that information concerning imminent death be provided to immediate and extended families; usually do not tell patient[2176] ✓ Per HIPAA, healthcare professional must obtain patient's permission to disclose health information to third parties ✓ Healthcare professional may ask patient who will make healthcare decisions for them if not themselves ✓ Health professional may discuss patient's terminal illness if applicable
Organ Donation	• Believe body should remain whole for burial; usually against organ donation[2177] • In cases where a patient needs an organ, believe that someone in family will provide it if he/she is able to do so[2178]

PERINATAL CARE

Baptism/Birth ceremony	• If practicing Roman Catholic parents, baptism is required, usually in church[2179]
Birth Process (Labor/ C-section/ Vaginal Birth)	• During labor mother remains active; delivers at hospital[2180] • During labor woman is often very vocal and expressive; usually asks for pain medication, asks God or family for assistance[2181] • If possible, both grandmothers of newborn are present and other females may support and coach[2182] • Prefer a natural delivery; a Cesarean section is often seen by elder family members as weakness when mother is unable to give birth on own and will restrict mother's capacity to provide infant care[2183]
Breastfeeding	• Highly promoted for all infants; mothers who have become familiar to the American cultural practices may utilize a combination of breastfeeding and bottle feeding[2184] • Not unusual for a toddler or preschooler to be on breast; weaning is done by child[2185]
Circumcision	• Generally male infants are not circumcised; female circumcision is not done[2186]
Contraception	• Roman Catholic church prohibits unnatural forms of birth control, only withdrawal or rhythm method allowed[2187] • Men may refuse condoms; they believe condoms are restrictive[2188]
Family/Father Involvement	• During labor and delivery, male partner, although supportive, waits outside birthing area[2189] • Postpartum, father is expected to continue to be loving and supportive, but sexual activity with new mother is prohibited[2190]
Genetic Conditions	• May believe condition is punishment from God; will care for child at home[2191] • "Husband, eldest person, mother and mother-in-law" tell new mother; problems are not shared with "outsiders"[2192] • The head of family decides if it is acceptable to share information with extended family[2193] ✓ Per HIPAA healthcare professional obtain patient's permission ✓ Patient's family may prefer for healthcare professional to inform father/ husband and elder family member first • If Roman Catholic, may want baptism for seriously ill newborn[2194]
Newborn Care	• Mothers bond with newborn after delivery by "holding and cuddling;" during 40 days post birth, grandmother is caregiver for newborn[2195] • If family is accustomed to US practices, father may actively contribute to infant care[2196]

Newborn Care (continued)	• May place a "black onyx charm in form of a hand" on newborn's wrist to protect newborn from "evil eye"[2197]
Post-Partum Care	• Grandmother helps family while mother recuperates and rests; mother's care for infant is limited to breastfeeding[2198] • Mother's first meals postpartum usually include warm soup and stews as well as lots of fluids to regain "strength and well-being"[2199] • Elder females may discourage mother from baths or shampoos during the first 40 days[2200] • Postpartum, father is expected to continue to be loving and supportive, but sexual activity with new mother is prohibited[2201]
Prenatal Care	• If financially feasible, will seek prenatal care early in pregnancy[2202]
Termination of Pregnancy	• Abortion prohibited in Roman Catholicism; however herbal remedies may be used secretly to cause abortion[2203]
PEDIATRICS	
Child/Teen Environment of Care	• May have special prayers and services for child or young person who dies; believe death of young or traumatic death indicates person was not prepared for death; special prayers will help "spirit go to heaven"[2204]

Latino: Mexican

Note: The following information is general. Specific beliefs and practices may vary. Details on page 12.

Legend: ✓ = Suggestions for Healthcare Professionals; ▶ = Significant Details or Exceptions.

♥ CARE OF THE PATIENT	
Beliefs	• Majority of people are Roman Catholics but may also believe in some type of witchcraft[2205]
	• Patriarchal society; elders and their opinions are respected; primarily seek care for illness[2206, 2207]
	• May believe in good health due to luck, a matter of keeping in balance or God-given[2208]
	• Illness results from hot/cold not being balanced or the result of not doing right[2209]
	• May believe that illness can be expected in life and must be tolerated[2210]
	• Prevent illness by "prayer, wearing medals or amulets," herbs[2211]
	• May seek healers and traditional medicines before or while utilizing medical care[2212]
	• Believe that when the "four body humors" are not balanced, illness occurs; cure comes from correcting the imbalance in these elements through addition or subtraction of "heat, cold, dryness, or wetness"[2213]
	✓ If patient refuses food or medication, healthcare professional may discuss what foods/medications he/she can take to restore balance
	• Many believe in maintaining health through hot/cold balance using hot foods for "cold" illness: "Hot foods include chocolate, eggs, oil, red meat, chilies, and onions. Cold foods include fresh vegetables, tropical fruits, dairy products, and fish or chicken"[2214]
	• Very social culture; family important, including extended family and godparents[2215]
	• Homosexuality generally not accepted[2216]
Blood	• Transfusions are acceptable; may be concerned about HIV[2217]
	• Blood taken for testing may cause concern; may not believe that blood will be replenished by body and person will be weaker[2218]
Communication	• English is often spoken by educated persons, however some Mexicans speak Chicano Spanish; recent immigrants use Spanish, but try to learn English[2219]
	• There are 62 languages used in Mexico; many recent immigrants speak Spanish, but are not literate in Spanish[2220]
	• Many have only an elementary level education and cannot read or write in Spanish; however many can read and write in English[2221]
	▶ Inquire if patient can read and write in English and/or Spanish

Communication (continued)	• May be suspicious of consent, especially written, if undocumented immigrant; fear they are "signing away their rights," and will be sent back to Mexico[2222]
	✓ Patient may prefer for healthcare professional to be Spanish-speaking or to be of the same ethnic group prior to giving consent
	• Will avoid eye contact with opposite gender and those considered in authority; extended direct eye contact can be misconstrued as a "challenge or intimidation;" gazing into another's eyes indicates an "intimate relationship"[2223]
	▸ Be warm and respectful in conversing with patient and look over patient's shoulder
	• When addressing a professional or elder, conventional persons "prefer the formal 'you' (usted) rather than the informal (tu)"[2224]
	✓ Healthcare professional may ask how patient would like to be addressed
	• Handshake is appropriate for stranger; family and close friends greet with hug; many females greet each other with kiss to each cheek[2225]
	• Patient and family may stand in respect when healthcare professional enters the room[2226]
	• Believe loudness to be impolite when addressing another; loudness may trigger disengagement and non-compliance[2227]
	✓ Patient may prefer healthcare professional to use non-confrontational tone when giving commands or making requests
	• Friendly conversations between friends and family may be loud[2228]
	• Intimate space may be up to 18 inches, depending on relationship; may maintain space of 9-12 feet with strangers[2229]
	• Women may use dramatic body language to express emotion; men are more stoic; however, some people may articulate less and maintain control over emotions[2230]
	• It is unacceptable to openly disagree with physician; it may appear patient agrees when he/she does not[2231]
	• Do not share family issues with non-family; typically communicate information about condition with "spouse, children, and selected members of extended family"[2232]
	• Touch "family and close friends," but it is not acceptable between others[2233]
	✓ Patient may prefer healthcare professional to inform patient why touch is needed
	✓ Healthcare professional obtain permission from patient before touching any area of patient's body, especially private areas
	• May not be on time for appointments; time focus is usually on present time; future is up to God[2234]
	▸ Stress the necessity of arriving on time for scheduled appointments

Communication (continued)	• May make social conversation first, before serious conversation with healthcare professional; may be polite and cautious, roundabout rather than frank; out of respect may agree with a provider's recommendation or prescription[2235] • Prefer to have interpreter who has "knowledge of regional differences in the Spanish language;" also someone who is same sex and near patient's age[2236] ✓ Healthcare professionals should avoid using relatives as interpreters to prevent sharing personal health information with relative ✓ Per HIPAA healthcare professional obtain patient's permission
Diet and Nutrition	• For many, lighter meal usually consumed in evening with big meal eaten during lunch[2237] ✓ Healthcare professional may consider meal sizes and times when planning medication schedule • Staples include "beans, rice, and tortilla"[2238] • High usage of salt and fat in diet[2239] • Traditionally use lard in cooking; some now reduce fat intake[2240, 2241] • Breads and pastries are often used for snacks[2242] • Have a preference for cool drinks in summer, especially fruit juices[2243] • Coffee is typically consumed for breakfast, on special occasions hot chocolate[2244] • Some Roman Catholics do not eat meat during Lent[2245]
Healing Environment	• Value modesty; uneasy revealing their bodies to someone of opposite sex[2246] ✓ Prevent unnecessary exposure of patient; present a cover for his/her lower extremities ✓ Patient may prefer privacy if bedpan or commode is used • When ill, patient makes every effort to remain clean; typical to bathe every day[2247] • Amulets and special clothing differ broadly; some examples include "crucifixes, scapulars, and religious medals"[2248] ✓ Patient may prefer to give permission before amulet or special clothing needs to be removed ✓ Patient may prefer amulet or special clothing to be handled with care and given to family • Patient is passive in self-care at hospital; may expect hospital staff to assist or may wait for family members[2249] • If patient perceives home care is a burden to family, may try to do self-care[2250] • Women are the primary caregivers, however some other family members may elect to be caregivers[2251]

Healing Environment (continued)	• Family members remain near patient, some may sleep close to patient who is elder or child; limited visiting hours may appear to family as a way "to hide something from family"[2252]
	• Touch, handshake, hugs are important in relationships; value physical presence[2253]
	• Patient may not follow directions if patient believes he/she has no control over illness[2254]
	• Elders and their opinions are respected[2255]
	• Need to gain confidence of patient in order to help patient; confidence building begins with formally using patient's correct surname and establishing rapport BEFORE discussing purpose of visit[2256]
	• It is unacceptable to openly disagree with physician; therefore, it may appear that the patient agrees when he/she does not[2257]
	• Family and Priest pray for patient[2258]
	✓ Healthcare professional clarify patient's understanding and wishes about his/her healthcare
Pain Management	• May refuse pain intervention if believes pain is due to wrongdoing he/she did[2259]
	• Pain is considered a sign of weakness, unlikely to express; but moaning is acceptable[2260]
	• May not pay attention to pain since "lack of stamina" is not acceptable and patient should practice "self-control"[2261]
	✓ Healthcare professional clarify patient's behavior regarding pain; discuss pain relief options and what patient has used in past for relief
	• Prior to seeking medical care, patients may utilize folk remedies such as herbal that a relative suggests; due to economics or legal status may not seek medical care[2262]
	• Also may seek healing by "visiting shrines or using spiritual healing or prayers"[2263]

END OF LIFE

Autopsy	• Autopsy acceptable[2264]
Death – Body Care	• Family may ask to view body before it is removed from room; some may want to participate in body preparation[2265]
	• Roman Catholics say the rosary the night before burial and a solemn mass of resurrection is said before interment[2266]
Death – Special Needs	• Patient may have religious items or rosary beads[2267]
	✓ Patient may prefer to have religious items close by
	• If patient is Roman Catholic, patient may request a visit to be anointed by the Priest[2268]

Death – Special Needs (continued)	✓ Patient may prefer healthcare professional to call Priest for sacrament of sick; if cannot reach Priest, call hospital Chaplain • Chaplain may still administer sacrament if patient dies before Priest arrives[2269] ✓ If Priest is on way, leave body in room until Priest arrives • Families of other faiths, including Protestants, may ask their Minister or Pastor to provide a service[2270] ✓ Patient's family may prefer extra time with deceased, to say good-bye
Death Process	• Members are compelled to visit in hospital or nursing home; anticipate many visitors as death involves extended family[2271] • Adult relatives, friends may wish to remain with dying, deceased[2272] ✓ Healthcare professional may locate a private place for family to gather with patient or nearby • Family may ask to have "lighted candles in room of dying patient"[2273] ✓ If possible, healthcare professional may offer electric candles • Mexican Americans express grief overtly, may pray the rosary[2274]
DNR	• May not want DNR in belief that there is hope for patient to get better[2275]
End-of-Life Discussion	• If there is serious or terminal illness, inform patient and family together and as soon as possible[2276] ✓ Family may prefer private space to grieve • Some may prefer to die at home; may accept hospice, but varies according to acculturation, physical, and financial support available to patient[2277] ✓ Per HIPAA, healthcare professional must obtain patient's permission to disclose health information to third parties ✓ Healthcare professional may ask patient who will make healthcare decisions for them if not themselves ✓ Health professional may discuss patient's terminal illness if applicable
Organ Donation	• If patient is practicing Roman Catholic, transplant may not be acceptable; believe in body integrity at interment[2278]

 PERINATAL CARE

Baptism/Birth ceremony	• Baptism is practiced for those who are of Roman Catholic faith[2279]
Birth Process (Labor /C-Section/ Vaginal Birth)	• If healthcare professional is male, Mexican female may refuse care[2280] • Favor natural delivery without medication; concern about effect of medication on mother and on baby[2281] • Mother may want to eat during labor[2282] • May perceive Cesarean section (C-S) as extreme[2283] ▶ If C-S is needed, clarify the rationale and results of undergoing C-S • Mother may desire a chubby baby; sees size as an indication of health[2284]

Contraception	• Birth control is acceptable; women may prefer pills or tubal ligation, although tubal ligation may cause "psychological issues" (ability to have children is seen as a very important part of being woman)[2285, 2286] • Mexican female may not accept any method that requires touching her "genitals;" may accept IUD[2287] • Men may not agree to birth control, especially condoms; may consider contraception that encourages women to have sexual relationships outside of marriage[2288]
Family/Father Involvement	• Mother very modest; may not be comfortable with father in delivery room[2289] • Husband may assume that his attendance at birth is not appropriate[2290] • If the father is accustomed to US practice, father may participate in delivery[2291] • Males generally do not participate in caring for baby[2292]
Fetal/End of Life	• For fetal death, mother may wish to see and hold fetus; photos may be acceptable as well as a lock of hair as remembrance[2293]
Genetic Conditions	• Believe that condition may be God's will, due to mother's lack of care or a hex[2294] • Usually open to counseling if recommended by provider, but may not want to undergo some testing; may have concerns that amniocentesis will lead to miscarriage[2295]
Neonatal Illness	• Discuss baby illness/ condition as soon as possible with parents if mother and father at hospital setting[2296] • New mothers consult with female family members regarding issues with baby; may search the Internet for information or ask healthcare professional, if available[2297] • If there are no other resources, some us traditional remedies[2298]
Neonatal/ Infant End of Life	• If Roman Catholic, parents may want baptism for seriously ill newborn[2299] • Believe that this is God's will, not mother's fault; accept death[2300]
Newborn Care	• May believe that blindness and deafness in newborns are associated with cutting the baby's hair or nails in the first 3 months[2301] ✓ Patient's family may prefer healthcare professional to obtain permission before cutting an infant's hair or nails • May follow practice of using "a key, coin or other metal object" on belly button to aid healing[2302] ✓ Healthcare professional should educate mother on how to prepare object to avoid infection • Family members may provide care for baby; grandmothers, aunts, and close female relatives may babysit[2303] • Baby may not be bathed for a few weeks to maintain balance in "hot and cold" theory[2304]

Newborn Care (continued)	• Babies are not permitted to cry for extended periods, in order to prevent umbilical hernia; may use a belt around baby's abdomen[2305] • Mother may wrap baby with many covers to protect from "bad air" and also to prevent others from looking at baby[2306] • Touch is important; believe that admiring a child but NOT touching may induce "evil eye," a folk illness[2307] ✓When assessing the infant, healthcare professional should touch the baby or pediatric patient to avoid concern about "evil eye"
Post-Partum Care	• Normally, women take 2-3 months to recuperate (la cuarentena – 40 days); viewed as "special time"[2308] • Post-partum woman is susceptible to illnesses; new mother avoids "strenuous physical activity" while family provides care and does housework for her[2309] • Generally family provides care for new mother and baby[2310] • Mother wears "an abdominal binder" to keep "air from entering the uterus"[2311] • May avoid tub bath; personal hygiene is very important[2312] • Mother may believe that "covering ears, head, shoulders, and feet can prevent blindness, mastitis, frigidity, or sterility"[2313] ✓Healthcare professional may identify which practices are harmless; respect the woman's belief • Sexual relations do not usually occur during the 40 days of recovery[2314]
Prenatal Care	• Mexican woman receives more attention during pregnancy than at any other time; it is a positive and natural condition[2315] • May refuse to seek prenatal care due to costs or doctor who is male[2316] • Other reasons for not seeking prenatal care may include: No insurance, financial issues, transportation, language barrier, undocumented immigrant, attendance at job, lack of someone to care for other children, necessity for pelvic exam[2317] ✓Patient may prefer healthcare professional to discuss the rationale and importance of the pelvic exam "before proceeding with history and physical examination" • Family and friends provide information and guide pregnant woman; prenatal care is usually sought for establishing due date or if there is a problem[2318] • Childbirth classes are rarely attended in belief that birth is natural situation and does not require preparation[2319] • May agree with providers' directions but not follow them; follow advice better when provided by someone who speaks her language or is of the same culture[2320] • May refuse to take prenatal vitamins which are considered "hot food"[2321] • Believe that mother's weight gain is not a problem; a healthy baby results if mother is "not thin or underweight"[2322]

Prenatal Care (continued)	• Avoid sexual relations toward end of pregnancy[2323] • In order to prevent birth deformities "safety pins, metal keys, or other metal amulets are worn"[2324]
Termination of Pregnancy	• More conservative do not accept abortion; level of acculturation and devotion to religious beliefs affect attitude toward abortion[2325] • Even when there is a problem with fetus, Mexicans do not opt for abortion; believe that God can heal fetus[2326] • In cases of incest or rape, abortion may be acceptable[2327]

PEDIATRICS

Child/Teen Environment of Care	• Although metamizole (a non-steroidal anti-inflammatory) is banned in US, it may be purchased in ethnic stores or Mexico and used for fever and pain; it has been linked to agranulocytosis and death in children[2328] • Recent immigrants learn English in US schools; once learned, English becomes language of choice for most children[2329] • Touch is important; believe that admiring a child but NOT touching may induce "evil eye," a folk illness[2330] ✓ When assessing the child, healthcare professional should touch the baby or pediatric patient to avoid concern about "evil eye"

Latino: Puerto Rican

Note: The following information is general. Specific beliefs and practices may vary. Details on page 12.

Legend: ✓ = Suggestions for Healthcare Professionals; ▶ = Significant Details or Exceptions.

♥ CARE OF THE PATIENT	
Beliefs	• Majority of population is Roman Catholic (85%)[2331]
	• May practice "Espiritismo, a blending of Indian, African, and Roman Catholic beliefs that deals with communication and use of evil and good spirits"[2332]
	• Puerto Ricans are extremely spiritual; heath care providers may be requested to communicate information with clergy or conventional faith healers[2333]
	• Causes for illness may be one of numerous reasons, for example, "seen as hereditary, punishment, caused by immoral behavior, failure to care for health, result of evil or negative environmental forces" in the individual[2334]
	• May believe in hot/cold system for good health; some seek folk healers[2335]
	• Most seek care only when ill; do not use healthcare services for preventative care[2336]
	• May use over-the-counter or traditional remedies for "mental health symptoms;" do not discuss mental status with others, which may make it difficult to obtain information[2337]
	• Gay or lesbian status is not discussed; most do not accept and consider this orientation a "stigma"[2338]
Blood	• May refuse blood (receiving/giving) due to concerns about HIV[2339]
	✓ Healthcare professional may want to cautiously review patient's attitude toward blood donation and transfusions
	✓ Clarify and correct misconceptions
Communication	• Use both Spanish and English in communication, although Spanish spoken mostly at home[2340]
	✓ Healthcare professional may want to provide information at slow pace to increase likelihood of understanding of English language
	• Education is highly valued but many leave high school before graduation; few continue education to become professionals[2341]
	• Interpersonal relationships are very important; very hospitable and caring[2342]
	• Puerto Ricans offer homemade foods as an expression of thanks and appreciation; refusal of foods may be insulting[2343]
	• Appropriate greeting for males involves a handshake; females tend to exchange embraces; close friends and family of both genders will generally exchange embrace[2344]

Communication (continued)	• Voice is pleasant sounding with Spanish accent; intonation often misunderstood as argumentative language[2345] • Commonly augment conversation with body language by using "hand, leg, head, and body gestures;" emotions are also articulated through touch[2346] • May nod "yes" and say "Aha!" during discussion, but this does not signify patient understands[2347] ✓When obtaining consent, healthcare professional may want to clarify understanding of information given ✓Patient may require time to read and communicate information to family • May not consider appointment is at fixed time; may arrive later than prescribed time and overstay visit with lengthy discussions[2348] • Develop "confianza" (trust) first so patient and family will be comfortable with discussions about health matters; most readily discuss health issues, except for "sexuality"[2349] • Formal greetings show esteem and consideration[2350] ✓Patient and family may prefer to be addressed as "Senora" or "Dona" for females, and "Don" or "Senor" for males • Puerto Ricans want to be perceived as "likeable, appealing, and fun-loving"[2351] • Expect direct eye contact; some may not look into eyes as sign of respect for other person; single women, due to modesty, may refrain from direct eye contact with men[2352] • Approachable in expressing their discomforts and physical issues with healthcare professionals[2353]
Diet and Nutrition	• Standard meal pattern is "three full meals a day"[2354] • Typical breakfast meal includes hot cereal cooked with toppings; less commonly may consume "corn pancakes or fritters"[2355] • Around noon, lunch is served, with dinner in early evening; traditional to have espresso at 10AM and 3PM[2356] ✓Healthcare professional may inquire about conventional foods and their nutritional content to help families with dietary practices that combine their standard or preferred selections • Diet includes various root foods which are believed to provide important nutrients[2357] • May find North American meals unappealing[2358] • Normally favor iced drinks; hot drinks preferred when experiencing colds or respiratory illness[2359] • Constipation and diarrhea are blamed on "harmful" food intake[2360]
Healing Environment	• Usually shampoo and shower daily except when ill; women do not shampoo during menstruation[2361] • If cannot use toilet, patient may refrain from passing a bowel movement[2362]

Healing Environment (continued)	• Prefer to do personal care on own or with little help from family member of same sex; in the home, family often offer support and care[2363]
	• Various herbal teas (home remedies) are used to "treat illness and promote health"[2364]
	✓ Healthcare professional may want to inquire about non-conventional therapies during routine health assessments and include in care if seen as harmless
	• May favor bathing with "a basin of water instead of taking a shower after surgery"[2365]
	• Family (nuclear and extended) regarded as very important; "all activities, decisions, social, and cultural standards conceived around family"[2366]
	• May seek advice from family and friends prior to seeking help from healthcare system[2367]
	• May consult elders before making decision as a "sign of respect; in some families oldest son and daughter are authorized to make healthcare decisions"[2368]
	• Husband's consent may be required in some women's health matters, particularly with older women[2369]
	• Men are expected to be decision-makers for the family, whereas women are caregivers[2370]
	• May find comfort in "Scripture readings, praise, and prayer"[2371]
	• During recovery, patient "assumes passive role," which may delay healing process[2372]
Pain Management	• As part of coping mechanism for pain, may be "very loud and outspoken"[2373]
	• Favor oral or intravenous medications for managing pain[2374]
	• Also use "herbal teas, heat, and prayer" to control pain[2375]
	• May seek advice from family and friends prior to seeking help from healthcare system[2376]

END OF LIFE

Autopsy	• Autopsy may be unacceptable, a "violation of the body"[2377]
Death – Special Needs	• Family may want to "touch and kiss" deceased before body is moved to morgue[2378]
	• Overt expressions of bereavement are common as some perceive lack of grief expression equates with lack of caring and respect for deceased[2379]
Death Process	• Ill person usually has family member stay with them 24/7[2380]
	• May expect all close family be in attendance when patient dies as well as at funeral[2381]
	• At death, spiritual leaders are anticipated to be with patient[2382]

Death Process (continued)	• May prefer that family spokesperson, rather than patient, be notified of impending death, usually in a private area and with clergy present[2383] ✓ Healthcare professional to obtain appropriate permission per HIPAA ✓ Patient may prefer for clergy to be present when receiving terminal news • Patient may desire closure with family before death so that spirit will be able to go into next life[2384] ✓ Healthcare professional may want to deliver terminal news to family in a private area; "allow time for the family to view, touch, and stay with the body before it is removed"
End-of-Life Discussion	• Patient may not be told of terminal illness, and this is seldom discussed within family; avoidance allows family to be positive[2385] ✓ Per HIPAA, healthcare professional must obtain patient's permission to disclose health information to third parties ✓ Healthcare professional may ask patient who will make healthcare decisions for them if not themselves ✓ Health professional may discuss patient's terminal illness if applicable
Organ Donation	• Organ donation acceptable; seen as an "act of goodwill and a gift of life"[2386] ✓ Calmly and carefully discuss organ donation ✓ Provide clear and precise information ✓ Priest or Minister may assist in discussion

PERINATAL CARE

Baptism/Birth Ceremony	• Baptism is practiced by those who are of Roman Catholic faith[2387]
Birth Process (Labor /C-Section/ Vaginal Birth)	• Women in labor prefer to give birth at the hospital; important to maintain modesty; "assume active, demanding role" during labor[2388] • Most "prefer bed position for labor"[2389] • Woman who undergoes a Cesarean section is seen as a "weak woman;" therefore, many do not want a Cesarean section[2390] ▸ Include education about Cesarean section early in pregnancy and reasons why it is sometimes a necessary "invasive intervention during labor" • Most ask for pain medication[2391]
Breastfeeding	• Breastfeeding mothers are encouraged to drink "lots of fluids such as chicken soup and milk; punches (beverages consisting of milk or fresh juices mixed with raw egg yolk and sugar) are consumed if feeling weak or tired"[2392] • Recommend against consumption of "hot foods such as chocolate, beans, lentils, and coffee" because they are believed to cause stomach irritability, flatus, and colic for mother and infant[2393] • May not understand the importance of breastfeeding as breastfeeding is thought of as a contributor to weight gain and unflattering changes to breast[2394]

Breastfeeding (continued)	✓ Healthcare professional may provide breastfeeding education; include maternal grandmothers and significant others who are influential for mother ✓ Healthcare professional my want to clarify beliefs
Circumcision	• Infant males often circumcised at birth; female circumcision not acceptable[2395]
Contraception	• Traditionally, women do not use birth control methods such as "foams, creams, and diaphragms;" these are seen as immoral by Roman Catholic church. "Only the rhythm method and sexual abstinence" are acceptable[2396] • Male may refuse condom use in belief that it is less manly and reduces male satisfaction; female may think male perceives her as "dirty" if he uses a condom[2397]
Family/Father Involvement	• Father is usually supportive during labor/delivery, but does not take an active role; may or may not be present depending on acculturation and age[2398]
Genetic Conditions	• Inform mother first if there are issues with the baby[2399] • Very stressful for family, frequently believe mother is at fault[2400] ✓ Healthcare professional may want to supply information about the causes of genetic defects to lessen guilt and stress for parents
Neonatal Illness	• Inform mother first if there are issues with the baby[2401] • If Roman Catholic, parents may want baptism for seriously ill newborn[2402]
Newborn Care	• New mother, with help from father, will care for baby; paternal grandmother of baby may provide assistance for several months[2403]
Post-Partum Care	• Traditionally "first meal after delivery is homemade chicken soup"[2404] • Women are encouraged to rest for the first 40 days after delivery; some may refrain from shampooing[2405]
Prenatal Care	• Although many women receive prenatal care, may not begin until later than usual in US culture[2406] • Women may receive gifts and good wishes, rest and eat well; males cater to women during their pregnancy and are "tolerant, understanding, and patient"[2407] • View exercise as unsuitable[2408] ✓ Healthcare professional may want to emphasize importance of exercise during pregnancy • Women often "refrain from sexual relations after second trimester; men may view this as time for extramarital sexual activity"[2409] ✓ Healthcare professional may discuss STDs and possible exposure to AIDS with husband

Termination of Pregnancy	• Abortion seen as unconventional in the past; accepted only when pregnancy placed life of mother at risk; however, many women now find it acceptable[2410]
	• If Roman Catholic, abortion is prohibited[2411]

 PEDIATRICS

Child/Teen Environment of Care	• May use small black rabbit foot, or small black fist (azabache) "to ward off evil; believe illness, misfortune, or death may result if rabbit foot or azabache is removed"[2412]
	• May use "amulet" to watch over child's health; also use "rosary and figures of saints" around the bed[2413]
	✓ Patient may prefer for healthcare professional to obtain permission before removing amulets or religious objects

Middle Eastern: Arab

Note: The following information is general. Specific beliefs and practices may vary. Details on page 12.

Legend: ✓ = Suggestions for Healthcare Professionals; ▶ = Significant Details or Exceptions.

♥ CARE OF THE PATIENT	
Beliefs	• Patriarchal society; family loyalty of greatest importance; do not want the patient to know seriousness of condition[2414] • Muslim Arab believes that mental illness is not possible if one is following faith tenets; mental illness is taboo[2415, 2416]
Blood	• Transfusion may be acceptable[2417]

Communication	• Silence may mean respect for healthcare professional or lack of understanding; may agree in order to be polite[2418]
	• Greeting:[2419]
	  ▶ Greet patient formally by title and first name
	  ▶ Handshake acceptable; touch between same gender
	• Left hand is used for "hygiene while right hand is used for eating;" may be offensive to hand patient something with left hand[2420]

Diet and Nutrition	• Do not mix hot and cold foods at same meal[2421] • Depending on faith, may eat meats; eat well cooked meats, avoid rare meat and raw fish[2422]
Healing Environment	• Family provides assistance to patient; someone remains with patient[2423] • Expect to rest when ill, view patient care as the responsibility of the healthcare worker and do not help with patient's personal care[2424, 2425] • May be willing to participate more actively in therapy if understand the reason for the therapy[2426] • Wash after toileting with running water; provide pitcher for patient[2427]
Pain Management	• Some use prayers and religious readings to cope with pain[2428] • Believe that he/she has low threshold for pain; may believe that relief should occur immediately after treatment or medication given[2429] • Consider injections better for pain relief; IV fluids indicate serious condition[2430] • Express pain to family non-verbally with loud noises; may exhibit less signs of pain with non-family[2431] • May avoid usual postoperative coughing and exercise to avoid pain[2432]
🏥 END OF LIFE	
Autopsy	• May not be acceptable; the body is considered holy[2433]

Death – Body Care	• After Muslim death, family member of like sex will prepare body in prescribed rites that include washing and rinsing dead body[2434, 2435]
Death – Special Needs	• Family may arrange for men to pray over patient who has died[2436] • May need a separate room for family to grieve; grief is expressed overtly and "uncontrollably"[2437]
Death Process	• Prefer to die in hospital where options to extend life are available[2438] • Muslim patients should be turned to face toward Mecca (Saudi Arabia)[2439]
DNR	• Death accepted as natural occurrence, however believe in providing heroics to extend life[2440] • Offering DNR option to family may cause them to mistrust professionals[2441]
End-of-Life Discussion	• Prefer discussion of serious matters be done with family spokesperson; family protects patient from serious information[2442] ✓ Per HIPAA, healthcare professional must obtain patient's permission to disclose health information to third parties ✓ Healthcare professional may ask patient who will make healthcare decisions for them if not themselves ✓ Health professional may discuss patient's terminal illness if applicable
Organ Donation	• Body should remain whole, therefore may not agree to organ donation[2443]
Withholding/Withdrawal	✓ See above "DNR" category

👤 PERINATAL CARE

Adoption	• For Muslim it is not acceptable to change surname or for child to lose connections with biological parents/family[2444]
Baptism/Birth Ceremony	• In Muslim family, father may "whisper call to prayer" in baby's ear[2445]
Birth Process (Labor/C-Section/ Vaginal Birth)	• Muslim mother keeps hair covered and remains in dress during labor, as long as possible[2446] • May express pain with loud nonverbal noises[2447] • May use low vocalization so that "strangers" cannot hear them[2448] • May withstand pain. Believe that God will reward that endurance[2449]
Breastfeeding	• May request that baby be cleaned before she breastfeeds, due to concern for mother's purity[2450] • Acceptable to breastfeed; may believe colostrum is not good for baby and wait until milk comes in[2451]
Circumcision	• Muslim requires circumcision[2452]
Contraception	• Muslims may use contraception in pill format for "preconception" but do not use "morning-after pill"[2453] • Acceptable within the married union[2454]

Family/Father Involvement	• Father not usually in attendance at birth[2455]
Genetic Conditions	• May view birth defects as a "test of faith"[2456]
Neonatal Illness	• Discussion of problems with baby should be with both mother and father, always providing hope to couple for restoration of health of baby[2457]
Newborn Care	• Parents may place amulet on clothing to protect newborn from "evil eye"[2458]
Post-partum Care	• Mother may expect complete bed rest after delivery; females in family take over mother's duties at home[2459]
Prenatal Care	• Mother is to rest and eat "well" during pregnancy; may not seek prenatal care because pregnancy is normal or because of the cost[2460] • Do not prepare for birth in advance; "deal with it when it happens"[2461]
Termination of Pregnancy	• Based on religious influence, abortion is not widely practiced[2462]
PEDIATRICS	
Child/Teen Environment of Care	• May view birth defects as a "test of faith;" most will mainstream child into daily family life, possibly pretending there is no problem[2463]

West Indian: Haitian

Note: The following information is general. Specific beliefs and practices may vary. Details on page 12.

Legend: ✓ = Suggestions for Healthcare Professionals; ▶ = Significant Details or Exceptions.

♥ CARE OF THE PATIENT

Beliefs	• Majority follow Roman Catholic or Protestant belief system[2464]
	  ▶ Frequently take communion
	  ▶ Believe prayer can bring about healing of body
	  ▶ Follow sacraments, but believe the sacrament of the sick indicates death is near
	  ▶ Many use traditional home remedies before seeking Western medical help
	• Believe in God and prayers[2465]
	• Matriarchal society with extended family[2466]
	• Follow folk medicine in addition to seeking physician's care; frequently will use leaves (which are thought to have "mystical powers") in clothing and on person[2467]
	• Some believe in voodoo – an illness believed to "originate supernaturally or magically is treated with voodoo medicine;" may seek herbs to treat usual illness or "evil eye"[2468, 2469]
	• Seek healthcare professional for acute illness[2470]

Blood	• Many believe that soul is associated with blood and are reluctant to give blood for testing[2471] • Due to the importance of blood, many are fearful of transfusions and the serious connotation of needing blood; also may be concerned about transmission of HIV/AIDS[2472]
Communication	• Touch in giving patient care is supportive to patient[2473] • Touch between friends in conversation is norm; may touch healthcare professional during discussion[2474] • May speak loudly and very emotionally[2475] • Eye contact with superior is considered rude[2476]
Diet and Nutrition	• May eat one meal per day[2477] • May not eat non-ethnic food; preferences include rice and beans, plantains[2478] • May follow "hot/cold theory" of balance to attain wellness[2479]
Healing Environment	• Supported by extended family[2480] • Family may wish to remain to do hands-on care[2481]

Healing Environment (continued)	• Often follow traditional remedies recommended by Priests and healers; may not seek healthcare until condition is advanced due to immigration status, poverty, and/or lack of education[2482] ✓ Healthcare professional may consider using educational material in video, audio, diagrams, and/or drawings; some may not be able to read • Based on personal experience or another Haitian's experience, may try "home remedies" including Haitian medication, some of which are made with roots and/or leaves; some produced in Europe[2483] • May agree by head movement, smile when do not comprehend instructions or discussion due to lack of education[2484] • May practice routine purging[2485]
Pain Management	• Many have a "very low pain threshold"[2486] • Expressive about pain, but may not localize it[2487] • Prefer parenteral route for pain medication[2488]

END OF LIFE

Autopsy	• Not promoted, but may accept if death was due to unnatural causes[2489]
Death – Body Care	• After death, family member gives last bath[2490] ✓ Healthcare professional may ask family about participation in post-mortem care
Death – Special Needs	• If patient is dying, family would like member who is authorized to know; then, authorized person will then let patient know if deems it appropriate to do so[2491]
Death Process	• Relatives, friends want to be present when death is close; family grieves overtly after patient's belongings removed from home[2492] • Deceased is buried within 24 hours of death[2493]
End-of-Life Discussion	✓ Per HIPAA, healthcare professional must obtain patient's permission to disclose health information to third parties ✓ Healthcare professional may ask patient who will make healthcare decisions for them if not themselves ✓ Health professional may discuss patient's terminal illness if applicable
Organ Donation	• Not promoted[2494] • Believe body should "remain whole for burial"[2495]

PERINATAL CARE

Birth Process (Labor/C-Section/ Vaginal Birth)	• Use midwife; during labor patient may "sing, pray, cry, or moan to call voodoo protector"[2496] • Deliver in "squatting or semi-seated position"[2497]

Birth Process (Labor/C-Section/ Vaginal Birth)(continued)	• Prefer normal delivery; "fear" surgical delivery[2498] • Generally do not request pain medication during labor[2499]
Breastfeeding	• Practiced after milk arrives[2500]
Circumcision	• Do not promote male circumcision in belief that it will limit sexual satisfaction[2501]
Contraception	• Traditional beliefs: God determines how many children a mother will bear; may not practice birth control[2502]
Family/Father Involvement	• Father usually not at delivery[2503]
Newborn Care	• Believe meconium should be eliminated and may give traditional laxative to baby while waiting for breast milk; use of home remedy to rid infant of meconium may produce diarrhea and lead to dehydration[2504] • When teaching pregnant or new mother, family may prefer healthcare professional to use the term "strong baby," which engages the mother's attention and interest more than "healthy baby"[2505]
Post-Partum Care	• Mother may practice traditional bath in hot water with herbs for first 3 days postpartum[2506] • Requires certain "cold" foods to restore balance to body[2507]
Prenatal Care	• May not seek prenatal care[2508] • Place emphasis on certain foods the new mother is allowed to eat during pregnancy and post delivery[2509] • Many not willing to discuss sexual matters with non-Haitian[2510] • Believe sexual intercourse is necessary to keep "birth canal lubricated for birth"[2511]
Termination of Pregnancy	• Up to the individual; most unlikely to discuss abortion, considered a private matter[2512]

West Indian: Jamaican

Note: The following information is general. Specific beliefs and practices may vary. Details on page 12.

Legend: ✓ = Suggestions for Healthcare Professionals; ▶ = Significant Details or Exceptions.

❤ CARE OF THE PATIENT	
Beliefs	• Religious beliefs are mostly Christian[2513] 　▶ Over 60 percent of the people belong to the Protestant churches 　▶ Over 34 percent belong to other religions, including spiritual cults and religions that are a combination of African cultural beliefs and Christianity • Special healing rituals include honoring ancestors, memorials, and giving thanks[2514] • Most believe in life after death[2515] • May seek help of traditional healers as well as modern medicine; promote wellness[2516] • Matriarchal society; family unit may include three generations: Grandmother, mother, and children; may or may not have father as part of the unit[2517, 2518] • May view illness as caused by germs, natural occurrence, or a medical treatment that "failed;" other sources of illness include punishment for sin of parent or ancestor or evil spirits[2519] • More accepting of physical illness than mental illness[2520]
Blood	• Blood transfusion is OK[2521]
Communication	• English is the official language of Jamaica; broken English, called Patois (patwa) is also widely spoken[2522] • Personal space should be observed[2523] • Customarily do not use touch with those they do not know[2524] • Avoids eye contact with those in authority; expects to be called by title and last name; may not understand or question healthcare professional about consents[2525] ✓ Healthcare professional greet patient formally with Mr. or Mrs. and last name, ex. Mr. Brown or Mrs. Patterson • May appear "shy" and reluctant to discuss information with caregiver; due to respect for health caregiver, may agree to instructions without understanding[2526] • Patient is unlikely to indicate he/she does not understand; will agree out of respect for provider[2527]
Diet and Nutrition	• Usually have big meal in middle of day; staples are carbohydrates (e.g., rice, yams, sweet potatoes), tropical fruits, cassava bread, with a small portion of protein (e.g., poultry, fish, beef, pork, goat)[2528]

Diet and Nutrition (continued)	• Most meals include rice; during illness drink only warm beverages[2529] • Traditionally, eat spiced food[2530] • Traditionally teas are taken for many minor conditions with specific leaves to treat each condition[2531] • May be at high risk for "diabetes, heart disease, and strokes" due to current tendency to eat diet of carbohydrates and foods "high in salt, sugar, and fat calories"[2532] • If Rastafarian, will not eat pork[2533]
Healing Environment	• Women make most healthcare decisions and take care of children[2534] • May use traditional healing before Western medicine[2535] • Greetings: Formally meet stranger using Mr., Mrs., or Miss or a title that designates the person's profession; shake hands and wish the person a "Good morning"[2536] • Greet family and friends with "simple nod or bow, handshake, hug, or kiss" expressing respect for the individual[2537] • Autonomous, believe that it is essential to make own decisions and depend on selves; may not be compliant if he/she believes healthcare professional discounts Jamaican's beliefs regarding healthcare[2538] • Family presence provides support when patient is told of serious or terminal illness[2539]
Pain Management	• Usually try traditional remedies such as "herbal teas, ointments, or balms," before Western medicine; may only take pharmaceuticals until symptoms are gone; prefer oral medications[2540] • Fear addiction to medications; may stop taking medicines as soon as pain or other symptoms are gone[2541]

END OF LIFE

Autopsy	• Usually will refuse, unless required[2542]
Death – Body Care	• No special rites or care given[2543]
Death – Special Needs	• Family may request to view body of deceased "as it was when individual died"[2544]
Death Process	• When death is near, family pray and "witness loved one's passing"[2545] • Death is accepted and natural for the very old; may believe death of younger person is due to having violated "cultural taboo," or from "spirits or envy"[2546]
End-of-Life Discussion	• If patient is "terminal, significant other(s) are to be told first" and they will decide when to tell patient[2547] ✓ Per HIPAA, healthcare professional must obtain patient's permission to disclose health information to third parties

End-of-Life Discussion (continued)	✓Healthcare professional may ask patient who will make healthcare decisions for them if not themselves ✓Health professional may discuss patient's terminal illness if applicable
Organ Donation	• May not agree to organ donations; believe keeping body whole is important[2548]

PERINATAL CARE

Baptism/Birth Ceremony	• "Christening" occurs shortly after birth when family's faith requires it[2549]
Birth Process (Labor/C-Section/Vaginal Birth)	• Encourage walking during labor; may be stoic with pain[2550] • Prefer normal delivery[2551] • Support system in labor may be very large; may want to have a large number of people at delivery[2552]
Breastfeeding	• Breastfeeding has been widely promoted and is preferred over bottle-feeding[2553] • Breastfeeding may end at 6 weeks and solids like porridge initiated[2554] • Temperature influences food given to baby; believe cold milk will give baby colic, and breast milk from mother who is hot is considered sour and not good for baby[2555]
Circumcision	• Not widely practiced[2556]
Contraception	• Birth control permitted; men reluctant to use condoms[2557] • May not be aware of contraception methods available in US[2558]
Family/Father Involvement	• Father may not go to prenatal visits or take childbirth education[2559] • Father does not usually attend birth[2560]
Genetic Conditions	• Seen as "God's will;" believe is "punishment for parents' sins"[2561] • Mother may be blamed for baby's condition[2562]
Neonatal Illness	• Prefer to have news given to father or grandparents so that they can be present with mother when provider gives her the news[2563] ✓Per HIPAA healthcare professional to obtain patient's permission
Newborn Care	• Mother typically has baby with her most of the time[2564] • A baby with colic may be given folk medicine tonic with high alcohol content[2565] • Believe that for good health babies and children need a cathartic and may give "laxative tonics;" during the purging, only liquids are taken[2566]
Post-partum Care	• May ask for beverages that are hot (temperature) after birth[2567] • May not consume dairy products; traditionally eat "salty, spicy" foods in post-partum period[2568]

Prenatal Care	• Modest and private; do not generally discuss sexual matters or anatomy; prefer same-sex caregiver[2569]
	• Traditionally, sexual experience starts at early age in both sexes; may have more than one partner[2570]
	• Usually seek prenatal care in second trimester; use traditional remedies even while pregnant; father does not usually go to childbirth classes[2571]
	✓ Healthcare professional may educate patient as to signs and symptoms for which she should go to medical doctor
	• Believe that mother's actions have effect on child's future[2572]
	• May not be concerned about weight gain as believes that more weight indicates healthier baby[2573]
	• Follows diet carefully during pregnancy to make sure the baby will receive proper nourishment[2574]
	• Traditional beliefs include specific instructions for certain foods and drinks (e.g., too much "milk, eggs, tomatoes, and green vegetables" will produce a baby that is too large for a vaginal birth); believe cravings should be satisfied for a healthy pregnancy and delivery[2575]
	✓ Healthcare professional provide education about good diet during pregnancy, including supplements
	• Due to separation from family, immigrant pregnant women may suffer stress routinely, and mental illness[2576]

 PEDIATRICS

Child/Teen Environment of Care	• Believe that for good health children need a cathartic and may give "laxative tonics;" during the purging, only liquids are taken[2577]

Disabilities

ALMOST 20 PERCENT OF AMERICANS – AND 42 PERCENT OF THOSE OVER AGE 65 – live with a disability.[2578] In its semiannual report, *Crossing the Quality Chasm*, the US Institute of Medicine (USIM) concluded that persons with disabilities are significantly more likely to be dissatisfied with their clinicians' focus on symptoms and diseases rather than on their overall health.[2579] The USIM observed that the American healthcare system fails many people, including persons with disabilities.[2580] The report outlines six guidelines for improving healthcare, ensuring healthcare that is:[2581]

- Safe (i.e., avoids injuring patients)
- Effective (i.e., based on scientific evidence of benefit)
- Patient-centered (i.e., respectful of patients' preferences, needs, and values)
- Timely (i.e., reduces waits and harmful delays)
- Efficient (i.e., avoids waste of equipment, supplies, ideas, and energy)
- Equitable (i.e., of equal quality, regardless of patients' personal characteristics)

A study conducted by the Boston Foundation, "Left Out in the Cold: Healthcare Experiences of Adults with Intellectual and Developmental Disabilities in Massachusetts," found that many disabled adults face longer waits than most patients, which prevents them from getting the best care for common adult conditions such as hypertension, heart disease, or thyroid disorders.[2582]

Reorienting the healthcare system to focus on the disabled patient's preferences and needs represents change that has already been implemented in many healthcare facilities; precedents established through legislative reform (Americans with Disabilities Act). This section outlines ways to personalize the level of care given to the disabled patient. Although there are several different types of disabilities, and each disabled patient's needs varies, this guide focuses on seven categories of disability:[2583]

- Autism
- Blind or Visually Impaired
- Cognitive /Mental Disability
- Deaf or Hard of Hearing
- Orthopedic Impairment (cerebral palsy, wheelchair bound, etc.)
- Speech or Language Impairment
- Traumatic Brain Injury

Etiquette based primarily on respect and courtesy is considered appropriate when interacting with people with disabilities.[2584] The table below lists common acceptable terminology as well as terms that should be avoided when dealing with a patient with a disability.[2585]

Common Terminology	Terms to Avoid
Intellectual disability	Retarded
Developmental disability	Handicapped
Cognitive disability	Disabled
Mental health issue or condition	Special
Person with a disability	Wheelchair bound
Visually impaired, blind	Crippled

Patients with physical disabilities may require assistance when showering or performing basic hygiene tasks. They may need a person to spot them while they bathe and wash their hair. When making decisions about healthcare, a person with a disability may seek advice from family and friends, guardians, or a power of attorney, before seeking help from healthcare professionals.[2586] Patients with cognitive disabilities may require an authorized guardian to make healthcare decisions such as blood transfusion or the proper pain management method.[2587]

Prenatal care is acceptable and encouraged. Screenings for disabilities may be acceptable in order to help educate and prepare the parent(s) for dealing with potential disability.[2588] The patient, as well as guardian when applicable, should be involved in these decisions.[2589] Mothers should be encouraged to bond with their child during breastfeeding. Lactation consultants should provide breastfeeding education.[2590] Additional support items may be needed based on the patient's specific disability.[2591] Vaginal birth may be possible, but will depend on the type and severity of the patient's disability.[2592] A C-section may be necessary if a patient cannot understand the expectations during the birth process.[2593]

Communication methods will vary based on a patient's individual disability.[2594] Use a sign language interpreter, a speech language pathologist, and/or a mental health counselor, when necessary.[2595]

General Tips for Communicating with People with Disabilities[2596]

- It is appropriate to offer to shake hands. People with limited hand use or who wear an artificial limb can usually shake hands.
- If you offer assistance, wait until the offer is accepted. Then listen to or ask for instructions.
- Treat adults as adults. Address people who have disabilities by their first names only when extending the same familiarity to all others.
- Relax. Don't be embarrassed if you happen to use common expressions such as "See you later," or "Did you hear about that?" that seem to relate to a person's disability.
- Don't be afraid to ask questions when you're unsure of what to do.

Tips for Communicating with Individuals with Speech Impairments[2597]

- If you do not understand something the individual says, do not pretend that you do. Ask the individual to repeat what he or she said and then repeat it back.

- Be patient. Take as much time as necessary.

- Try to ask questions which require only short answers or a nod of the head.

- Concentrate on what the individual is saying.

- Do not speak for the individual or attempt to finish her or his sentences.

If you are having difficulty understanding the individual, consider writing as an alternative means of communicating, but first ask the individual if this is acceptable.

Autism

Note: The following information is general. Specific beliefs and practices may vary. Details on page 12.

Legend: ✓ = Suggestions for Healthcare Professionals; ▶ = Significant Details or Exceptions.

♥ CARE OF THE PATIENT	

Barriers to Healthcare	• In the past, arbitrary discriminatory insurance practices existed, such as:
	  ▶ Denial of service for conditions deemed pre-existing
	  ▶ Stricter limits for conditions in terms of treatment duration
	• These discriminatory practices have changed with passage of the 2010 Health Care Reform Act[2598]
	  ▶ Much higher out-of-pocket costs for mental and behavioral health care than for other medical care

Common Medical Issues	• Accompanying conditions may include:[2599]
	  ▶ Epilepsy, hyperactivity, intellectual disability, fragile X syndrome, hearing loss, cerebral palsy, and vision loss
	  ▶ GI problems such as chronic constipation or diarrhea are common

Communication Tips	• Patients may have problems using and understanding language, interpreting facial expressions or emotion[2600]
	• Patient may have difficulty differentiating between emotions being exuded, for example, happy, sad, angry may all seem the same[2601]
	• Patient may have developed speech but communicate through non-verbal methods such as gestures, repetitive body movements[2602] (flapping hands or rocking) or writing[2603]
	• Patient may excel consistently at certain mental tasks (for example, counting, measuring, art, music, and memory)[2604]
	• Patient may be preoccupied, usually with lights, moving objects, or parts of objects[2605]
	• Patient may have echolalia where he/she repeats words or phrases over and over[2606]
	• Sign language is an alternative communication method for young children[2607]
	  ▶ Limit distractions; consider moving to a quiet or private location
	• Speak clearly, using short, succinct sentences[2608]
	• Word choice is important so that patient does not misinterpret an event to be worse than it really is[2609]
	  ▶ For example, when starting an IV, instead of saying. "This will hurt," say, "You will feel a slight pinch"
	• Be prepared to repeat what you say, orally or in writing[2610]
	• Observe caregivers' communication and note how patient responds[2611]

Diet and Nutrition	• Biomedical treatments include implementing a gluten-free and/or casein free (GFCF) diet as well as food allergy testing[2612]
	
	• A combination of methods:[2613]
	
	  ▸ Eating a therapeutic diet to heal the gut
	
	  ▸ Add nutrients such as vitamins to replace nutrients that have not been absorbed due to GI issues

Healing Environment	• Change in environment can be a stress trigger resulting in tantrums or physical aggression. Slowly introduce new people and objects[2614]
	
	• Consistency in care is very important[2615]
	
	  ▸ Having the same nurse care for the patient may be beneficial
	
	• To perform procedures or make an assessment, distract the patient with a favorite object or television show[2616]
	
	• Offer rewards for doing routine tasks like opening his/her mouth to take oral medications[2617]
	
	• If the patient is NPO use a sticker to mark the chart. G-tube feedings may be used instead of food[2618]
	
	• Patient may be hypersensitive or hyposensitive[2619]
	
	• Very important to explain what is going to happen and where before touching the patient[2620]
	
	• If a patient is hypersensitive to tactile stimuli, pay close attention to anything that touches him/her, i.e., an IV, gown, bandages, sheets, or medical devices[2621]
	
	• Patient may exhibit loud crying or no reaction at all[2622]
	
	• Loud noises tend to agitate autistic patients[2623, 2624]
	
	  ▸ Limit auditory and stimuli to familiar sounds, like music or movies, when possible
	
	• Patient may also have heightened sense of taste or an aversion to certain textures[2625, 2626]
	
	  ▸ A speech therapist or occupational therapist may need to work with patient to overcome feeding difficulties by working on swallowing techniques
	
	  ▸ If the guardian or family members cannot manage the day-to-day care, a long-term care facility may be an option for the patient
	
	• Establish safety within a new environment[2627]
	
	• Pad the side rails of a stretcher or bed[2628]
	
	• After a surgical procedure, some physicians may choose to keep an autistic patient sedated longer than a patient who is not autistic[2629, 2630]
	
	  ▸ This can help to reduce post-operative anxiety
	
	  ▸ If the patient is extubated, an extra nurse may be helpful for possible anesthesia emergency or to soothe the patient

Treatment Management	*The following treatments may be recommended by healthcare providers. No endorsement of any of the following is implied by its being listed here;* • Stimulant drugs may be used to treat hyperactivity and Attention Deficit Hyperactivity Disorder[2631] • Antidepressants used to treat depressive disorders, anxiety disorders; other medications/treatments prescribed for ADHD, bedwetting, smoking cessation, and obsessive compulsive disorder (OCD), the latter being used to control repetitive behaviors[2632] • Anticonvulsants may be used to treat seizures[2633] • Mood stabilizers traditionally used to treat bipolar disorder (BD)[2634, 2635, 2636] ▸ Improves mood, affective instability, impulsivity, and aggression, as well as seizure control

END OF LIFE

End-of-Life Discussion	✓ Per HIPAA, healthcare professional must obtain patient's permission to disclose health information to third parties ✓ Healthcare professional may ask patient who will make healthcare decisions for them if not themselves ✓ Health professional may discuss patient's terminal illness if applicable

PERINATAL CARE

Child/Teen Environment of Care	• Psychostimulants, used to treat Attention Deficit Hyperactivity Disorder (ADHD) in children, at higher doses have been found to increase stereotypic behavior and irritability in children[2637] • Antidepressants such as SSRIs have been used as the medication of choice when treating both autistic and non-autistic children[2638] • Antipsychotic medications have been found to increase stereotypical behavior and irritability in children[2639] • Antipsychotic medications have also been shown to improve over-activity and inattention[2640] • Atypical antipsychotic medications "help control aggression, hyperactivity, irritability, self-injury, and tantrums"[2641] • Side effects are noted at higher doses[2642]

Blind or Visually Impaired

Note: The following information is general. Specific beliefs and practices may vary. Details on page 12.

Legend: ✓ = Suggestions for Healthcare Professionals; ▶ = Significant Details or Exceptions.

♥ CARE OF THE PATIENT

Barriers to Healthcare	• Lack of comprehensive healthcare reform/affordable access[2643] • Affordable access would increase the proportion of individuals who adhere to ocular health screening recommendations[2644] • Adults view ocular health as separate from routine health checkups, for example with a PCP, and place less value because ocular procedures are not routinely covered by health insurance[2645]

Common Medical Issues	• Age-related macular degeneration (AMD)[2646, 2647]
	  ▶ Loss of central vision, peripheral vision stays intact
	  ▶ Metamorphopsia (object distortion), central scotomas (depressed vision), increased glare sensitivity, and decreased color vision
	• Cataract symptoms include decreased visual acuity, color perception, and glare disability[2648]
	• Diabetic retinopathy symptoms include decreased visual acuity, color perception, light/dark adaptation. May also have glare disability, distortion, and scotomas[2649]
	• Glaucoma[2650]
	  ▶ Initial loss of peripheral vision, difficulty functioning in dim light, decreased contrast sensitivity, glare disability, and decreased dark, light adaptation

Communication Tips	• Sign language and Braille are communication methods[2651]
	• May use a white long or support cane, others may use a dog, and others may not use Braille or a mobility aid at all[2652]
	• Speak to the individual when you approach him or her, stating clearly who you are; speak in a normal tone of voice[2653]
	  ▶ Using words such as blind, visually impaired, seeing, looking, and watching television is acceptable in conversation
	  ▶ Using descriptive language, including references to color, patterns, and the like is also OK
	• When referring to patients with disabilities, refer to the person first, then the disability, for instance, "The patient in 439 who is blind"[2654]
	• Tell the individual when you are leaving[2655]
	• Be descriptive when giving directions; verbally give the person information that is visually obvious to individuals who can see[2656]
	• If you are offering a seat, gently place the individual's hand on the back or arm of the chair so that the person can locate the seat[2657]

Communication Tips (continued)	• Stay in one place, if possible, when you speak. It is hard for a blind person to try to face a speaker who is constantly moving around[2658] • Verbalize and demonstrate procedures before they are performed[2659] • If the patient has a companion, avoid using that person as a go-between. Address your questions and comments directly to the patient[2660] • For the newly blinded patient, whether vision loss is caused by accident, illness, or is incidental to the hospital admission, staff should consult with state and local blindness service delivery agencies to ensure immediate services and continuity of care after discharge[2661]
Diet and Nutrition	• Vitamins A, C & E, beta carotene, and zinc[2662; 2663] ▸ High dose regimen (five to 15 times dietary intake) • Lack proper nutrition because of obstacles when shopping for and preparing food, or eating in restaurants[2664] • May need nutritional services to teach them about proper food intake and assistive services once discharged[2665] • A diabetic diet may be appropriate for patients with diabetes[2666]

Healing Environment	• Family member or guardian may be visually impaired and may require auxiliary aids or services[2667]
	  ▸ For example, a parent or guardian who is blind may be required to grant consent for his or her child's surgery. The contents of the form must be communicated effectively. In most cases, read the consent form to the individual or provide the form in Braille
	• Never touch or distract a service dog without first asking the owner[2668]
	• Patients with visual impairment may not react normally to light or movement. He/she may have "roaming eyes" that may or may not indicate emergent neurological problems[2669]
	• Do not leave doors ajar[2670] Tell the visually impaired or blind patient if you move any furniture or equipment[2671]
	• When moving a person into a hospital room, let him examine the furnishings in the room[2672]
	• Orient the person to the controls of the bed, paging system, TV and radio. Give other directions that are important[2673]
	• Do not touch or remove mobility canes unless requested to do so. Do not interfere with guide dogs[2674]
	• If you leave a person alone in an unfamiliar area be sure he or she is near something to touch[2675]
	  ▸ Staff should be aware of the range of abilities of persons with vision loss and the availability of equipment and devices that can make self-care possible, e.g., talking thermometers, blood pressure and glucose monitoring equipment, and dosage measuring devices
	• Be sure your patient can perform all self-care tasks required after he leaves the hospital or center[2676]

| Treatment Management | • For glaucoma patients, topical ocular medications (i.e., prostaglandins, beta blockers, adrenergics, cabonic anhydrase inhibitors, and miotics), oral medications, laser therapy, and filtering surgery[2677, 2678] |

 END OF LIFE

| End-of-Life Discussion | ✓ Per HIPAA, healthcare professional must obtain patient's permission to disclose health information to third parties
✓ Healthcare professional may ask patient who will make healthcare decisions for them if not themselves
✓ Health professional may discuss patient's terminal illness if applicable |

 PEDIATRICS

| Child/Teen Environment of Care | • The American Diabetes Association recommends that children with diabetes have an initial ophthalmologic exam after age ten if they have had diabetes for three to five years, followed by annual exams[2679] |

Cognitive/Learning Disabilities

Note: The following information is general. Specific beliefs and practices may vary. Details on page 12.

Legend: ✓ = Suggestions for Healthcare Professionals; ▶ = Significant Details or Exceptions.

CARE OF THE PATIENT	

Barriers to Healthcare	• Lack of knowledge of the nature and health needs of people with learning disabilities[2680, 2681]
	• Lack of access to adequate training in the dental needs of groups with disabilities[2682]
	• A patient's limited communication skills; i.e., limited or absent reading and verbal skills[2683]
	  ▶ Limits how advice can be adhered to or causes delay in making new appointments for follow-up and additional care
	• Difficulties in communication and gaining proper consent[2684, 2685]
	  ▶ Individuals with learning disabilities have had bad healthcare experiences and often avoid seeking health care when necessary
	• Problems assessing needs and providing care[2686, 2687]
	• Poor discharge planning[2688]

Common Medical Issues	• Other coexisting disabilities such as: Mobility problems, cerebral palsy, seizure disorders, vision impairment, hearing loss, and attention-deficit/hyperactivity disorder (ADHD)[2689]
	• At least a third of people with Down syndrome can expect to develop Alzheimer's disease[2690]
	• Depression[2691]
	• Oral health is often poor. Toothache may manifest itself as challenging behavior. High prevalence of dental cavities and toothlessness for intellectually disabled[2692]
	• Gastrointestinal (GI) problems[2693, 2694]
	  ▶ Constipation significantly correlated with lack of mobility, cerebral palsy, the use of anticonvulsants, benzodiazepines, proton pump inhibitors, and poor nutrition
	  ▶ GI reflux disease
	• Respiratory disease[2695]
	  ▶ Greater incidence, main cause of death
	  ▶ More problems with aspiration pneumonia, dysphagia, and gastroesophageal disorders
	  ▶ Epilepsy is more common, as is trauma and fractures sustained during seizures

Common Medical Issues (continued)	• Unintentional injuries[2696]
	  ▸ Mobility and sensory impairments
	  ▸ Greater risk of fracture because of greater risk of osteoporosis
	• Non-accidental injury[2697]
	  ▸ Greater incidence of being physically and sexually abused
	• Gastroesophageal (GO) reflux disease may be unnoticed[2698, 2699, 2700, 2701, 2702]
	  ▸ Manifestations of haematemesis, rumination, dental erosions, and hand-mouthing (putting whole hand in mouth)
	  ▸ If left untreated, there is an increased risk of esophageal carcinoma
	• Many families and caregivers of people with intellectual disability may ask for them to receive lifelong contraception or have surgery to regulate fertility[2703]
	  ▸ There is little guidance for providers in this area.
	• Menstrual problems in women with intellectual disabilities are either the same as other women or are related to inappropriate behavior[2704]

Communication Tips	• Indicators that a person has a learning disability[2705, 2706]
	  ▸ Difficulty in providing sequential history, poor planning, and sequencing abilities
	  ▸ Providing irrelevant information, repetition of phrases in conversation
	  ▸ Difficulty understanding questions and responding quickly, lack of understanding or vagueness
	  ▸ Inability to deal with more than one question at a time
	  ▸ Difficulty in following straightforward instructions
	  ▸ Difficulty in understanding abstract concepts, such as time, distance, or directions
	  ▸ Confusion about times of appointments
	• Provider behaviors that may improve communication[2707, 2708, 2709, 2710]
	  ▸ Leveling: Physical posturing that results in the patient having a comparable eye level
	  ▸ Using declarative sentences
	  ▸ Using open-ended questions
	  ▸ Provide corrective feedback
	  ▸ Removing distracting objects
	  ▸ Removing distracting individuals
	• Sample open-ended questions which may help determine whether a patient is currently being treated for a learning disability[2711]
	  ▸ How do you spend your day?
	  ▸ What kinds of places do you visit?
	  ▸ Do you see other nurses and doctors?

Diet and Nutrition	• Normalization of hyperhomocysteine (HHcy) slows Alzheimer's progress[2712]

Healing Environment	• Refer to care packages (if applicable)[2713]
	  ▸ Contact designated individual(s) after proper consent is gained
	  ▸ Communicate discharge/admission decisions
	• Properly document intervention steps and their outcomes[2714]
	• Practitioners are not allowed to document that the patient has a learning disability, but will need to find proper ways to communicate this information[2715]
	• Patients with learning disabilities have increased healthcare needs that often result in higher mortality rate in hospitals[2716]
	• Practitioners should assume that more than one condition exists until evidence rules this possibility out[2717]
	• Unaccompanied people with learning disabilities may require additional assistance to understand the healthcare process[2718]
	✓ Healthcare professional may want to consider fast-tracking the patient (multitasking to shorten a patient's treatment time)
	• Check for available health records that may aid in assessing patient, including a health management/action plan[2719, 2720]
	• When possible, explain what to expect from the healthcare process; how investigations, diagnosis and treatment will be handled[2721]
	• Provide patient education leaflets to help patient and his/her family understand what is going on[2722]
	• A holistic approach to healthcare is needed, assessing both physical and mental well-being[2723]
	✓ Healthcare professional should communicate this approach to all person(s) who will come in contact with the patient
	• Involve both the patient and his/her family members when possible[2724]
	✓ Healthcare professional should follow HIPAA policies to protect the patient's rights
	• When possible, have one nurse handle the patient[2725]

Importance of Consent	• Adults with learning disabilities have the same right to exercise choice and control over their own health care as other patients[2726]
	• Patients must be involved in discussions about examination, treatment, and care[2727]
	• Guidelines to follow:[2728]
	  ▸ Have a clear understanding of the legal requirement for consent
	  ▸ Understand that no one can consent on behalf of a patient with a learning disability, and healthcare professionals need to have a clear understanding of the legal requirement for consent and develop ways in which to inform and gain valid consent
	  ▸ Be aware of the issue of incapacity

Treatment Management	• There is no evidence to support any benefit in using antipsychotic drugs to treat behavior[2729]
	• When prescribing medications for patients who are already taking several medications, good practice should be consulted so that unnecessary medications can be discontinued and side effects minimized[2730]
	• Methods of conveying physical state, e.g., pain or discomfort[2731]
	▸ Vocal and non-language (e.g., crying or screaming may indicate pain, laughing does not mean absence of pain)
	▸ Sign language, gestures, and body movement (e.g., grimacing, clenching teeth, pacing, rocking)
	▸ Scales of pain and pictures or images of pain
	▸ Inflicting self-harm (e.g., picking at fingernails, pulling out hair)
	▸ Display aggressive behavior (e.g., biting, pinching, punching, pushing, scratching, or kicking), which may be a way for the patient to attract or reject attention
	▸ Functional limitations (e.g., reluctance to bear weight on a limb, inability to lift or carry everyday item)
	▸ Show physiological changes (e.g., sweating or altered breathing)
	▸ Pain-reducing behaviors (e.g., going to bed early to rest)

 PEDIATRICS

Child/Teen Environment of Care	• Approximately 4 to 6 percent of all students are classified as having specific learning disabilities (SLD) in our nation's public schools[2732]
	• Evaluation is the first step in diagnosing a child or teen with a learning disability. It involves gathering information from a variety of sources about a child's functioning and development in all areas[2733]

Deaf or Hard of Hearing

Note: The following information is general. Specific beliefs and practices may vary. Details on page 12.

Legend: ✓ = Suggestions for Healthcare Professionals; ▶ = Significant Details or Exceptions.

CARE OF THE PATIENT	
Barriers to Healthcare	• Provider's lack of knowledge of Americans with Disabilities Act (ADA)[2734] • Illegible written communication by practitioners[2735] • Difficulty with TTY telephone communication[2736] • Lack of practitioners with ASL skills[2737]
Communication Tips	• American Sign Language (ASL) and Braille are communication methods[2738] • ASL may be primary language spoken and English may be a second language[2739] ▶ Familiar medical terminology such as "bowel" or "glaucoma" may not have a direct translation or may be new terms • Use of ASL interpreter when medical information is given[2740] • Text messaging, using pictures or typing on a computer may be acceptable[2741] • Patient may have some hearing or use a cochlear implant[2742] • Gain the person's attention before starting a conversation (i.e., tap the person gently on the shoulder or arm)[2743] • Look directly at the individual, face the light, speak clearly, in a normal tone of voice, and keep your hands away from your face. Many deaf or hard of hearing persons can read lips[2744] • Maintain eye contact and use short, simple sentences[2745] • If the individual uses a sign language interpreter, speak directly to the person, not the interpreter[2746] • For newly deaf patients or children, communicate with pictures - Print on Palm (POP) - where you draw letters on a person's palm to spell out words (for those familiar with the written alphabet), or use the one hand manual alphabet[2747] • If the patient responds solely to the interpreter and disregards healthcare professional, it could be a sign of hostility toward the provider. Be sensitive when trying to determine the source of hostility or discomfort[2748] • In an emergency, the universal sign for communicating is to draw the letter X on the back of the person with the fingertips[2749] • There are personal alert systems that convert sounds from sources such as a smoke alarm or telephone into vibrations that can be felt by a person who is deaf[2750]

Common Medical Issues	• Increased risk for cardiovascular disease[2751] • Three times more likely to have high cholesterol, instances of obesity, hypertension, thyroid gland diseases, and respiratory diseases[2752] • Twice as likely to get diabetes, heart disease, and gastrointestinal diseases[2753] • At an elevated risk for sexually transmitted diseases because of inferior sexual education and communication within the hearing community[2754] • Many studies suggest that deaf people experience anxiety and depression at higher rates than their hearing counterparts[2755] • Studies suggest a higher suicide rate[2756] • Substance abuse problems are also prevalent in deaf teenagers struggling to adjust and cope with everyday frustrations[2757] ✓ Health professional may watch for signs of emotional distress, offer open and honest opinions and referrals for drug abuse, substance abuse, mental health clinics, or suicide resources[2758]
Diet and Nutrition	• Needs to consume the recommended intake of fruits and vegetables because of higher risk of cardiovascular disease[2759]
Healing Environment	• Keep a file with common phrases and closed questions (questions that can be answered with yes or no). Have file readily available to use with deaf patients on admission to the hospital[2760] • Produce a short video in ASL to orient the patient to the department's environment - funding can come from grants or charities[2761] • Closed-captioned television[2762] • Have an interpreter available at all times[2763] ▸ Should be present to ensure effective communication with patient, especially when explaining a medical procedure or process • Avoid inserting an intravenous needle into the patient's hands because this can impede communication[2764] • Provide visual alarms in all public and common-use areas, including restrooms, where audible alarms are provided[2765] • Evacuation procedures should include specific measures to ensure the safety of patients and visitors who are deaf or hard of hearing[2766]

END OF LIFE

End of Life Discussion	✓ Per HIPAA, healthcare professional must obtain patient's permission to disclose health information to third parties ✓ Healthcare professional may ask patient who will make healthcare decisions for them if not themselves ✓ Health professional may discuss patient's terminal illness if applicable

Orthopedic Impairment

Note: The following information is general. Specific beliefs and practices may vary. Details on page 12.

Legend: ✓ = Suggestions for Healthcare Professionals; ▶ = Significant Details or Exceptions.

❤ CARE OF THE PATIENT	
Barriers to Healthcare	• Inaccessible environments[2767] • Bias, rejection, and discrimination[2768] • Difficulties living independently[2769] • Limited or non-existent transportation[2770] • Difficulties finding jobs[2771] • Affordability[2772] • Lack of health insurance[2773] • Social rejection by people without disabilities[2774]

Common Medical Issues	• Common medical issues include:[2775]
	  ▶ Congenital anomaly
	  ▶ Disease
	  ▶ Other causes such as cerebral palsy and amputations
	  ▶ Neuromotor (brain and spinal cord) impairments
	  ▶ Seizure disorders
	  ▶ Cerebral palsy
	  ▶ Spinal cord disorders
	  ▶ Polio
	  ▶ Muscular dystrophy
	  ▶ Multiple sclerosis
	  ▶ Muscular/skeletal conditions
	  ▶ Juvenile arthritis
	  ▶ Limb deficiencies
	  ▶ Skeletal disorders

Communication Tips	• If a patient uses a wheelchair: • If possible, put yourself at the wheelchair user's eye level[2776] • Do not lean on a wheelchair or any other assistive device[2777] • Never patronize people who use wheelchairs by patting them on the head or shoulder[2778] • Do not assume the individual wants to be pushed —ask first[2779] • Offer assistance if the individual appears to be having difficulty opening a door[2780] • If you telephone the individual, allow the phone to ring more times than usual to allow extra time for the person to reach the telephone[2781]

Healing Environment	• An accessible environment[2782]
	  ‣ Remove physical barriers, provide clear paths throughout the space
	  ‣ Ensure floor is clear of all obstacles
	  ‣ Keep support devices close to patient
	  ‣ Add support equipment in the patient's room (e.g., support bars in the bathroom)
	• Physical therapy, occupational therapy, and massage therapy[2783]
	• Alternative therapy such as acupuncture[2784]
	• Use of robotics, advanced technology, or artificial limbs to aid in movement and improve ability to perform day-to-day tasks[2785]
	• If the guardian or family members are not able to manage the day-to-day care, long-term care facilities may be option for the patient[2786]

Treatment Management	• The treatment plan offered for pain and injury may include:[2787]
	  ‣ Medications
	  ‣ Physical therapy
	  ‣ Occupational therapy
	  ‣ Psychological support
	  ‣ Braces
	  ‣ Injections of muscles, bursae, joints
	  ‣ Interventional procedures, including epidural and facet injections
	  ‣ Electromyography

END OF LIFE

End-of-Life Discussion	✓ Per HIPAA, healthcare professional must obtain patient's permission to disclose health information to third parties ✓ Healthcare professional may ask patient who will make healthcare decisions for them if not themselves ✓ Health professional may discuss patient's terminal illness if applicable

PEDIATRICS

Child/Teen Environment of Care	• A child's chronic illness can affect families in ways such as:[2788]
	  ‣ Fatigue
	  ‣ Low vitality
	  ‣ Restricted social lives
	  ‣ Preoccupation with decisions related to the child's illness
	• Some families find that seeking out others with similar problems is helpful[2789]
	• Depending on the severity of the impairment, the child may be considered for special-needs classes in school[2790]

Speech and Language Impairment

Note: The following information is general. Specific beliefs and practices may vary. Details on page 12.

Legend: ✓ = Suggestions for Healthcare Professionals; ▶ = Significant Details or Exceptions.

♥ CARE OF THE PATIENT

Barriers to Healthcare	• Patient may struggle with reading, have difficulty understanding and expressing language, and misunderstand social cues[2791]

Common Medical Issues	• Patient may have or develop feeding or swallowing disorders[2792]
	• Feeding disorders include problems gathering food and getting ready to suck, chew, or swallow[2793]
	• Swallowing disorders, also known as dysphagia, can occur at different phases of the swallowing process[2794]
	   ▶ Oral phase: Sucking, chewing, and moving food or liquid into the throat
	   ▶ Pharyngeal phase: Starting to swallow, squeezing food down the throat, and closing off the airway to prevent food or liquid from entering the airway (aspiration) or to prevent choking
	   ▶ Esophageal phase: Relaxing and tightening the openings at the top and bottom of the feeding tube in the throat (esophagus) and squeezing food through the esophagus into the stomach
	• A patient may stutter or have difficulty articulating words. Speech impairment affects spoken language[2795]
	• Patient may have:[2796]
	   ▶ Aphasia - which is often the result of a neurological deficit. Aphasia can be classified as:
	   ✓ Receptive (the patient cannot interpret spoken words),
	   ✓ Expressive (the patient cannot communicate verbally),
	   ✓ Global (the patient cannot understand or communicate spoken words)
	   ▶ Apraxia (facial grimaces or unusual movements may accompany speech, such as groping to produce sounds, syllables, and words; difficulty planning and sequencing movements for speech within the brain; speech may be unintelligible or not understandable), etc.[2797]
	   ▶ Voice disorders affect the sound of the voice itself (i.e., hoarseness, breathy voice, strained/tense voice). Such disorders are often caused by changes in the shape of the vocal cords (e.g., swelling of vocal cords, growths on the vocal cords such as vocal nodules)[2798]

Communication Tips	• People with severe speech or language problems rely on augmentative and alternative communication methods (AAC)[2799]
	  ▸ Unaided communication - a person's body (e.g., gestures, body language, or sign language)
	  ▸ Aided communication systems - use of tools or equipment in addition to the user's body (e.g., paper and pencil, communication books or boards, devices that produce voice or written output)

Diet and Nutrition	• Patient may develop eating and swallowing disorders (e.g., dysphagia)[2800] ▸ For example, decrease in speech may create lack of nourishment if the patient is unable to request food • Patient may need to work with a speech-language pathologist to learn to eat and swallow properly[2801]

Healing Environment	• Perform special tests, if necessary, to evaluate swallowing, such as:[2802]
	  ▸ Modified barium swallow – patient eats or drinks food or liquid with barium in it, and then the swallowing process is viewed on an X-ray
	  ▸ Endoscopic assessment – a fiber optic endoscope is passed transnasally and permits inspection of swallowing mechanisms and functions.[2803]
	• The speech language pathologist may work as part of a feeding team. Other team members may include:[2804]
	  ▸ Occupational therapist
	  ▸ Physical therapist
	  ▸ Physician or nurse
	  ▸ Dietitian or nutritionist
	  ▸ Developmental specialist
	• Speech therapy may help patients learn to better communicate[2805]
	• Speech therapy may help patients control facial and oral movement, which may help to improve speech[2806]
	  ▸ Medical devices or computer technology may be used to help patients learn to mimic proper speech patterns

END OF LIFE

End-of-Life Discussion	✓ Per HIPAA, healthcare professional must obtain patient's permission to disclose health information to third parties ✓ Healthcare professional may ask patient who will make healthcare decisions for them if not themselves ✓ Health professional may discuss patient's terminal illness if applicable

PEDIATRICS

Child/Teen Environment of Care	• Signs and symptoms of feeding and swallowing difficulty in children:[2807]

- Signs and symptoms of feeding and swallowing difficulty in children:[2807]
  - ▸ Arching or stiffening of the body during feeding
  - ▸ Irritability or lack of alertness during feeding
  - ▸ Refusing food or liquid
  - ▸ Failure to accept different textures (pureed foods or crunchy cereals)
  - ▸ Long feeding times (e.g., more than 30 minutes)
  - ▸ Difficulty chewing
  - ▸ Difficulty breastfeeding
  - ▸ Coughing or gagging during meals
  - ▸ Excessive drooling or food/liquid coming out of the mouth or nose
  - ▸ Difficulty coordinating breathing with eating and drinking
  - ▸ Increased stuffiness during meals
  - ▸ Gurgly, hoarse, or breathy voice quality
  - ▸ Frequent spitting up or vomiting
  - ▸ Recurring pneumonia or respiratory infections
  - ▸ Less than normal weight gain or growth
- Children may show signs of:[2808]
  - ▸ Dehydration or poor nutrition
  - ▸ Aspiration (food or liquid entering the airway) or penetration (food or liquid entering the airway above the level of the vocal folds)
  - ▸ Pneumonia or repeated upper respiratory infections that can lead to chronic lung disease
  - ▸ Embarrassment or isolation in social situations involving eating

Traumatic Brain Injury

Note: The following information is general. Specific beliefs and practices may vary. Details on page 12.

Legend: ✓ = Suggestions for Healthcare Professionals; ▶ = Significant Details or Exceptions.

♥ CARE OF THE PATIENT	
Barriers to Healthcare	• Reaching maximum payouts for insurance[2809] • Higher insurance premiums[2810] • Ethnic barriers to access of proper care[2811] • Language, lack of insurance for immigrants, fear of new healthcare system[2812]

Common Medical Issues	• Cognitive symptoms may include:[2813]
	  ▶ Short-term memory loss and/or long-term memory loss
	  ▶ Trouble concentrating and processing information
	  ▶ Communication difficulties
	  ▶ Spatial disorientation
	  ▶ Organizational problems and impaired judgment
	• Physical symptoms may include:[2814]
	  ▶ Seizures
	  ▶ Muscle spasticity
	  ▶ Double vision or low vision, even blindness
	  ▶ Loss of smell or taste
	  ▶ Pain, headaches, or migraines
	  ▶ Balance problems
	• Depression[2815]

Communication Tips	• Language problems vary[2816]
	• Some communication barriers include:[2817]
	  ▶ Word-finding difficulty
	  ▶ Poor sentence formation
	  ▶ Lengthy and often faulty descriptions or explanations
	• Reading and writing abilities are often worse than persons without traumatic brain injury[2818]
	• Simple and complex mathematical abilities are often affected[2819]

Communication Tips (continued)	• Speech can also be affected:[2820]
	
	  ▸ Dysarthria – patient's speech may be slow, slurred, and difficult or impossible to understand
	
	  ▸ Patient may experience dysphagia (problems swallowing)
	
	  ▸ Apraxia of speech also common, where the patient's speech muscles are unimpaired but the patient still experiences difficulty saying words correctly in a consistent manner
	
	✓ Present information slowly, but don't raise your voice as if that will help the information get through
	
	✓ Explain what you will do prior to beginning any procedure

Diet and Nutrition	• A nutritionist/dietitian may be needed to treat the patient for feeding and swallowing difficulties[2821] • Patients should be given nutritional supplementation through a gastric feeding tube as soon as possible, for it can improve their chances of survival by as much as four-fold[2822] • A saturated-fat diet aggravates the outcome of traumatic brain injury on hippocampal plasticity and cognitive function by reducing brain-derived neurotrophic factor. Consult with dietician for diet recommendations[2823] • If no swallowing difficulties are present, pecans may help to protect neurological function, as it is among the top fifteen dietary sources of antioxidants including Vitamin E[2824] ✓ If patient has physical impairments, may need assistance preparing food on tray or feeding self
Healing Environment	• Assessment is a continual, ongoing process[2825] • Immediately following the injury, a neurologist or another physician may conduct an informal, bedside evaluation of attention, memory, and the ability to understand and speak[2826] • Once the patient is in a stable physical condition, a speech-language pathologist may evaluate cognitive and communication skills[2827] • A neuropsychologist may evaluate other cognitive and behavioral abilities. Occupational therapists may assess cognitive skills related to the individual's ability to perform "activities of daily living" (ADL) such as dressing or preparing meals[2828] • An audiologist may assess hearing[2829] • Treatment may focus on re-orienting a patient to person, place, time, and situation[2830] • The rehab process may last several months to a year, as necessary[2831]

END OF LIFE

End-of-Life Discussion	✓ Per HIPAA, healthcare professional must obtain patient's permission to disclose health information to third parties
	✓ Healthcare professional may ask patient who will make healthcare decisions for them if not themselves
	✓ Health professional may discuss patient's terminal illness if applicable

Generations

GENERATIONAL NAMES ARE BORN FROM POPULAR CULTURE. THEY ARE DEFINED BY historic events, rapidly changing social or demographic trends, and the dawn of a new era. For the purpose of this section, generations were classified and defined in one of four categories: Traditional/ Silent, Baby Boomers, Generation X (aka "Gen Xers"), and the Millennials. Each category is outlined in the table below:[2832]

Generational Title	Born	Today's Age	Population in the US (in millions)*	% of the Population
Traditional/Silent	1925 to 1945	66 to 86	34	11.1%
Baby Boomers	1946 to 1964	47 to 65	79	25.9%
Generation X	1965 to 1980	31 to 46	65	21.3%
Millennials	1981 to 1995	19 to 30	60	19.6%

*Note: There is a fifth generational category, Gen 2020, which describes individuals born after 1995. For the sake of this document, only the aforementioned categories (four) will be addressed. Because of a lack of availability of data, the Gen 2020 category was not included in this guide. At the time when the population data was taken from the US Census Bureau, there were approximately 305 million people living in the United States.

Traditional/Silent

Members of the *Traditional/Silent* generation are children of the Great Depression, The New Deal, World War II, and the Korean War – many of these events were followed on the radio.[2833] The "Silent" label refers to conformist and civic attitudes.[2834] This generation tends to focus on advancement with a view toward the past, yet is cautious of untried initiatives, and these attitudes may be interpreted as reluctance to change. Medical concerns and untreated depression among older adults can have a devastating effect on their ability to concentrate.[2835]

The *Traditional* generation has seen tremendous change in their lifetime, especially as related to gender and racial equality and drug-free workplace initiatives.[2836] Feeling respected for their contributions and historical knowledge is important for this group, who would prefer not to be marginalized as ineffective because they may lack the technological skills of later generations.[2837]

Some issues that patients of the Traditional/Silent generation will more likely struggle with may include respect for diversity and consequences of lifestyle behaviors, including the effects of smoking and alcoholism.[2838]

Baby Boomers

The term *Baby Boomers* refers to the great spike in birth rate during the post-war era until 1964, which almost coincides with the introduction of the birth control pill.[2839] This is the generation of the Salk Vaccine, the Civil Rights Act, the cold war, the birth control pill, the Peace Corps, the moon landing, the assassinations of JFK, RFK, and MLK, the founding of NOW, Woodstock, the Vietnam War, and the Kent State shootings – many of these events being broadcast or rebroadcast on television.[2840] Valuing personal gratification and seeking high achievement, Boomers dedicate 100 percent to whatever they perceive to be the task at hand, and will expect nothing less from anyone else.[2841]

Some issues that patients of the Baby Boomer generation will more likely struggle with may include nontraditional styles of younger generations and the paradigm shift of technological advances replacing human interaction.[2842]

Generation X

Generation X or "Gen Xers" were previously called the "Baby Bust" generation.[2843] The events that marked this generation were Intel's first computer chip, electronic mail delivery (e-mail), personal computers (PCs), AIDS/HIV. Then there was the Challenger explosion, replayed in full color on TV.

As a group, Gen Xers are resourceful and comfortable with diversity and accepting of change.[2844] Gen Xers are usually a highly independent, outspoken, adaptable and fearless group of individuals who are competent and willing risk takers.[2845]

Some issues that a patient of the Gen Xer generation will more likely struggle with include conflict resolution, multigenerational communication and cooperation, and balancing work and life.[2846]

Millenial/Gen Y

The *Millennial* generation is named for those who will come of age during the new millennium.[2847] This generation has been described as the best educated generation – and they know it. Events that have marked this generation include the dissolution of the Soviet Union, the Oklahoma City bombing, Columbine massacre, 9/11, Hurricane Katrina, the Virginia Tech massacre (some of them covered by TV in real time), the banking meltdown and subsequent depression, and the BP oil spill – events that could be viewed on cell phones or described via text message, or uploaded through social networking sites.[2848] The "live for today" mindset is characteristic of Millennials, and can have a negative impact on both present and future circumstances. Credit problems from unplanned and spontaneous spending, accidents, unsafe health behaviors, and legal problems related to episodes of impulsive violence, risk taking, and substance use are significant issues for this generation.[2849]

Some issues that a patient of the Millennial generation are more likely to struggle with include consequences of their lifestyle or risk-taking behavior.[2850]

The most detailed study to date of the 18 to 29 year old Millennials generation finds this group will most likely be the most educated in American history. But the 50 million Millennials also have the highest share that are unemployed or out of the workforce in almost four decades, according to a 2010 study released by the Pew Research Center.[2851]

A 2009 Thomson-Reuters study found that, "It is important for healthcare professionals, employers, and policy makers to consider how the economy and healthcare policies affect demographic segments differently," said Gary Pickens, chief research officer for the Healthcare and Science business of Thomson Reuters and lead author of the study. "Clearly, the age groups that represent the largest slice of the employer-sponsored insurance landscape – Baby Boomers and Generation X – are most susceptible to the ebbs and flows of the economy."[2852]

Traditional/Silent Generation (1925 to 1945)

Note: The following information is general. Specific beliefs and practices may vary. Details on page 12.

Legend: ✓ = Suggestions for Healthcare Professionals; ▶ = Significant Details or Exceptions.

♥ CARE OF THE PATIENT

Barriers to Healthcare	• Affordability of health insurance[2853] • Increasing cost of medication[2854] • Transportation to and/from healthcare facilities[2855] • This generation is not likely to seek mental health services. Reducing the stigma of mental illness and facilitating linkages with mental health professionals are critical for this generation[2856] • Being on a fixed income[2857]
Common Medical Issues	• Chronic disease common to this age group include chronic obstructive pulmonary disease, diabetes, osteoporosis, high blood pressure, high cholesterol, and cardiovascular disease[2858] • Diseases of aging, i.e., signs of dementia or Alzheimer's as well as illness related to smoking or alcoholism may begin to appear or are progressing[2859] • Depression[2860] • Substance abuse, especially alcohol[2861] • Increased rates of suicide[2862] • Long-term alcohol abuse will have affected physical health[2863]
Communication Tips	• Traditionalists are private, the "silent generation"[2864] • Don't expect members of this generation to share their thoughts immediately, or to share their feelings[2865] • For the Traditionalist, an educator's word is his/her bond, so it's important to focus on words rather than body language or inferences[2866] • Face-to-face or written communication is preferred[2867] • Don't waste their time, or let them feel as though their time is being wasted[2868]
Defining Generational Characteristics	• Conservative[2869] • Hardworking[2870] • Respects authority[2871] • Struggles with respect for diversity[2872] • Past-oriented and may be reluctant to embrace change[2873]
Diet and Nutrition	• Usually regimented in type of foods consumed, typically not open to foods that are new and foreign[2874] • More likely to restrict diet because of health concerns[2875]

Healing Environment	• Privacy and comfort are important[2876] • May request religious leader or prayer with a Chaplain[2877] • May prefer being at home to being in a hospital or strange setting[2878] • Struggle with accepting their condition, and may be reluctant to make lifestyle changes for better health[2879] • Treatment compliance depends on affordability of medications as well as the cost of a treatment[2880] • Illness, treatment, or the side effects of treatment may keep those who are still working out of work for a few days or for a period of time[2881] • Believes depression is an embarrassment and should be addressed quietly, alone, and out of the public eye[2882] • Misuse of alcohol may become more pronounced to reduce the stress of unmanaged mental health issues or as a strategy to avoid uncomfortable relationships[2883]
Pain Management	• Chronic pain is a multidimensional experience that transcends several domains of functioning. Elderly patients are particularly vulnerable to several pain-related illnesses[2884] • Several assessment instruments and treatment options are available for evaluating and managing pain[2885]

END OF LIFE

Death Process	• May prefer to be at home[2886] ✓ Patient may want healthcare professional to be direct, usually in a private area and with clergy present ✓ Healthcare professional may ask for clergy to be present when delivering terminal status news ✓ Per HIPAA healthcare professional to obtain patient's permission
End-of-Life Discussion	• Patient may want to discuss within his/her family to allow finally to be prepared[2887] ✓ Per HIPAA, healthcare professional must obtain patient's permission to disclose health information to third parties ✓ Healthcare professional may ask patient who will make healthcare decisions for them if not themselves ✓ Health professional may discuss patient's terminal illness if applicable
New Parent/Caregivers	• Some grandparents find themselves acting as primary parents due to new responsibility of caring for young children[2888] • The new parent role can be overwhelming, as grandparents delve into child care, after-school programs, sporting events, enrichment activities, medical insurance, healthcare, school enrollment, custody, and legal issues and investigate the assistance options available[2888]

New Parent/Caregivers (continued)	• Many grandparents are on a fixed income and may not be able to afford additional costs associated with raising a child such as child care, insurance, healthcare and providing for the basic needs of the child[2889]
	• Challenged when trying to enroll children in school because of proof of guardianship or custody[2890]
	• Grandparents may not feel as though they can keep up with the child, due to health concerns or simply because children are so active[2891]
	• Traditionals may feel out of touch with what is happening in today's educational system and unable to keep up with or understand today's technology[2892]
	• Becoming a grandparent/parent again can be very trying, but there are options available in many communities as this issue becomes more prevalent[2893]

Baby Boomers (1946 to 1964)

Note: The following information is general. Specific beliefs and practices may vary. Details on page 12.

Legend: ✓ = Suggestions for Healthcare Professionals; ▶ = Significant Details or Exceptions.

♥ CARE OF THE PATIENT	
Barriers to Healthcare	• Increasing cost of healthcare[2894] • Increasing costs of insurance[2895] • Prolonged recession[2896] • Recession impacting affordability of and provision of services to this group[2897]
Common Medical Issues	• Having to balance work and parenting and caring for older parents present a myriad of stressors. Challenges and dilemmas for many Baby Boomers can be felt as financial and marital stress and contribute to fatigue[2898] • Medical and cosmetic advancements have helped Baby Boomers delay the aging process[2899] • Health consequences of lifestyle choices may now be appearing for this generation[2900] • Common issues include diabetes, high cholesterol, high blood pressure, heart and lung disease, overweight and obesity[2901] • Screenings for breast, colon, and prostate cancers have resulted in better treatment options earlier in the disease process, and more Baby Boomers may be receiving care for these illnesses[2902] • Medical issues will result from years of drug abuse as the aging hippie generation continues to use alcohol, marijuana, and other illicit drugs[2903]
Communication Tips	• Baby Boomers are the "show me" generation; body language is important when communicating[2904] • Speak in an open, direct style, but avoid controlling language[2905] • Answer questions thoroughly and expect to be pressed for details[2906] • Present options to demonstrate flexibility in your thinking[2907]
Defining Generational Characteristics	• Believe in equality for all people and right to individual choice[2908] • Feels optimistic about opportunities[2909] • Value challenge and change[2910] • Goal-oriented[2911] • Adaptive to diversity[2912]
Diet and Nutrition	• Baby Boomers believe in balanced meals, consumption of fruits and vegetables, and avoidance of fats[2913] • They care less about natural and organic choices and specific functional foods than younger consumers do[2914]

Diet and Nutrition (continued)	• Baby Boomers have a mental list of foods to be avoided; for instance, trans-fats[2915]
Healing Environment	• As they age, Baby Boomers seek spirituality[2916] • Baby Boomers are now facing their own mortality and considering what legacy they will leave[2917] • A mid-life crisis for previous generations has turned into a mid-life quest by boomers, with many conducting a spiritual re-assessment and searching for meaning[2918] • More likely to seek behavioral healthcare services[2919] • Readily use mental health services and psychiatric medications[2920] • This generation is known for pursuing activities and spending money on self-improvement services[2921] • Mental health services framed in the context of self-improvement and coaching will help to improve access to mental health services[2922] • Receptive to prevention programs designed to minimize health risk[2923]
Pain Management	• The aches and pains of aging and postsurgical pain relief may result in more frequent prescriptions for pain medications and the risks associated with addictive medications[2924]

END OF LIFE

End-of-Life Discussion	✓ Patient may want to discuss within his/her family to allow finally to be prepared[2925] ✓ Per HIPAA, healthcare professional must obtain patient's permission to disclose health information to third parties ✓ Healthcare professional may ask patient who will make healthcare decisions for them if not themselves

PERINATAL CARE

Breastfeeding	• Believes breastfeeding is important, but also believes in a woman's right to choose[2926] ✓ Healthcare professional may supply patient with breastfeeding education; include maternal grandmothers and significant others who are influential for mother
New Parent/Caregivers	• Some Baby Boomers are the primary caretakers for their children, grandchildren, and/or aging parents[2927] • Baby Boomers more likely to relocate from their immediate families for job opportunities; caring for aging parents often is done at a distance[2928] • Open to both domestic and international adoption[2929] • Baby Boomers are part of the "sandwich generation" or multigenerational households. Caregivers of parents and children[2930]

New Parent/Caregivers (continued)	• Pew Research Center found that since the start of the recession in 2007, 49 million Americans (just over 16 percent of the population, including a rising number of seniors) lived in multi-generation households[2931] • In 2008, about 20 percent of adults 65 and older were living in households with at least two generations under one roof[2932] • The biggest factor in creating new multigenerational households was the number of young adults in the 25 to 34 age group that moved in with their parents or older relatives. The percentage of young adults ages 25 to 34 who were living in multigenerational households in 2008 was about the same as the percentage of people who were 65 and older[2933] • The increase in young adults living in multigenerational households was dramatic (from 11 percent in 1980 to 20 percent in 2008) while the increase among older people was more gradual (from 17 percent in 1980 to 20 percent in 2008)[2934]
Termination of Pregnancy	• Strong belief in individual choice and freedom of choice[2935]

Generation X (1965 to 1980)

Note: The following information is general. Specific beliefs and practices may vary. Details on page 12.

Legend: ✓ = Suggestions for Healthcare Professionals; ▶ = Significant Details or Exceptions.

CARE OF THE PATIENT

Barriers to Healthcare	• Cost and lack of insurance[2936] • Highest unemployment in economic downturns[2937] • 3.5 times less likely to seek care due to cost to uninsured[2938] • Will have to overcome financing issues in order to guarantee best healthcare options[2939]

Common Medical Issues	• Gen Xers have children at a higher rate than recent generations[2940]
	• Gen Xers face smoking-related health issues[2941]
	  ▶ Highest prevalence of smoking rates at 25.6 percent for ages 25 to 44
	  ▶ The smoking rate for men in this age group is 28.4 percent
	  ▶ The smoking rate for women in this age group is 22.8 percent
	• Eating disorders are common in both men and women[2942]
	• Depression and anxiety are issues for many of this generation due to the many stressors related to upbringing and social expectations[2943]
	• Divorce rates, which climbed quickly during their developmental years and on into young adulthood, have contributed to the incidence of depression among this group[2944]
	• Delayed treatment for depression is normal because there is a fear of being viewed as weak and less competitive if not able to handle your own problems[2945]
	• Confusion and anxiety related to developing meaningful intimacy also are issues for this generation[2946]
	• Substance abuse issues – drug experimentation and alcohol (binge drinking) are prevalent among Gen Xers[2947]

Communication Tips	• Use e-mail as a primary communication tool[2948] • Talk in short sound bites to keep their attention[2949] • Ask them for their feedback and provide them with regular feedback[2950] • Share information with them on a regular basis and strive to keep them in the loop[2951] • Use an informal communication style[2952]
Defining Generational Characteristics	• Family-oriented[2953] • Values their contribution and likes feedback and recognition[2954] • Highly adaptive – likes change[2955] • Independent[2956]

Defining Generational Characteristics (continued)	• Immediate access to information[2957]
Diet and Nutrition	• Called the "organic" generation[2958] ▸ The perceived healthfulness of a product is an important factor, i.e., more likely to choose naturally grown foods over chemically enhanced or treated • Gen Xers are far less satisfied with their health status and behaviors than their elders or the Millennial generation, a fact that's related to their search for "better for you" items on restaurant menus[2959] • Many Gen Xers are parents, so they are interested in healthier options for their children[2960]
Healing Environment	• Gen Xers have an awakened spirituality[2961] • They are interested in spiritual topics, as exhibited by their fascination with the supernatural programs like the "X-Files" and "Outer Limits"[2962] • Interested in God, but not necessarily interested in organized religion[2963]
Pain Management	• Most likely to be open-minded about alternative pain management options[2964]

END OF LIFE

End-of-Life Discussion	✓ Per HIPAA, healthcare professional must obtain patient's permission to disclose health information to third parties ✓ Healthcare professional may ask patient who will make healthcare decisions for them if not themselves ✓ Health professional may discuss patient's terminal illness if applicable

PERINATAL CARE

Birth Process (Labor /Cesarean Section/ Vaginal Birth)	• C-sections are becoming more commonplace because they don't interfere with mom's schedule[2965]
Breastfeeding	• Breastfeeding viewed as inconvenience long-term[2966]
Prenatal Care	• Important as long as it doesn't interrupt a schedule[2967]
Termination of Pregnancy	• Abortion was legalized In this generation; thus, became a method of birth control[2968]

Millennials/Generation Y (1981 to 1995)

Note: The following information is general. Specific beliefs and practices may vary. Details on page 12.

Legend: ✓ = Suggestions for Healthcare Professionals; ▶ = Significant Details or Exceptions.

CARE OF THE PATIENT

Barriers to Healthcare	• Affordability of health insurance[2969] • Increasing cost of medication[2970] • Job stability due to the recession[2971]
Common Medical Issues	• Millennials have few medical issues that are prevalent[2972] • Millennials are generally not ill and do not see a doctor often, with 1.5 visits per year; this is below average[2973] • Medical issues are more for routine or preventive care[2974] • Women in this age group tend to see their OB/GYN annually[2975] • Emergency room visits are higher for this group than other age groups because of automobile and sporting accidents[2976] • Many Millennials access the ER for routine medical care of illness such as sinusitis[2977] ▶ The higher than average rate of emergency room visits suggests that Millennials are more likely to wait until a health issue becomes severe instead of seeing a primary care physician when symptoms first appear ▶ Emergency room visits for routine medical care also may suggest that Millennials are unfamiliar with how to use their medical benefit plans, have not identified or developed a relationship with a primary care physician, and/or lack health insurance coverage • Drug abuse – alcohol (binge drinking), illicit drugs, drug experimentation[2978] • Hospital admissions for this age group, in rank order, are related to childbirth, psychosis, tobacco-use disorders, depressive disorders, and alcohol- or drug-related conditions[2979]
Communication Tips	• Use action words and challenge them at every opportunity[2980] • They will resent it if you talk down to them[2981] • They prefer electronic forms of communication – e-mail or texting[2982] • Seek their feedback constantly and provide them with regular feedback[2983] • Use humor and create a fun learning environment, and don't take yourself too seriously[2984] • Challenge them to be a part of the process by finding alternate solutions, which helps to keep them engaged[2985]
Defining Generational Characteristics	• Respect must be earned; it is not freely granted based on age, authority, or title[2986]

Defining Generational Characteristics (continued)	• Adapt rapidly to change[2987] • Crave change and challenge[2988] • Creative mindset[2989] • Significantly value diversity, intolerance of bias[2990]
Diet and Nutrition	• Millennials are the largest users of natural and organic foods, but are less likely to avoid specific items, such as trans fats[2991] • While the majority of Millennials say freshly prepared food is important, they're slightly less enthusiastic than older consumers[2992] • Millennials are also less concerned about healthy choices[2993]
Healing Environment	• Religion is losing this generation because they perceive that it invokes disagreement and violence, and encourages negativity and separation between people[2994] • Millennials consider themselves to be more spiritual and far less religious than generations before them[2995] • This young generation is particularly at risk for suicide, increased incidences of eating disorders; sexual dysfunction and adjustment disorders are less frequently occurring, but do occur within this population[2996] • Emerging adulthood is a time of significant transition, both socially and psychologically[2997] • Anxiety disorders are most often reported by young people and are the most common reason for seeking mental health services[2998] • The early twenties is a time of psychological developmental, in which more chronic mental illnesses such as bipolar disorder, major depression, and thought disorders first appear[2999] • Because their peers condone binge drinking and misuse of alcohol, Millennials may not perceive their alcohol use as a source for concern and are not likely to seek help[3000]
Pain Management	• The most often prescribed drug categories for this group, ranked in order of frequency, are: Anti-inflammatory medicines, antibiotics, asthma and respiratory medicines, pain medicines, steroids, psychiatric medicines, and antihistamines and allergy medicines[3001]

END OF LIFE

End-of-Life Discussion	✓ Per HIPAA, healthcare professional must obtain patient's permission to disclose health information to third parties ✓ Healthcare professional may ask patient who will make healthcare decisions for them if not themselves ✓ Health professional may discuss patient's terminal illness if applicable

References

(Endnotes)

RELIGIONS AND CHRISTIAN DENOMINATIONS

1   "U.S. Religious Landscape Survey," Pew Research Center, accessed January 17, 2012, http://religions.pewforum.org/reports.

2   S. Sorajjakool, M.F. Carr, and J.J. Nam, *World Religions for Healthcare Professionals* (New York: Routledge, 2010).

3   L. Dossey, *Healing Words: The Power of Prayer and the Practice of Medicine* (San Francisco, CA: Harper Collins, 1993).

4   "National Advisory Council For Complementary and Alternative Medicine Minutes of the Seventeenth Meeting," Department of Health and Human Services National Institutes of Health National Center for Complementary and Alternative Medicine, updated June 4, 2004, http://nccam.nih.gov/about /naccam /minutes/2004junemin.pdf.

5   "Prayer and Spirituality in Health: Ancient Practices, Modern Science," *CAM at the NIH*, XII, no. 1 (Dec. 2005), http://www.jpsych.com/pdfs/NCCAM%20-%20Prayer%20and%20Spirituality%20in%20Health.pdf.

6   "Spirituality Emerges as Point of Debate in Mind-Body Movement," Religion Link, updated Feb. 13, 2006, http://www.religionlink.com/tip_060213.php.

7   "Major Religions of the World Ranked by Number of Adherents," Adherents.com, accessed January 17, 2012, http://www.adherents.com/Religions_By_Adherents.html.

8   "Religious Composition of the U.S.—U.S. Religious Landscape Survey," Pew Forum on Religion & Public Life, accessed January 17, 2012, http://religions.pewforum.org/pdf/affiliations-all-traditions.pdf.

9   Sorajjakool et al., *World Religions for Healthcare Professionals*.

10   "Christianity Today - General Statistics and Facts of Christianity," About.com, accessed January 17, 2012, http://christianity.about.com/od/denominations/p/christiantoday.htm.

11-15 Sorajjakool et al., *World Religions for Healthcare Professionals*.

16   "Muslim Population in the World," Muslim Population.com, accessed January 17, 2012, http://www.islamicpopulation.com/.

17-28 Sorajjakool et al., *World Religions for Healthcare Professionals*.

29-30 "Fundamental Beliefs," Seventh-day Adventist Church, accessed December 20, 2011, http://www.adventist.org/beliefs/fundamental/index.html.

31   The Secretariat, General Counsel of Seventh-day Adventists, *Seventh-day Adventist Church Manual* (Hagerstown, MD: Review and Herald Publishing Association, 2010), 119–122.

32   "Fundamental Beliefs," Seventh-day Adventist Church, accessed December 20, 2011, http://www.adventist.org/beliefs/fundamental/indcx.html.

33-34 "Health," Seventh-day Adventist Church, accessed December 20, 2011, http://www.adventist.org/mission-and-service/health.html.

35-36 "Fundamental Beliefs," Seventh-day Adventist Church, accessed December 20, 2011, http://www.adventist.org/beliefs/fundamental/index.html.

37   E.G. White, *The Ministry of Healing* (Nampa, ID: Pacific Press Publishing Association, 1942), 122, 127, 254–257, 275–276.

38   "Guidelines for Sabbath Observance," Seventh-day Adventist Church, accessed December 20, 2011, http://www.adventist.org/beliefs/other-documents/other-doc6.html.

39   "Religious Views on Organ, Tissue, and Blood Donation," Donate Life NM.org, accessed December 20, 2011, http://www.donatelifenm.org/religiousviews.htm#sda.

40   The Secretariat, General Counsel of Seventh-day Adventists, *Seventh-day Adventist Church Manual* (Hagerstown, MD: Review and Herald Publishing Association, 2010), 91.

41   E.G. White, *Counsels on Health* (Nama, ID: Pacific Press Publishing Association, 1951), 127–31.

42-43   "What Foods Are On the 7th Day Adventist Diet?" Livestrong.com, accessed December 20, 2011, http://www.livestrong.com/article/441583-what-foods-are-on-the-7th-day-adventist-diet/.

44   R.E. Spector, *Cultural Diversity in Health & Illness* (New York: Appleton & Lange, 1996).

45   White, *Ministry of Healing*, 222–275.

46   J.A. Shelly, *Spiritual Care: A Guide for Caregivers* (Downers Grove, IL: InterVarsity Press, 2000), 25.

47   The Secretariat, *Seventh-day Adventist Church Manual*, 77–78.

48   The Secretariat, *Seventh-day Adventist Church Manual*, 73.

49   White, *Ministry of Healing*, 222–275.

50   Ministerial Association, General Conference of Seventh-day Adventists, *Adventists Believe... A Biblical Exposition of 27 Fundamental Doctrines* (Hagerstown, MD: Review & Herald Publishing Association, 1988).

51   Shelly, *Spiritual Care*, 25.

52   "Trust Services and Planned Giving," Chesapeake Conference of Seventh-day Adventists, accessed December 21, 2011, http://www.ccosda.org/article.php?id=48.

53   Spector, *Cultural Diversity*, 157.

54   "After Death: Religious Needs of Patients in Sickness, Dying, and Death," SWAHS Pastoral Care and Chaplaincy Services, last updated December 21, 2011, http://www.wsahs.nsw.gov.au/services/pastoralcare/relneeds.htm.

55   E.R. DuBose, ed., The Park Ridge Center for the Study of Health, Faith, and Ethics, "Seventh-day Adventist Tradition," in *Religious Beliefs & Health Care Decisions—A Quick Reference to 15 Religious Traditions and their Application in Health Care* (n.p. Chicago?: The Center In Chicago, 1995).

56   The Secretariat, *Seventh-day Adventist Church Manual*, 165.

57-58   "A Statement of Consensus on Care for the Dying," Seventh-day Adventist Church, accessed December 20, 2011, http://adventist.org/beliefs/statements/main-stat6.html.

59   DuBose, "Seventh-day Adventist Tradition," in *Religious Beliefs & Health Care Decisions*.

60   "A Statement of Consensus on Care for the Dying," Seventh-day Adventist Church, accessed December 20, 2011, http://adventist.org/beliefs/statements/main-stat6.html.

61   The Secretariat, *Seventh-day Adventist Church Manual*, 73.

62   Ministerial Association, *Adventists Believe*, 188–89.

63   M.M. Andrews and J.S. Boyle, *Transcultural Concepts in Nursing Care*, 2nd ed. (New York: Lippincott, 1995), 404.

64   M.A. Shah, *Transcultural Aspects of Perinatal Health Care: A Resource Guide* (Tampa, FL: National Perinatal Association, 2004), 291.

65   "Seventh-day Adventists: Infant Circumcision," AllExperts.com, updated April 28, 2009, http://en.allexperts.com/q/Seventh-Day-Adventists-2318/2009/4/infant-circumcision.htm.

66   "Birth Control: A Seventh-day Adventist Statement of Consensus," Seventh-day Adventist Church, accessed December 20, 2011, http://adventist.org/beliefs/statements/main-stat6.html.

67-68   "Guidelines on Abortion," Seventh-day Adventist Church, accessed December 20, 2011, http://www.adventist.org/beliefs/guidelines/main-guide1.html.

69 Andrews and Boyle, *Transcultural Concepts*, 400.

70-71 Shah, *Transcultural Aspects of Perinatal Health Care,* 291.

72 "Considerations on Assisted Human Reproduction," Seventh-day Adventist Church, accessed December 20, 2011, http://adventist.org/beliefs/other-documents/other-doc10.html.

73 "Guidelines on Abortion," Seventh-day Adventist Church, accessed December 20, 2011, http://www.adventist.org/beliefs/guidelines/main-guide1.html.

74-76 M. Good and P. Good, *20 Most Asked Questions About the Amish and Mennonites*, rev. ed. (Intercourse, PA: Good Books, 1995), 7–8, 16, 46.

77 R.H. Seitz, *Amish Values: Wisdom that Works* (Harrisburg, PA: RB Books, Seitz and Seitz, Inc., 1995), 52.

78 A. Beachy, E. Hershberger, R. Davidhizar, G. Davidhizar, and J.N. Giger, "Cultural Implications for Nursing Care of the Amish," *Journal of Cultural Diversity* 4, no. 4 (1997): 121.

79 Andrews and Boyle, *Transcultural Concepts,* 172.

80 Good and Good, *20 Most Asked Questions,* 58.

81 "Food Intake, Dietary Practices, and Nutritional Supplement Use Among the Amish," C. Carter, OhioLINK, accessed December 21, 2011, http://drc.ohiolink.edu/handle/2374.OX/5155.

82 Beachy et al., "Cultural Implications," *Journal of Cultural Diversity*, 124–*25*.

83-84 N.L. Fisher, *Cultural and Ethnic Diversity: A Guide for Genetics Professionals* (Baltimore, MD: Johns Hopkins University Press, 1996), 183.

85 Good and Good, *20 Most Asked Questions,* 62–65.

86 E. Randall-David, *Strategies for Working with Culturally Diverse Communities and Clients* (Washington, DC: Association for the Care of Children's Health, 1989), 39.

87 Beachy et al., "Cultural Implications," *Journal of Cultural Diversity*, 121.

88 Beachy et al., "Cultural Implications," *Journal of Cultural Diversity*, 123.

89 Andrews and Boyle, *Transcultural Concepts,* 169–172.

90 "Amish Kapps, Traditional Head Coverings for Amish Women," Suite 101.com, Sarah Tennant, updated June 11, 2008, http://sarah-tennant.suite101.com/amish-kapps-a56816.

91 Seitz, *Amish Values,* 56.

92 Beachy et al., "Cultural Implications," *Journal of Cultural Diversity*, 122.

93 Beachy et al., "Cultural Implications," *Journal of Cultural Diversity*, 120–23.

94 "Religion and Organ and Tissue Donation," The Gift of a Lifetime, accessed December 12, 2011, http://www.organtransplants.org/understanding/religion/.

95 Beachy et al., "Cultural Implications," *Journal of Cultural Diversity*, 120.

96 D.B. Kraybill, S.M. Nolt, and D.L. Weaver-Zercher, *The Amish Way: Patient Faith in a Perilous World*, (San Francisco: John Wiley & Sons, Inc., 2010), 169.

97 S. Obernberger, "When Love and Abuse are not Mutually Exclusive," *Issues in Law and Medicine* 355 (Spring 1997).

98 Fisher, *Cultural and Ethnic Diversity*, 189–190.

99 Kraybill et al., *The Amish Way*, 172–173.

100 Kraybill et al., *The Amish Way*, 171–172.

101 Kraybill et al., *The Amish Way*, 172–173.

102 Good and Good, *20 Most Asked Questions,* 66–69.

103-104   Beachy et al., "Cultural Implications," *Journal of Cultural Diversity*, 123.

105   "Religion and Organ and Tissue Donation," The Gift of a Lifetime, accessed December 12, 2011, http://www. organtransplants.org/understanding/religion/.

106   Kraybill et al., *The Amish Way*, 171.

107   Fisher, *Cultural and Ethnic Diversity*, 190.

108   Good and Good, *20 Most Asked Questions,* 56.

109   Good and Good, *20 Most Asked Questions,* 16.

110   J. Lipson and S. Dibble, eds. *Culture and Clinical Care* (San Francisco, CA: UCSF Nursing Press, 2005), 199.

111   Beachy et al., "Cultural Implications," *Journal of Cultural Diversity*, 123.

112   Fisher, *Cultural and Ethnic Diversity*, 187.

113   "Do Amish Use Birth Control?" Amish America, accessed December 22, 2011, http://amishamerica.com/do-amish-use-birth-control/.

114   Beachy et al., "Cultural Implications," *122–124.*

115   K.A. Granju, "The Culture of Childbirth," *CityPages*, May 1, 1999, http://www.citypages.com/1999-05-01/feature/the-culture-of-childbirth/.

116   Randall-David, *Strategies for Working with Culturally Diverse,* 36.

117   Beachy et al., "Cultural Implications," *123.*

118-119   Fisher, *Cultural and Ethnic Diversity*, 186.

120   DuBose, "The Anabaptist Tradition," in *Religious Beliefs & Health Care.*

121   Beachy et al., "Cultural Implications," *123.*

122   L.D. Purnell and B.J. Paulanka, *Guide to Culturally Competent Health Care* (Philadelphia, PA: F. A. Davis Company, 2009), 43.

123   Beachy et al., "Cultural Implications," *Journal of Cultural Diversity*, 122–124.

124   Fisher, *Cultural and Ethnic Diversity*, 187.

125   Kraybill et al., *The Amish Way*, 171.

126   M. Yehieli and M.A. Grey, *Health Matters: A Pocket Guide for Working with Diverse Cultures and Underserved Populations* (Yarmouth, ME: Intercultural Press, Inc., 2005), 44.

127   Beachy et al., "Cultural Implications," *Journal of Cultural Diversity*, 120.

128   N.L. Fisher, *Cultural and Ethnic* Diversity, 187.

129-130   F.S. Mead, S.S. Hill, and C.D. Atwood, "Baptist Churches" in *Handbook of Denominations in the United States*, 13th ed., (Nashville, TN: Abingdon Press, 2010).

131   "American Baptist Policy Statement on Health, Healing, and Wholeness," General Board of the American Baptist Churches, updated June 1991, http://www.abc-usa.org/LinkClick.aspx?fileticket=kA7QkBgFPIE%3D&tabid=199.

132   "Baptist," Patheos.com, accessed December 26, 2011, http://www.patheos.com/Library/Baptist.html.

133   "Blood Transfusions," Baptist Health and Wellness Center, accessed December 26, 2011, http://community.e-baptisthealth.com/health-info/content/ped/eng/hematology/trans.html.

134   G.C. White, *Believers and Beliefs: A Practical Guide to Religious Etiquette for Business and Social Occasions* (New York: Berkley Publishing Group, 1997), 161.

135   C. Young and C. Koopsen, *Spirituality, Health, and Healing* (Sudbury, MA: Jones and Bartlett Publishers, 2006), 45, 126, 158.

136   Ibid., 47.

137   W.D. Hale, R.G. Bennett, *Building Healthy Communities Through Medical-Religious Partnerships* (Baltimore, MD: Johns Hopkins University Press, 2000), 78–79.

138   S. Gellar, "Religious Attitudes and the Autopsy," *Archives of Pathology & Laboratory Medicine* 108 (1984): 494.

139-140 "After Death: Religious Needs of Patients in Sickness, Dying, and Death," SWAHS Pastoral Care and Chaplaincy Services, accessed December 26, 2011, http://www.wsahs.nsw.gov.au/services/pastoralcare/relneeds.htm.

141   C.B. Rosdahl and M.T. Kowalski, *Textbook of Basic Nursing* (Philadelphia, PA: Lippincott Williams & Wilkins, 2008), 127.

142   White, *Believers and Beliefs*, 162.

143   "Religion and Organ and Tissue Donation," http://www.organtransplants.org/understanding/religion/.

144   J.M. Luce and T.A. Raffin, "Withholding and Withdrawal of Life Support From Critically Ill Patients," *Western Journal of Medicine* 167, no. 6 (December 1997): 411–416.

145-146 White, *Believers and Beliefs*, 161–162.

147   "Circumcision," Baptist Hospital East, accessed December 26, 2011, http://baptisteast.adam.com/content.aspx?productId=14&pid=14&gid=000133.

148   W. Flint, *Alabama Baptists: Southern Baptists in the Heart of Dixie* (Tuscaloosa, AL: University of Alabama Press, 1998), 532.

149   "What Do Baptists Believe About Abortion?" Answers.com, accessed December 26, 2011, http://wiki.answers.com/Q/What_do_Baptists_believe_about_abortion.

150   A. Abyad, "The Role of Different Faiths and Their Attitudes Toward Death," *Healing Ministry* (Jan/Feb, 1996): 23.

151   Andrews and Boyle, *Transcultural Concepts*, 363, 376–77.

152   "The Noble Eightfold Path," The Bigview.com, accessed December 26, 2011, http://www.thebigview.com/buddhism/eightfoldpath.html.

153-154 White, *Believers and Beliefs*, 11–14.

155   Spector, *Cultural Diversity*, 244.

156   Spector, *Cultural Diversity*, 153.

157   White, *Believers and Beliefs*, 15.

158   "Guidelines for Health Care Providers Interacting with Muslim Patients and their Families," 1999, International Strategy and Policy Institute, last modified June 10, 2006, http://www.ispi--usa.org/guidelines.htm.

159   J. Gillman, "Religious Perspectives on Organ Donation," *Critical Care Nursing Quarterly* 22, no.3 (1999): 19–29.

160-161 White, *Believers and Beliefs*, 12–15.

162   Spector, *Cultural Diversity*, 153.

163   Andrews and Boyle, *Transcultural Concepts*, 363–77.

164   White, *Believers and Beliefs*, 11.

165   "Guidelines for Health Care Providers," http://www.ispi--usa.org/guidelines.htm.

166   Gellar, "Religious Attitudes," *Archives of Pathology & Laboratory Medicine*, 494.

167   Abyad, "Role of Different Faiths," *Healing Ministry*, 24.

168   "Guidelines for Health Care Providers," http://www.ispi--usa.org/guidelines.htm.

169   White, *Believers and Beliefs*, 16.

170   J.G. Lipson, S. Dibble, and P.A. Minarik, eds., *Culture and Nursing Care: A Pocket Guide* (San Francisco, CA: UCSF Nursing Press, 1996), B-7.

171   Abyad, "Role of Different Faiths," *Healing Ministry*,24.

172   White, *Believers and Beliefs*, 16.

173   "Guidelines for Health Care Providers," http://www.ispi--usa.org/guidelines.htm.

174   Spector, *Cultural Diversity*, 153.

175-176   "Buddhism and Organ Donation," *Mingkok Buddhist News*, last modified August 31, 2011, http://mingkok. buddhistdoor.com/en/news/d/22456.

177   White, *Believers and Beliefs*, 17.

178   Spector, *Cultural Diversity*, 153.

179   P.D. Numrich, "The Buddhist Tradition," in *Religious Beliefs & Health Care*.

180-181   Lipson et al., *Culture and Nursing* Care, B-7.

182-183   Andrews and Boyle, *Transcultural Concepts*, 363–77.

184   Lipson et al., *Culture and Nursing* Care, B-7.

185   "Church of Christ, Scientist," ReligionFacts, accessed December 26, 2011, http://www.religionfacts.com/a-z-religion-index/christian_science.htm.

186-187   White, *Believers and Beliefs*, 18–20.

188   Andrews and Boyle, *Transcultural Concepts*, 381–82.

189   White, *Believers and Beliefs*, 21.

190   White, *Believers and Beliefs*, 18–20.

191   "Church of Christ, Scientist," ReligionFacts, accessed December 26, 2011, http://www.religionfacts.com/a-z-religion-index/christian_science.htm.

192-194   Mead et al., "Church of Christ, Scientist (Christian Science)" in *Handbook of Denominations*.

195   Andrews and Boyle, *Transcultural Concepts*, 384.

196   "Sunday Church Services and Wednesday Testimony Meetings," Christian Science.com, accessed December 26, 2011, http://christianscience.com/church-of-christ-scientist/the-mother-church-in-boston-ma-usa/sunday-church-services-and-wednesday-testimony-meetings.

197   Andrews and Boyle, *Transcultural Concepts*, 383–385.

198   White, *Believers and Beliefs*, 22.

199   M.B. Eddy, *Science and Health* (Boston, MA: Christian Science Publishing Society, 1902), 74.

200   "Christian Science Church Beliefs and Practices," J. Zavada, About.com Christianity, accessed December 26, 2011, http://christianity.about.com/od/christianscience/a/christsciencebeliefs.htm.

201   R. Peel, *Health and Medicine in the Christian Science Tradition* (New York: Crossroad Publications, 1986), 73.

202   "Faith Traditions and Health Care," Pennsylvania Medicine Pastoral Care and Education, revised June 2003, http://www.uphs.upenn.edu/pastoral/pubs/traditions.html.

203   Andrews and Boyle, *Transcultural Concepts*, 384.

204   S. Salimbene, *What Language Does Your Patient Hurt In?*, 2nd ed. (Amherst, MA: Diversity Resources, Inc., 2005), 210.

205   Lipson et al., *Culture and Nursing* Care, B-10.

206   "Faith Traditions and Health Care," http://www.uphs.upenn.edu/pastoral/pubs/traditions.html.

207   D. Harris-Abbott, ed., "The Christian Science Tradition," in *Religious Beliefs and Health Care*.

208   "Faith Traditions and Health Care," http://www.uphs.upenn.edu/pastoral/pubs/traditions.html.

209-210   White, *Believers and Beliefs*, 23.

211   Andrews and Boyle, *Transcultural Concepts*, 384.

212   "Faith Traditions and Health Care," http://www.uphs.upenn.edu/pastoral/pubs/traditions.html.

213   Andrews and Boyle, *Transcultural Concepts*, 383–385.

214   Lipson et al., *Culture and Nursing* Care, B-10.

215   "Religion and Organ and Tissue Donation," http://www.organtransplants.org/understanding/religion/.

216   Andrews and Boyle, *Transcultural Concepts*, 384–385.

217   "Faith Traditions and Health Care," http://www.uphs.upenn.edu/pastoral/pubs/traditions.html.

218   White, *Believers and Beliefs*, 23.

219   Peel, *Health and Medicine in the Christian Science Tradition*, 72.

220   "What is the Birth Practice in Christian Scientist?" All About Cults, accessed December 26, 2011, http://www.allaboutcults.org/birth-practice-in-christian-scientist-faq.htm.

221-222   Andrews and Boyle, *Transcultural Concepts*, 384.

223-224   D. Harris-Abbott, "The Christian Science Tradition," in *Religious Beliefs and Health Care*.

225   "Faith Traditions and Health Care," http://www.uphs.upenn.edu/pastoral/pubs/traditions.html.

226   B.J. Kramer, "Health and Aging of Urban American Indians," *Western Journal of Medicine* 157, no. 3 (September 1992): 281–85.

227   Salimbene, *What Language*, 210.

228   "Doctrinal and Ethical Positions, Church of the Nazarene," D. Bratcher, ed., *CRI/Voice*, Appendix, Chapter V, 903, "Current Moral and Social Issues," section 4, "Articles of Faith," last modified November 11, 2011, http://www.crivoice.org/creednazarene.html .

229   Bratcher, "Doctrinal and Ethical Positions, Church of the Nazarene," section 1, "Articles of Faith," http://www.crivoice.org/creednazarene.html .

230   "Church of the Nazarene Beliefs and Practices," J. Zavada, About.com.Christianity, accessed December 4, 2011, http://www.christianity.about.com/od/Nazarene-Church/a/Nazarene-Beliefs.htm.

231   Bratcher, "Doctrinal and Ethical Positions, Church of the Nazarene," section 2, "Articles of Faith," http://www.crivoice.org/creednazarene.html .

232   D. Blevins, C. Lewis, Jr., F. Moore, R. Samples, and J. Stone, eds., *Manual Church of the Nazarene 2005–2009*, Kansas City, MO: Nazarene Publishing House,2005), http://sermons.logos.com/submissions/107737-Manual-Church-Of-The-Nazarene-2005-2009-manual2005-2009-Church-#content =/submissions/107737.

233   Blevins et al., *Manual Church of the Nazarene*.

234   Blevins et al., *Manual Church of the Nazarene*.

235   Blevins et al., *Manual Church of the Nazarene*.

236   Bratcher, "Doctrinal and Ethical Positions, Church of the Nazarene," section 18, "Articles of Faith," http://www.crivoice.org/creednazarene.html .

237-247   Blevins et al., *Manual Church of the Nazarene*.

248-252   Bratcher, "Doctrinal and Ethical Positions, Church of the Nazarene," section 36, "Sanctity of Life," http://www.crivoice.org/creednazarene.html .

253   Bratcher, "Doctrinal and Ethical Positions, Church of the Nazarene," section 903.1, "Current Moral and Social Issues," http://www.crivoice.org/creednazarene.html .

254   Blevins et al., *Manual Church of the Nazarene*.

255-258   "Doctrinal and Ethical Positions, Church of the Nazarene," D. Bratcher, ed., *CRI/Voice*, Appendix, Chapter V, 903, "Current Moral and Social Issues," section 16, "Articles of Faith," last modified November 11, 2011, http://www.crivoice.org/creednazarene.html .

259-261   Blevins et al., *Manual Church of the Nazarene*.

262-265   Bratcher, "Doctrinal and Ethical Positions, Church of the Nazarene," section 36, "Sanctity of Life," http://www.crivoice.org/creednazarene.html .

266-267   Blevins et al., *Manual Church of the Nazarene*.

268-269   Bratcher, "Doctrinal and Ethical Positions, Church of the Nazarene," section 36, "Sanctity of Life," http://www.crivoice.org/creednazarene.html .

270   "The Holy Scriptures," The Episcopal Church Visitors' Center, accessed December 26, 2011, http://www.episcopalchurch.org/visitors_11564_ENG_HTM.htm.

271   S. Matlins and A. Magida, eds., "Episcopalian and Anglican" in *How to Be a Perfect Stranger: A Guide to Etiquette in Other People's Religious Ceremonies* (Woodstock, VT: SkyLight Paths Publishing, 2011), 87.

272   "The Creeds," The Episcopal Church Visitors' Center, accessed December 26, 2011, http://www.episcopalchurch.org/visitors_11838_ENG_HTM.htm.

273   "The Sacraments," The Episcopal Church Visitors' Center, accessed December 26, 2011, http://www.episcopalchurch.org/visitors_10850_ENG_HTM.htm

274   "The Ministry," The Episcopal Church Visitors' Center, accessed December 26, 2011, http://www.episcopalchurch.org/visitors_11748_ENG_HTM.htm.

275   "God the Father," The Episcopal Church Visitors' Center, accessed December 26, 2011, http://www.episcopalchurch.org/visitors_11773_ENG_HTM.htm.

276   "Evangelism," The Episcopal Church, accessed December 27, 2011, http://www.episcopalchurch.org/congdev/2020home.html.

277   "What is the Episcopal Church About?" Episcopal Church Visitors' Center, accessed December 27, 2011, http://www.episcopalchurch.org/visitors_16976_ENG_HTM.htm?menupage=49678.

278   "Religion and Organ and Tissue Donation," The Gift of a Lifetime, accessed December 27, 2011, http://www.organtransplants.org/understanding/religion/.

279   "Churchgoers – How Different Are Your Beliefs From the Next Church Over?" Straight Dope Message Board, last updated January 23, 2006, http://boards.straightdope.com/sdmb/archive/index.php/t-355383.html.

280   C. Young and C. Koopsen, *Spirituality, Health, and Healing* (Sudbury, MA: Jones and Bartlett Publishers, 2006), 45, 126, 158.

281   DuBose, "The Episcopal Tradition," in *Religious Beliefs & Health* Care. with

282   "Advance Directives," Episcopal Diocese of Michigan, accessed December 27, 2011, http://edomi.org/index.php/resources/people-resources/advance-directives.

283   "Religions and the Autopsy," E.C. Burton, K.A. Collins, and S.A. Gurevitz, Medscape Reference, accessed December 27, 2011, http://emedicine.medscape.com/article/1705993-overview#aw2aab6b7.

284   "After Death: Religious Needs of Patients in Sickness, Dying, and Death," SWAHS Pastoral Care and Chaplaincy Services, accessed December 26, 2011, http://www.wsahs.nsw.gov.au/services/pastoralcare/relneeds.htm.

285   L. White, *Foundations of Nursing*, (New York: Thomson Delmar, 2005), 211.

286   Ibid., 212.

287   DuBose, "The Episcopal Tradition," in *Religious Beliefs and Health Care*.

288   "Anglican Afterlife and Salvation," Patheos.com, accessed December 27, 2011, http://www.patheos.com/Library/Anglican/Beliefs/Afterlife-and-Salvation?offset=0&max=1.

289-290   DuBose, "The Episcopal Tradition," in *Religious Beliefs and Health Care*.

291   "Religion and Organ and Tissue Donation," The Gift of a Lifetime, accessed December 27, 2011, http://www. organtransplants.org/understanding/religion/.

292   "Episcopal Church Offers Resources for End-of-Life Issues," Episcopal News Service Archive, accessed December 27, 2011, http://www.episcopalchurch.org/3577_60370_ENG_HTM.htm.

293   Matlins and Magida, *How to Be a Perfect Stranger,* 91.

294   "Holy Baptism," The Episcopal Church Visitors' Center, accessed December 26, 2011, http://www. episcopalchurch.org/visitors_11674_ENG_HTM.htm.

295   "History of Circumcision," History of Circumcision.net, accessed January 31, 2012, http://www. historyofcircumcision.net/.

296   "Positions on Social Issues: Birth Control, Death Penalty, Children," Episcopal Diocese of New York, accessed December 27, 2011, http://www.dioceseny.org/pages/322.

297   DuBose, "The Episcopal Tradition," in *Religious Beliefs and Health Care.*

298   "In Vitro Fertilization," ivf-worldwide, accessed December 27, 2011, http://www.ivf-worldwide.com/Education/ christianity.html.

299-300 "Abortion: Where Do the Churches Stand?" E.L. Ohlhoff, National Right to Life, updated September 12, 2000, http:// www.pregnantpause.org/people/wherchur.htm.

301   "Religions in India," A. Daniel, accessed December 5, 2011, http://adaniel.tripod.com/religions.htm.

302   "Four Facts of Hinduism," Kauai's Hindu Monastery, accessed December 5, 2011, http://www.himalayanacademy. com/basics/fourf/.

303   "Hinduism and Medicine," A. Sukumaran, 1999, accessed December 5, 2011, http://www.angelfire.com/az/ ambersukumaran/medicine.html.

304-308 "Nine Beliefs of Hinduism," Kauai's Hindu Monastery, accessed December 5, 2011, http://www. himalayanacademy.com/basics/nineb/.

309   "Glossary-'Four Traditional Goals,'" Kauai's Hindu Monastery, accessed December 5, 2011, http://www. himalayanacademy.com/resources/lexicon/.

310   D. Thakrar, R. Das, and A. Sheikh, eds., *Caring for Hindu Patients* (Abingdon, UK: Radcliffe Publishing, 2008), 14.

311   A. Abyad, "The Role of Different Faiths and Their Attitudes Toward Death," *Healing Ministry* (Jan/Feb, 1996): 23.

312   "Nine Beliefs of Hinduism," http://www.himalayanacademy.com/basics/nineb/.

313-314 M.M. Andrews and J.S. Boyle, *Transcultural Concepts in Nursing Care,* 5th ed. (New York: Lippincott, 1995), 386.

315   J. Ramakrishna and M.J. Weiss, "Health, Illness, and Immigration—East Indians in the United States," in "Cross-cultural Medicine a Decade Later," ed. J. Barker and M.M. Clark, special issue, *Western Journal of Medicine*, 157, no.3 (1992): 267. http://www.ncbi.nlm.nih.gov/pmc/articles/PMC1011274/?page=1.

316   "Glossary-'Namaskara,'" Kauai's Hindu Monastery, accessed December 5, 2011, http://www.himalayanacademy. com/resources/lexicon/

317-318 "India—Language, Culture, Customs and Etiquette," Kwintessential, accessed December 6, 2011, http://www. kwintessential.co.uk/resources/global-etiquette/india-country-profile.html.

319   J.N. Giger and R.E. Davidhizar, *Transcultural Nursing, Assessment and Intervention* (St. Louis, MO: Elsevier Mosby, 2008), 543.

320   "Hindus: Dietary Guidelines," Ethnicity Online—Cultural Awareness in Healthcare, accessed December 5, 2011, http://www.ethnicityonline.net/hindu_diet.htm

321   Giger and Davidhizar, *Transcultural Nursing,* 555.

322   Ibid., 553.

323   G.C. White, *Believers and Beliefs: a Practical Guide to Religious Etiquette for Business and Social Occasions* (New York: Berkley Publishing Group, 1997).

324-325   "Hinduism and Medicine," http://www.angelfire.com/az/ambersukumaran/medicine.html.

326-327   G.C. White, *Believers and Beliefs*.

328-329   Giger and Davidhizar, *Transcultural Nursing,* 553.

330   Ibid., 556.

331   "Culture and Customs of India," Adventure Travellers Club, accessed December 5, 2011, http://www.nepaltravellers.com/Culture_and_Customs.htm.

332   Abyad, "The Role of Different Faiths," *Healing Ministry,* 21.

333   S. Singh, A. Karafin, A. Karlin, A. Mahapatra, A. Thomas, and R. Wlodarski, *South India,* (Melbourne: Lonely Planet, 2007), 517.

334-336   "Hindus—Physical Examinations," Ethnicity Online, accessed December 5, 2011, http://www.ethnicityonline.net/hindu_examinations.htm.

337   S. Thrane, "Hindu End of Life: Death, Dying, Suffering, and Karma: Professional Care Issues," *Journal of Hospice and Palliative Nursing* 12, no. 6 (2010): 337.

338-340   "Hinduism and Medicine," http://www.angelfire.com/az/ambersukumaran/medicine.html.

341   Ramakrishna and Weiss, "Health, Illness, and Immigration," *Western Journal of Medicine,* 266.

342   Editors of *Hinduism Today* Magazine, *What is Hinduism? Modern Adventures Into a Profound Global Faith,* (Kapaa, HI: Himalayan Academy, 2007), 351.

343   G.A. Galanti, *Caring for Patients From Different Cultures,* 4th ed. (Philadelphia, PA: University of Pennsylvania Press, 2008), 57.

344   "Rituals Related to Death in Hindu Family," Religious Portal—All About Hinduism, accessed December 5, 2011, http://www.religiousportal.com/HinduDeathRituals.html.

345   Editors of *Hinduism Today* Magazine, *What is Hinduism?* , 351.

346   S. Thrane, "Hindu End of Life," *Journal of Hospice and Palliative Nursing,* 337.

347   "Rituals Related to Death in Hindu Family," http://www.religiousportal.com/HinduDeathRituals.html.

348   "Hinduism and Medicine," http://www.angelfire.com/az/ambersukumaran/medicine.html

349   S. Thrane, "Hindu End of Life," *Journal of Hospice and Palliative Nursing,* 337.

350   "Hinduism and Medicine," http://www.angelfire.com/az/ambersukumaran/medicine.html.

351   S. Firth, *Dying, Death and Bereavement in a British Hindu Community,* (n.p. Belgium?, Peeters, Bondgenotenlaan, Leuven, 1997), 86.

352   "Rituals Related to Death in Hindu Family," http://www.religiousportal.com/HinduDeathRituals.html.

353   "Death: Hindu Rites, Rituals, and Preparations for Funerals," Dr. P.C. Shah and Prof. B. Sanwal, accessed December 5, 2011, http://www.hcclondon.ca/Hindu%20Death%20Rites%20&%20Rituals.pdf.

354   Firth, *Dying, Death, and Bereavement,* 58, 62.

355   "Hinduism and Medicine," http://www.angelfire.com/az/ambersukumaran/medicine.html.

356   "Rituals Related to Death in Hindu Family," http://www.religiousportal.com/HinduDeathRituals.html.

357   C. D'Avanzo, *Pocket Guide to Cultural Health Assessment* (St. Louis, MO: Elsevier Mosby, 2008), 101.

358   G.C. White, *Believers and Beliefs: a Practical Guide to Religious Etiquette for Business and Social Occasions* (New York: Berkley Publishing Group, 1997), 36.

359   "Glossary-'soul,'" Kauai's Hindu Monastery, accessed December 5, 2011, http://www.himalayanacademy.com/resources/lexicon/.

360   "Glossary-'death,'" Kauai's Hindu Monastery, accessed December 5, 2011, http://www.himalayanacademy.com/resources/lexicon/.

361   "Funeral Rites Across Different Cultures," Funeral_Rites_website.doc, accessed December 6, 2011, www.egfl.org.
        uk/export/sites/egfl/.../Furneral_Rites_website.doc

362   S. Thrane, "Hindu End of Life," *Journal of Hospice and Palliative Nursing*, 337.

363-364 J.G. Lipson, S. Dibble, and P.A. Minarik, eds., *Culture and Nursing Care: A Pocket Guide* (San Francisco,
        CA: UCSF Nursing Press, 1996), B-12.

365   "Hinduism and Medicine," http://www.angelfire.com/az/ambersukumaran/medicine.html.

366   S. Thrane, "Hindu End of Life," *Journal of Hospice and Palliative Nursing*, 337.

367   L. Bregman, *Religion, Death, and Dying, Volume 3, Bereavement and Death Rituals*, (Santa Barbara,
        CA: Greenwood Publishing Group, 2010), 160.

368   "Hindus—Physical Examinations," Ethnicity Online, accessed December 5, 2011, http://www.ethnicityonline.net/
        hindu_examinations.htm.

369   "Hindus: Birth, Babies, and Motherhood," Ethnicity Online, accessed December 6, 2011, http://www.
        ethnicityonline.net/hindu_birth.htm.

370   G.C. White, *Believers and Beliefs*, 34.

371   Ramakrishna and Weiss, "Health, Illness, and Immigration," *Western Journal of Medicine*, 266.

372   D. Thakrar, R. Das, A. Sheikh, eds., *Caring for Hindu Patients* (Abingdon, UK: Radcliffe Publishing, 2008),
        55–64.

373   "Hinduism and Medicine," http://www.angelfire.com/az/ambersukumaran/medicine.html.

374-375 M.M. Andrews and J.S. Boyle, *Transcultural Concepts in Nursing Care*, 5th ed. (New York: Lippincott, 1995), 386.

376   "Hinduism vs. Buddhism," Oppapers.com, accessed December 6, 2011, http://www.oppapers.com/essays/
        Hinduism-Vs-Buddhism/141221.

377   J.G. Lipson, S. Dibble, and P.A. Minarik, eds., *Culture and Nursing Care: A Pocket Guide* (San Francisco,
        CA: UCSF Nursing Press, 1996), B-12.

378   E.B. Kelly, *Gene Therapy* (Santa Barbara, CA: Greenwood Publishing Group), 117.

379   Lipson et al., *Culture and Nursing* Care, B-12.

380   "Beliefs and Facts About Foods During Pregnancy in India," IndiaCurry.com, accessed December 6, 2011, http://
        www.indiacurry.com/women/pregnancytaboo.htm.

381   G.C. White, *Believers and Beliefs,* 34.

382   "IVF Concept in Different Religions," In Vitro Fertilization IVF, accessed December 6, 2011, http://in-vitro-
        fertilization.eu/different-religious-concepts-in-vitro-fertilization-assisted-reproduction/.

383   "Hinduism and Medicine," http://www.angelfire.com/az/ambersukumaran/medicine.html.

384   E. Buchanan, *Parent/Teacher Handbook: Teaching Children Ages 10 to 12 Everything They Need to
        Know About Their Christian Heritage* (Nashville, TN: Broadman and Holman Publishers, 2006), 44.

385   A. Sarker, *Understand My Muslim People* (Newberg, OR: Barclay Press, 2004), 155–100.

386   G. ElGindy, "Death and Dying Across Cultures," *Minority Nurse* (Spring 2004), http://www.minoritynurse.com/
        hospice-end-life-care/death-and-dying-across-cultures.

387   Sarker, *Understand My Muslim People*, 35.

388   Buchanan, *Parent/Teacher Handbook*, 44.

389   Sarker, *Understand My Muslim People*, 71.

390   Buchanan, *Parent/Teacher Handbook*, 44.

391   F.S. Mead, S.S. Hill, C.D. Atwood, "Islam" in *Handbook of Denominations in the United States*, 13th ed.,
        (Nashville, TN: Abingdon Press, 2010).

392   M.M. Andrews and J.S. Boyle, *Transcultural Concepts in Nursing Care*, 5th ed. (New York: Lippincott, 1995), 387.

393   Abyad, "The Role of Different Faiths," *Healing Ministry*, 23.

394   "Muslim Prayer Rugs and The Way They're Used," TDL Cluster Blog, accessed December 6, 2011, http://www.tdlcluster.org/shopping-and-product-reviews/muslim-prayer-rugs-and-the-way-theyre-used/.

395   "Taharat and Najasat," S.M. Rizvi, Islamic-Laws, accessed December 6, 2011, http://www.islam-laws.com/taharatandnajasat.htm.

396   "Basic Tenets of Faith," S.M.S. Al-Munajjid, Islamic Q and A, accessed December 6, 2011, http://islamqa.com/en/ref/20207/amulets.

397   K. Hedayat, "When the Spirit Leaves: Childhood Death, Grieving, and Bereavement in Islam," *Journal of Palliative Medicine* 9, no. 6 (2006).

398   A. Clarfield, M. Gordon, H. Markwell, and S. Alibhai, "Ethical Issues in End-of-Life Geriatric Care: The Approach of Three Monotheistic Religions—Judaism, Catholicism, and Islam," *Journal of American Geriatric Society* 51, no.8 (2003): 1152.

399   K.M. Hedayat and R. Pirzadeh, "Issues in Islamic Biomedical Ethics: A Primer for the Pediatrician," *Pediatrics* 108, no. 4 (2001): 969.

400   "Islamic Medical Ethics," IMANA Ethics Committee, accessed December 6, 2011, http://www.isna.net/Leadership/pages/Islamic-Medical-Ethics.aspx.

401-402   "Prohibition of Free-Mixing Between Men and Women," IslamCan.com, accessed December 6, 2011, http://www.islamcan.com/youth/prohibition-of-free-mixing-between-men-and-women.shtml.

403   "Islamic Dietary Laws and Practices," The Islamic Bulletin, accessed December 6, 2011, http://www.islamicbulletin.org/newsletters/issue_2/dietarylaws.aspx.

404   "Taboo Table Offerings," Etiquette International, accessed December 6, 2011, http://www.etiquetteinternational.com/Articles/TableOfferings.aspx.

405   B. Khoda, *Islamic Duas: A Compilation of Prayers* (n.p.[Iran?]: A Duas Publishing Project, duas.org), 494.

406   "What is Ramadan?" About.com Islam, accessed December 6, 2011, http://islam.about.com/od/ramadan/f/ramadanintro.htm.

407   Hedayat and Pirzadeh, "Issues in Islamic Biomedical Ethics," *Pediatrics*, 968.

408   "Muslim-Dietary Guidelines," Ethnicity Online, accessed December 6, 2011, http://www.ethnicityonline.net/islam_diet.htm.

409   "Muslim Medicine and Health Care," A.F. Yousif, accessed December 6, 2011, http://www.truthandgrace.com/muslimmedicine.htm.

410   N. Sarhill, S. LeGrand, R. Islambouli, M.P. Davis, and D. Walsh, "The Terminally Ill Muslim: Death and Dying from the Muslim Perspective," *American Journal of Hospice & Palliative Medicine* 18, no. 4 (July/August, 2001): 252.

411   "Using Alcohol or Gelatin Derived from Pork as Medicine," IslamWeb, accessed December 6, 2011, http://www.islamweb.net/emainpage/index.php?page=showfatwa&Option=Fatwald&Id=90894.

412-414   J.D. Andrews, *Cultural, Ethic and Religious: Reference Manual for Health Care Providers*, (Winston-Salem, NC: Jamarda Resources, 1995), 41.

415   M.M. Andrews and J.S. Boyle, *Transcultural Concepts in Nursing Care*, 5th ed. (New York: Lippincott, 1995), 357.

416   Sarhill et al., "The Terminally Ill Muslim," *American Journal of Hospice & Palliative Medicine*, 252.

417-418   Andrews, *Cultural, Ethic and* Religious, 41–42.

419-420   "Guidelines for Health Care Providers Interacting with Muslim Patients and their Families," International Strategy and Policy Institute, last updated June 10, 2006, http://www.ispi-usa.org/guidelines.htm.

421   Abyad, "The Role of Different Faiths," *Healing Ministry*, 23.

422   Andrews, *Cultural, Ethic and* Religious, 41–42.

423   "The Five Pillars of Wisdom," Islam for Children, accessed December 6, 2011, http://atschool.eduweb.co.uk/
           carolrb/islam/fivepillars.html.

424   "Tayammum / Dry Ablution," Qul.org, accessed January 31, 2012, http://www.qul.org.au/library/a-guide-on-
           praying/conducting-tayammum.

425   "Etiquettes of Reading and Handling the Qur'an al-Kareem," Mas'ud Ahmed Khan's Home Page, accessed
           December 6, 2011, http://www.themodernreligion.com/basic/quran/etiquette.html.

426   "Guidelines for Health Care Providers Interacting with Muslim Patients and their Families," International Strategy
           and Policy Institute, last updated June 10, 2006, http://www.ispi-usa.org/guidelines.htm.

427   Clarfield et al., "Ethical Issues in End-of-Life Geriatric Care," *Journal of American Geriatric Society*, 1152.

428   "Guidelines for Health Care Providers Interacting with Muslim Patients and their Families," International Strategy
           and Policy Institute, last updated June 10, 2006, http://www.ispi-usa.org/guidelines.htm.

429   A. McKennis, "Caring for the Islamic Patient," *AORN Journal* 69, no. 6 (June 1999): 1185–96.

430   D. Biema, "Kingdom Come," *Time*, (August 4, 1997), 38–39.

431   "Religious Diversity-Practical Points for Health Care Providers," Penn Medicine, revised April 20, 2007, http://
           www.uphs.upenn.edu/pastoral/resed/diversity_points.html.

432-433   Clarfield et al., "Ethical Issues in End-of-Life Geriatric Care," *Journal of American Geriatric Society*, 1152.

434   Sarhill et al., "The Terminally Ill Muslim," *American Journal of Hospice & Palliative Medicine,* 253.

435   "Religious Diversity-Practical Points for Health Care Providers," Penn Medicine, revised April 20, 2007, http://
           www.uphs.upenn.edu/pastoral/resed/diversity_points.html.

436   Abyad, "The Role of Different Faiths," *Healing Ministry*, 23.

437   Sarhill et al., "The Terminally Ill Muslim," *American Journal of Hospice & Palliative Medicine*, 252.

438   "Religious Diversity-Practical Points for Health Care Providers," Penn Medicine, revised April 20, 2007, http://
           www.uphs.upenn.edu/pastoral/resed/diversity_points.html.

439   "Islam," Encyclopedia of Death and Dying, accessed January 31, 2012, http://www.deathreference.com/Ho-Ka/
           Islam.html.

440-441   K. Hedayat, "When the Spirit Leaves," *Journal of Palliative Medicine*.

442   Abyad, "The Role of Different Faiths," *Healing Ministry*, 23.

443   "Guidelines for Health Care Providers Interacting with Muslim Patients and their Families," International Strategy
           and Policy Institute, last updated June 10, 2006, http://www.ispi-usa.org/guidelines.htm.

444   Sarhill et al., "The Terminally Ill Muslim," *American Journal of Hospice & Palliative Medicine*, 252.

445   Ibid., 251–253.

446   J. Klossig, "Cross-Cultural Medicine a Decade Later: The Effect of Values and Culture on Life-Support Decisions,"
           Western Journal of Medicine 157, no. 3 (September 1992): 318.

447   Hedayat and Pirzadeh, "Issues in Islamic Biomedical Ethics," Pediatrics, 967.

448   "Muslim Medicine and Health Care," A.F. Yousif, accessed December 6, 2011, http://www.truthandgrace.com/
           muslimmedicine.htm.

449-451   Hedayat and Pirzadeh, "Issues in Islamic Biomedical Ethics," *Pediatrics*, 967.

452-453   K. Hedayat, "When the Spirit Leaves," *Journal of Palliative Medicine*.

454-455   A.R. Gatrad, "Muslim Customs Surrounding Death, Bereavement, Postmortem Examinations, and Organ
           Transplants," *British Medical Journal* 309 (August 1994): 521–23.

456   J. Klessig, "Cross-Cultural Medicine," *Western Journal of Medicine*, 318.

457   Clarfield et al., "Ethical Issues in End-of-Life Geriatric Care," *Journal of American Geriatric Society*, 1152.

458   M.S.M. Takrouri and T.M. Halwani, "An Islamic Medical and Legal Prospective of Do Not Resuscitate Order in Critical Care Medicine," *Internet Journal of Health* 7, no. 1 (2008).

459-460   Clarfield et al., "Ethical Issues in End-of-Life Geriatric Care," *Journal of American Geriatric Society*, 1152.

461   B.B. Ott, J. Al-Khaduri, and S. Al-Junaibi, "Preventing Ethical Dilemmas: Understanding Islamic Health Care Practices," *Pediatric Nursing* 29, no. 3 (2003).

462   M. Crawshaw and M. Balen, eds., *Adopting After Infertility* (Philadelphia, PA: Jessica Kingsley Publishers, 2010), 112.

463   "Muslims: Birth, Babies, and Motherhood," Ethnicity Online, accessed December 6, 2011, http://www.ethnicityonline.net/islam_birth.htm.

464   "If Husband Can Be Present," Islamhelpline, accessed December 6, 2011, http://www.islamhelpline.com/node/4425.

465   "Life Cycle Observances in Islam," Exploring Religions, accessed December 6, 2011, http://uwacadweb.uwyo.edu/religionet/er/islam/islife.htm.

466   "General Guidelines," Boston University School of Medicine, Boston Healing Landscape Project, accessed December 6, 2011, http://www.bu.edu/bhlp/Resources/Islam/health/guidelines.html.

467   Hedayat and Pirzadeh, "Issues in Islamic Biomedical Ethics," *Pediatrics*, 967.

468-469   "Muslim Medicine and Health Care," A.F. Yousif, accessed December 6, 2011, http://www.truthandgrace.com/muslimmedicine.htm.

470   "Male Circumcision in Islam," Islamic Forum; IslamicBoard.com, September 22, 2008, http://www.islamicboard.com/health-science/134271551-male-circumcision-islam.html.

471   Hedayat and Pirzadeh, "Issues in Islamic Biomedical Ethics," *Pediatrics*, 969.

472   "Contraception and Abortion in Islam," D.C. Maguire, accessed December 6, 2011, http://www.religiousconsultation.org/islam_contraception_abortion_in_SacredChoices.htm.

473   "If Husband Can Be Present," Islamhelpline, accessed December 6, 2011, http://www.islamhelpline.com/node/4425.

474-476   K. Braun, J.H. Pietsch, and P.L. Blanchette, *Cultural Issues in End-Of-Life Decisions* (Thousand Oaks, CA: Sage Publications, 2000), 206.

477   "Muslim Medicine and Health Care," A.F. Yousif, accessed December 6, 2011, http://www.truthandgrace.com/muslimmedicine.htm.

478-481   M. Chichester, "Multicultural Issues in Perinatal Loss," *Association of Women's Health, Obstetric, and Neonatal Nurses: Lifelines* 9, no. 4 (August 2005): 318.

482   Andrews, *Cultural, Ethic and* Religious, 42.

483   Ibid., 41–42.

484-486   "Guidelines for Health Care Providers Interacting with Muslim Patients and their Families," International Strategy and Policy Institute, last updated June 10, 2006, http://www.ispi-usa.org/guidelines.htm.

487-488   A. Sheikh and A. Gatrad, *Caring for Muslim Patients: Death and Bereavement* (Abingdon, Oxon: Radcliffe Medical Press, 2000), 104.

489   "What Do They Believe?" Jehovah's Witnesses Official Web Site, accessed December 7, 2011, http://www.watchtower.org/e/jt/article_03.htm.

490-491   "Jehovah's Witnesses," Patheos.com, accessed December 7, 2011, http://www.patheos.com/Library/Jehovahs-Witnesses.html.

492   "Religious Diversity-Practical Points for Health Care Providers," Penn Medicine Pastoral Care and Education, revised April 20, 2007, http://www.uphs.upenn.edu/pastoral/resed/diversity_points.html.

493   "Jehovah's Witnesses," http://www.patheos.com/Library/Jehovahs-Witnesses.html.

494   "Religious Diversity," Penn Medicine, http://www.uphs.upenn.edu/pastoral/resed/diversity_points.html.

495   "Jehovah's Witnesses," http://www.patheos.com/Library/Jehovahs-Witnesses.html.

496-497   "Religious Diversity," Penn Medicine, http://www.uphs.upenn.edu/pastoral/resed/diversity_points.html.

498   "Jehovah's Witnesses—Position Overview—Bloodless Medicine & Surgery," Penn Medicine, accessed December 7, 2011, http://www.pennmedicine.org/health_info/bloodless/000206.html.

499   "Family Care and Medical Management for Jehovah's Witnesses," Watchtower Bible and Tract Society of Pennsylvania (1992), Chapter 3.

500   Ibid., Chapter 7.

501   Andrews, *Cultural, Ethic and Religious*, 60.

502   "Jehovah's Witnesses," AllExperts, updated August 20, 2006, http://en.allexperts.com/q/Jehovah-s-Witness-1617/Diet.htm.

503   "Highlights of the Beliefs of Jehovah's Witnesses," Tower Watch Ministries, accessed December 7, 2011, http://www.towerwatch.com/Witnesses/Beliefs/their_beliefs.htm.

504-506   "Faith Traditions and Health Care," Pennsylvania Medicine Pastoral Care and Education, revised June 2003, http://www.uphs.upenn.edu/pastoral/pubs/traditions.html.

507   DuBose, "The Jehovah's Witness Tradition," in *Religious Beliefs & Health Care*.

508-510   "Faith Traditions and Health Care," http://www.uphs.upenn.edu/pastoral/pubs/traditions.html.

511   "Customs and Religious Protocols," A Memory Tree, accessed December 7, 2011, http://www.amemorytree.co.nz/customs.php.

512-514   "Faith Traditions and Health Care," http://www.uphs.upenn.edu/pastoral/pubs/traditions.html.

515   "Religious Diversity," Penn Medicine, http://www.uphs.upenn.edu/pastoral/resed/diversity_points.html.

516   J. Gillman, "Religious Perspectives on Organ Donation," *Critical Care Nursing Quarterly* 22, no.3 (1999): 26.

517   "Faith Traditions and Health Care," http://www.uphs.upenn.edu/pastoral/pubs/traditions.html.

518-519   "Jehovah's Witness—Rites of Passage," AllExperts, updated June 5, 2005, http://en.allexperts.com/q/Jehovah-s-Witness-1617/Rites-Passage.htm.

520   "Family Care and Medical Management for Jehovah's Witnesses," Watchtower Bible and Tract Society of Pennsylvania (1992), Chapter 3.

521   "Do Jehovah's Witnesses Practice Circumcision?" Yahoo!Answers, accessed December 6, 2011, http://answers.yahoo.com/question/index?qid=20080920181032AA82nwp.

522-523   "Faith Traditions and Health Care," http://www.uphs.upenn.edu/pastoral/pubs/traditions.html.

524   DuBose, "The Jehovah's Witness Tradition," in *Religious Beliefs & Health Care*.

525   "Infertility—The Choice, The Issues," Jehovah's Witness Official Web Site, accessed December 7, 2011, http://www.watchtower.org/e/20040922/article_02.htm.

526   "What are Jehovah's Witness Beliefs About Birth Control?" Answers.com, accessed December 7, 2011, http://wiki.answers.com/Q/What_are_Jehovah%27s_witnesses_beliefs_about_birth_control.

527   "Family Care and Medical Management for Jehovah's Witnesses," Watchtower Bible and Tract Society of Pennsylvania (1992), Chapter 3.

528   "What are Jehovah's Witness Beliefs About Birth Control?" Answers.com, accessed December 7, 2011, http://wiki.answers.com/Q/What_are_Jehovah%27s_witnesses_beliefs_about_birth_control.

529-531   "Judaism—Beliefs and Practices," Religious Tolerance, accessed December 8, 2011, http://www.religioustolerance.org/judaism.htm.

532   F.S. Mead, S.S. Hill, C.D. Atwood, "Judaism" in *Handbook of Denominations in the United States*, 13th ed., (Nashville, TN: Abingdon Press, 2010).

533   "Afterlife," J. Telushkin, Jewish Virtual Library, accessed December 8, 2011, http://www.jewishvirtuallibrary.org/jsource/Judaism/afterlife.html.

534   "Do We Own our Bodies, or are They Only on Loan?" Aish.com, accessed December 8, 2011, http://www.aish.com/ci/sam/48960576.html.

535   "Judaism, Health, and Vegetarianism," JVNA, accessed December 8, 2011, http://jewishveg.com/jh.html.

536   "Afterlife," Telushkin, Jewish Virtual Library, http://www.jewishvirtuallibrary.org/jsource/Judaism/afterlife.html.

537   "When and Why Do We Wear a Kippah?" Aish.com, accessed December 8, 2011, http://www.aish.com/jl/m/pb/48949686.html.

538   M.A. Shah, *Transcultural Aspects of Perinatal Health Care: A Resource Guide* (Tampa, FL: National Perinatal Association, 2004), 205.

539   "Religious Diversity," Penn Medicine, http://www.uphs.upenn.edu/pastoral/resed/diversity_points.html.

540   L. Purnell and B. Paulanka, *Guide to Culturally Competent Health Care*, (Philadelphia, PA: F.A. Davis Company, 2009), 266–67.

541   Ibid., 267.

542   "Kashrut: Jewish Dietary Laws," Judaism101, accessed December 8, 2011, http://www.jewfaq.org/kashrut.htm.

543   "Religious Diversity," Penn Medicine, http://www.uphs.upenn.edu/pastoral/resed/diversity_points.html.

544   "Kashrut: Jewish Dietary Laws," Judaism101, accessed December 8, 2011, http://www.jewfaq.org/kashrut.htm.

545   "Jews: Dietary Guidelines," Ethnicity Online, accessed December 8, 2011, http://www.ethnicityonline.net/judaism_diet.htm.

546   "Kashrut: Jewish Dietary Laws," Judaism101, accessed December 8, 2011, http://www.jewfaq.org/kashrut.htm.

547   J. Leichter, "Lactose Tolerance in a Jewish Population," *Digestive Diseases and Sciences* 16, no. 12: 1123–1126, http://www.springerlink.com/content/lh25036588434651/.

548   "Sick Visiting," Something Jewish, last updated March 23, 2007, http://www.somethingjewish.co.uk/articles/2257_sick_visiting.htm,.

549   M.E. O'Brien, *A Nurse's Handbook of Spiritual Care: Standing on Holy Ground* (Sudbury, MA: Jones and Bartlett, 2004), 45.

550   A. Steinberg and F. Rosner, *Encyclopedia of Jewish Medical Ethics: A Compilation of Jewish Medical Law* (Jerusalem, Israel: Feldheim Publishers, 2003), 323.

551   W.S. Tseng and J. Streltzer, *Cultural Competence in Health Care, Volume 877* (New York: Springer Science and Business Media, 2008), 56.

552   S. Hoffman, *Mental Health, Psychotherapy and Judaism* (New York: Golden Sky, 2011), vi.

553-555 "Religious Diversity," Penn Medicine, http://www.uphs.upenn.edu/pastoral/resed/diversity_points.html.

556   O'Brien, *A Nurse's Handbook*, 45.

557   W. Frankel, World Jewish Congress, *Survey of Jewish Affairs* (Cranbury, NJ: Associated University Presses, 1988), 239.

558   J.N. Giger and R.E. Davidhizar, *Transcultural Nursing, Assessment and Intervention* (St. Louis, MO: Elsevier Mosby, 2008), 554.

559   Tseng and Streltzer, *Cultural Competence in Health* Care, 56.

560   A. Clarfield, M. Gordon, H. Markwell, and S. Alibhai, "Ethical Issues in End-of-Life Geriatric Care: The Approach of Three Monotheistic Religions—Judaism, Catholicism, and Islam," *Journal of American Geriatric Society* 51, no.8 (2003): 1150.

561   "Religious Diversity," Penn Medicine, http://www.uphs.upenn.edu/pastoral/resed/diversity_points.html.

562   B.B. Kadden and B. Kadden, *Teaching Jewish Life Cycle: Traditions and Activities*, (Denver, CO: A.R.E. Publishing, Inc. 1997), 102.

563   J. Klessig, "Cross-Cultural Medicine ," *Western Journal of Medicine,*318.

564   "Religious Diversity," Penn Medicine, http://www.uphs.upenn.edu/pastoral/resed/diversity_points.html.

565   "Living Judaism: Judaism's Perspective on Organ Donation After Death," G. Loeb, The Philadelphia Jewish Voice, accessed December 8, 2011, http://www.pjvoice.com/v38/38700judaism.aspx.

566   "Religious Diversity," Penn Medicine, http://www.uphs.upenn.edu/pastoral/resed/diversity_points.html.

567   "Autopsy," A. Scheib, Jewish Virtual Library, accessed December 8, 2011, http://www.jewishvirtuallibrary.org/jsource/Judaism/autopsy.html.

568   "Medical Informed Consent in Jewish Law—from the Patient's Side," D. Eisenberg, MD, Jewish Law Articles, accessed December 8, 2011, http://www.jlaw.com/Articles/MedConsent.html.

569   "Religious Diversity," Penn Medicine, http://www.uphs.upenn.edu/pastoral/resed/diversity_points.html.

570   C. D'Avanzo, *Pocket Guide to Cultural Health Assessment* (St. Louis, MO: Elsevier Mosby, 2008), 348.

571   "Dying," My Jewish Learning, accessed December 8, 2011, http://www.myjewishlearning.com/life/Life_Events/Death_and_Mourning/Dying.shtml.

572   "Religious Diversity," Penn Medicine, http://www.uphs.upenn.edu/pastoral/resed/diversity_points.html.

573   C. D'Avanzo, *Pocket Guide to Cultural Health Assessment* (2008), 348.

574   E. Macdonald, *Difficult Conversations in Medicine* (New York: Oxford, 2004), 142.

575-576   A. Abyad, "The Role of Different Faiths and Their Attitudes Toward Death," *Healing Ministry* (Jan/Feb, 1996): 24.

577   "Religious Diversity," Penn Medicine, http://www.uphs.upenn.edu/pastoral/resed/diversity_points.html.

578-579   J. Klessig, "Cross-Cultural Medicine," *Western Journal of Medicine*, 319.

580   "The Sanctity of Life: A Jewish Approach to End of Life Challenges," The Curious Jew, updated September 14, 2008, http://curiousjew.blogspot.com/2008/09/sanctity-of-life-jewish-approach-to-end.html.

581   "Religious Diversity," Penn Medicine, http://www.uphs.upenn.edu/pastoral/resed/diversity_points.html.

582   Shah, *Transcultural Aspects of Perinatal Health Care*, 197.

583-586   Ibid., 194.

587   "Planning a Brit Milah: What to Do Besides Calling the Mohel," G. Robinson, InterfaithFamily, accessed December 8, 2011, http://www.interfaithfamily.com/life_cycle/pregnancy_and_birth_ceremonies /Planning_a_Brit_Milah_What_To_Do_Besides_Calling_the_Mohel.shtml.

588   "Faith Traditions and Health Care," http://www.uphs.upenn.edu/pastoral/pubs/traditions.html.

589-590   Shah, *Transcultural Aspects of Perinatal Health Care*, 190.

591   Ibid., 193.

592   "Childbirth in Jewish Law," Jewish Women's Health, accessed December 8, 2011, http://www.jewishwomenshealth.org/article.php?article=20.

593   Shah, *Transcultural Aspects of Perinatal Health Care*, 200.

594-595   Chichester, "Multicultural Issues in Perinatal Loss," 316.

596-597   Shah, *Transcultural Aspects of Perinatal Health Care*, 192.

598   "Jewish Burial Customs," Star of David Memorial Chapels, Inc., accessed December 8, 2011, http://jewish-funeral-home.com/Jewish-burial-customs.html.

599   Shah, *Transcultural Aspects of Perinatal Health Care*, 200.

600   Chichester, "Multicultural Issues in Perinatal Loss," 316.

601   Shah, *Transcultural Aspects of Perinatal Health Care*, 200.

602   Chichester, "Multicultural Issues in Perinatal Loss," 316.

603   Shah, *Transcultural Aspects of Perinatal Health Care*, 196.

604   Ibid., 194.

605   Ibid., 195.

606-607   Ibid., 194.

608-609   Ibid., 195.

610   "Jewish Childrearing Related Questions," Faqs.org, last updated April 10, 1996, http://www.faqs.org/faqs/judaism/FAQ/12-Kids/.

611-612   Shah, *Transcultural Aspects of Perinatal Health Care*, 191.

613   "The Preembryo in Halacha," Rabbi Y. Breitowitz, Jewish Law Articles, accessed December 8, 2011, http://www.jlaw.com/Articles/preemb.html.

614-615   Shah, *Transcultural Aspects of Perinatal Health Care*, 191.

616   J.D. Andrews, *Cultural, Ethic and Religious: Reference Manual for Health Care Providers* (Winston-Salem, NC: Jamarda Resources, 1995), 68.

617   Shah, *Transcultural Aspects of Perinatal Health Care*, 192.

618-619   F.S. Mead, S.S. Hill, C.D. Atwood, "Lutheran Churches" in *Handbook of Denominations in the United States*, 13th ed., (Nashville, TN: Abingdon Press, 2010).

620   J. Moltmann, *God in Creation: A New Theology of Creation and the Spirit of God* (Minneapolis, MN: Augsburg Fortress, 1993), 16.

621   Moltmann, *God in Creation*, 231.

622   Mead et al., "Lutheran Churches" in *Handbook of Denominations*.

623   M.E. Marty, *Health and Medicine in the Lutheran Tradition* (New York: Crossroad Publishing Co., 1986), 154.

624   G. Gassmann and S.H. Hendrix, *Fortress Introduction to the Lutheran Confessions* (Minneapolis, MN: Augsburg Fortress, 1999), 96.

625   "Life Thoughts in the Church Year," Lutherans for Life, accessed December 9, 2011, http://www.lutheransforlife.org/media/life-thoughts-in-the-church/.

626   H.C. Alleman and W.H. Dunbar, *Lutheran Teacher Training Series for the Sunday School, Volume 1* (Philadelphia, PA: Lutheran Publication Society, 1909), 170.

627   "Religious Views on Organ, Tissue, and Blood Donation," New Mexico Donor Services, accessed December 8, 2011, http://www.donatelifenm.org/religiousviews.htm#lutheran.

628   "Prayer: Fasting," Evangelical Lutheran Church in America, accessed January 31, 2012, http://www2.elca.org/prayer/resources/fasting.html.

629   Marty, *Health and Medicine in the Lutheran Tradition*, 160–61.

630   "How Can We Provide for Communion of the Ill, Homebound, and the Imprisoned?" Evangelical Lutheran Church of America, accessed December 8, 2011, https://www.elca.org/Growing-In-Faith/Worship/Learning-Center/FAQs/Communion-Distribution-Outside.aspx.

631   D. Harris-Abbott, ed., "The Lutheran Tradition," in *Religious Beliefs and Health Care*.

632   "The Basics on Advance Directives—Thy Will Be Done," J. Lamb, May 26, 2010, http://www.lutheransforlife.org/article/the-basics-on-advance-directives-thy-will-be-done/.

633   S. Gellar, "Religious Attitudes and the Autopsy," *Archives of Pathology & Laboratory Medicine* 108 (1984): 494.

634   "Funerals," Evangelical Lutheran Church of America, accessed December 12, 2011, https://www.elca.org/Growing-In-Faith/Worship/Learning-Center/FAQs/Funerals.aspx.

635   "Pastoral Care Religious Needs of Patients in Sickness and Death," SWAHS Pastoral Care and Chaplaincy Services, accessed December 12, 2011, http://www.wsahs.nsw.gov.au/services/pastoralcare/relneeds.htm.

636   Marty, *Health and Medicine in the Lutheran Tradition*, 160–61.

637   L. White, *Foundations of Nursing*, (New York: Thomson Delmar, 2005), 212.

638   D. Harris-Abbott, "The Lutheran Tradition," in *Religious Beliefs and Health Care*.

639   "Organ Donation," Evangelical Lutheran Church of America, accessed December 12, 2011, http://www.elca.org/What-We-Believe/Social-Issues/Resolutions/1989/CA89,-p-,07,-p-,72-Organ-Donation.aspx.

640   "End of Life Decisions," Evangelical Lutheran Church of America, accessed December 12, 2011, http://www.elca.org/What-We-Believe/Social-Issues/Messages/End-of-Life-Decisions.aspx.

641   White, *Foundations of Nursing*, 212.

642   Mead et al., "Lutheran Churches" in *Handbook of Denominations*.

643   White, *Foundations of Nursing*, 212.

644   "Are most Lutherans circumcised at birth?" Yahoo!Answers, accessed December 12, 2011, http://answers.yahoo.com/question/index?qid=20110426210543AAPEL05.

645-647   D. Harris-Abbott, "The Lutheran Tradition," in *Religious Beliefs and Health Care*.

648   "Lutheran Report Gives Biblical Response to Stem Cell, Cloning, In-Vitro Fertilization," The Christian Post, December 6, 2005, http://www.christianpost.com/news/lutheran-report-gives-biblical-response-to-stem-cell-cloning-in-vitro-fertilization-3969/.

649   Marty, *Health and Medicine in the Lutheran Tradition*, 149.

650   "Abortion," Evangelical Church in America, updated September 4, 1991, http://www.elca.org/What-We-Believe/Social-Issues/Social-Statements/Abortion.aspx.

651   D. Harris-Abbott, "The Lutheran Tradition," in *Religious Beliefs and Health Care*.

652-653   M. Good and P. Good, *20 Most Asked Questions About the Amish and Mennonites*, rev. ed. (Intercourse, PA: Good Books, 1995), 7–8, 16, 46.

654   J.C. Wenger, *The Doctrines of the Mennonites* (Mennonite Publishing House, 1950), 27–28.

655   J.B. Toews, *The Story of the Early Mennonite Brethren* (Fresno, CA: Centers for Mennonite Brethren Studies, 2002), 85.

656   J. Witte, *God's Joust, God's Justice: Law and Religion in the Western Tradition* (Grand Rapids, MI: Eerdmans Publishing Co., 2006), 216–217.

657   "Religious Views on Organ Donation," Gift of Life Donor Program, accessed December 12, 2011, http://www.donors1.org/learn/religion/#16.

658   "Mennonite Patients," Tripod, accessed December 12, 2011, http://members.tripod.com/mattmiller_16/id44.htm.

659   Good and Good, *20 Most Asked Questions*, 62–66.

660   A. Beachy, E. Hershberger, R. Davidhizar, G. Davidhizar, and J.N. Giger, "Cultural Implications for Nursing Care of the Amish," *Journal of Cultural Diversity* 4, no. 4 (1997):121.

661   "Mennonite Patients," http://members.tripod.com/mattmiller_16/id44.htm.

662   "Choices at the End of Life," C. Kennel-Shank, *Mennonite Weekly Review*, accessed December 12, 2011, http://www.mennoweekly.com/2011/1/24/choices-end-life/.

663   "Mennonite Patients," http://members.tripod.com/mattmiller_16/id44.htm.

664   "What Do Mennonites Believe About Death and Dying?" Third Way Café, accessed December 12, 2011, http://www.thirdway.com/menno/faq.asp?f_id=7.

665   Good and Good, *20 Most Asked Questions*, 66–69.

666   J.N. Hertzler, *Ask Third Way Café: 50 Common and Quirky Questions About Mennonites* (Telford, PA: Cascadia Publishing House, 2009), 24.

667   Ibid., 27.

668   "What We Believe," Tangent Mennonite Church, accessed December 12, 2011, http://www.tangentmennonite.org/faith.html.

669   "Choices at the End of Life," C. Kennel-Shank, http://www.mennoweekly.org/2011/1/24/choices-end-life/.

670   Hertzler, *Ask Third Way Café*, 24.

671   "Choices at the End of Life," C. Kennel-Shank,http://www.mennoweekly.org/2011/1/24/choices-end-life/?page=2.

672   DuBose, "The Anabaptist Tradition," in *Religious Beliefs and Health Care*.

673   "Baptism, Age at," Global Anabaptist Mennonite Encyclopedia Online, accessed December 12, 2011, http://www.gameo.org/encyclopedia/contents/B369ME.html.

674   Good and Good, *20 Most Asked Questions*, 62–65.

675   "Dedication of Infants," Global Anabaptist Mennonite Encyclopedia Online, accessed December 12, 2011, http://www.gameo.org/encyclopedia/contents/D39ME.html.

676   "Mennonite Patients," http://members.tripod.com/mattmiller_16/id44.htm.

677   "Empty Arms," Third Way Café, accessed December 12, 2011, http://www.thirdway.com/AW/?Page=5668%7CEmpty+Arms.

678   D.O. Doheny, D. de Leon, D. Raymond, "Genetic Testing and Genetic Counseling" in *Dystonia: Etiology, Clinical Features and Treatment* (Philadelphia, PA: Lippincott Williams & Wilkins, 2004), 23–31.

679   DuBose, "The Anabaptist Tradition," in *Religious Beliefs and Health Care*.

680   "Baptism, Age at," Global Anabaptist Mennonite Encyclopedia Online, accessed December 12, 2011, http://www.gameo.org/encyclopedia/contents/B369ME.html.

681-682 "Mennonite Patients," http://members.tripod.com/mattmiller_16/id44.htm.

683-686 Mead et al., "United Methodist Church" in *Handbook of Denominations*.

687-688 "What Happens after a Person Dies?" People of the United Methodist Church, accessed January 18, 2012, http://www.umc.org/site/apps/nlnet/content3.aspx?c=lwL4KnN1LtH&b=4746357&ct=3008067.

689   "Religion and Organ and Tissue Donation," The Gift of a Lifetime, accessed December 12, 2011, http://www.organtransplants.org/understanding/religion/.

690-694 "What United Methodists Believe," First United Methodist Church, accessed December 12, 2011, http://www.siouxcityfirst.com/283125.

695   S. Gellar, "Religious Attitudes and the Autopsy," *Archives of Pathology & Laboratory Medicine* 108 (1984): 494.

696-699 "What United Methodists Believe," http://www.siouxcityfirst.com/283125.

700   J. Gillman, "Religious Perspectives on Organ Donation," *Critical Care Nursing Quarterly* 22, no.3 (1999): 26.

701   "What United Methodists Believe," http://www.siouxcityfirst.com/283125.

702-703 Mead et al., "United Methodist Church" in *Handbook of Denominations*.

704   "Christian Parents and the Circumcision Issue," J.E. Peron, *Many Blessings* 3 (Spring 2000), accessed December 12, 2011, http://www.clrp.org/pages/cultural/peron1/.

705-706 DuBose, "The United Methodist Tradition," in *Religious Beliefs and Health Care*.

707   R.M. Reeb and S.T. McFarland, "Emergency Baptism," *Journal of Christian Nursing*: 12, no. 2 (Spring 1995), 26–27.

708   DuBose, "The United Methodist Tradition," in *Religious Beliefs and Health Care*.

709   "In Vitro Fertilization," IVF Worldwide, accessed December 12, 2011, http://www.ivf-worldwide.com/Education/christianity.html.

710   "Abortion," The People of the United Methodist Church, accessed January 31, 2012, http://archives.umc.org/interior.asp?mid=1732..

711-712   Mead et al., "Latter-day Saints (Mormons)" in *Handbook of Denominations*.

713   "Sacrament Mormonism," Why Mormonism, updated July 3, 2008, http://whymormonism.org/33/sacrament_mormonism.

714   "Mormon Beliefs," MormonBeliefs.org, accessed December 12, 2011, http://www.mormonbeliefs.org/.

715   "Do Mormons Believe in the Resurrection?" MormonBeliefs.org, accessed December 12, 2011, http://www.mormonbeliefs.org/mormon_beliefs/mormon-doctrine-salvation/do-mormons-believe-in-the-resurrection.

716   "Mormon Beliefs," http://www.mormonbeliefs.org/.

717   Mead et al., "Latter-day Saints (Mormons)" in *Handbook of Denominations*.

718   "Spiritual Gifts in the Mormon Church," MormonBeliefs.org, accessed December 12, 2011, http://www.mormonbeliefs.org/mormon_beliefs/thoughts-mormon-beliefs/spiritual-gifts-the-mormon-church.

719   Mead et al., "Latter-day Saints (Mormons)" in *Handbook of Denominations.*

720   "Mormon Rites," MormonBeliefs.org, accessed December 12, 2011, http://www.mormonbeliefs.org/mormon_beliefs/mormon-beliefs-culture/mormon-rites.

721   "Prayer," MormonBeliefs.org, accessed December 12, 2011, http://www.mormonbeliefs.org/mormon_beliefs/mormon-doctrine-salvation/mormon-beliefs-prayer.

722   "Mormon Missionaries," MormonBeliefs.org, accessed December 12, 2011, http://www.mormonbeliefs.org/mormon_missionaries.

723   "Will Mormons Do Blood Transfusions?" ChaCha, accessed December 12, 2011, http://www.chacha.com/question/will-mormons-do-blood-transfusions.

724   "Laws of Health," MormonBeliefs.org, accessed December 12, 2011, http://www.mormonbeliefs.org/mormon_beliefs/mormon-beliefs-laws-of-health.

725   "Mormon Beliefs," http://www.mormonbeliefs.org/.

726   "Fasting," MormonBeliefs.org, accessed December 12, 2011, http://www.mormonbeliefs.org/mormon_beliefs/mormon-beliefs-culture/fasting.

727   "Mormon Underwear," MormonBeliefs.org, accessed December 12, 2011, http://www.mormonbeliefs.org/mormon_temples/mormon-underwear.

720   "A Lay Clergy: The Value of Service," MormonBeliefs.org, accessed December 12, 2011, http://www.mormonbeliefs.org/mormon_beliefs/mormon-beliefs-culture/a-lay-clergy-the-value-of-service.

729   "Laws of Health," MormonBeliefs.org, accessed December 12, 2011, http://www.mormonbeliefs.org/mormon_beliefs/mormon-beliefs-laws-of-health.

730   W.J. Wood, "Advance Directives: Religious, Moral, and Theological Aspects," *The Elder Law Journal* (1999), https://litigation-essentials.lexisnexis.com/webcd/app?action=DocumentDisplay&crawlid=1&srctype=smi&srcid=3B15&doctype=cite&docid=7+Elder+L.J.+457&key=bc39b2fabc06c96b649a1b0f65085b68.

731   S. Gellar, "Religious Attitudes and the Autopsy," *Archives of Pathology & Laboratory Medicine* 108 (1984): 494.

732-733   "Latter-Day Saints," About.com, accessed December 12, 2011, http://lds.about.com/od/basicsgospelprinciples/p/death.htm.

734   "Do Mormons Believe in the Resurrection?" MormonBeliefs.org, accessed December 12, 2011, http://www.mormonbeliefs.org/mormon_beliefs/mormon-doctrine-salvation/do-mormons-believe-in-the-resurrection.

735   "Latter-Day Saints," About.com, http://lds.about.com/od/basicsgospelprinciples/p/death.htm.

736-738   C. Krohm and S.K. Summers, *Advance Health Care Directives: A Handbook for Professionals* (Chicago: American Bar Association, 2002), 128.

739   "Mormons and Organ Donation," BBC Religions, accessed December 12, 2011, http://www.bbc.co.uk/religion/religions/mormon/socialvalues/organ_donation.shtml.

740   Krohm and Summers, *Advance Health Care Directives*, 128.

741   M.A. Shah, *Transcultural Aspects of Perinatal Health Care: A Resource Guide* (Tampa, FL: National Perinatal Association, 2004), 248.

742-743   "Mormon Rites," MormonBeliefs.org, accessed December 12, 2011, http://www.mormonbeliefs.org/mormon_beliefs/mormon-beliefs-culture/mormon-rites.

744   Shah, *Transcultural Aspects of Perinatal Health Care*, 254.

745-747   Ibid., 250.

748   Ibid., 251.

749   "Circumcision in the United States of America," Circlist.com, accessed December 12, 2011, http://www.circlist.com/rites/usa.html.

750   "Birth Control," LDS.net, accessed December 12, 2011, http://mormon.lds.net/birth-control.

751   Shah, *Transcultural Aspects of Perinatal Health* Care, 251.

752   Ibid., 250.

753   Ibid., 252.

754   Ibid., 249.

755   D. Harris-Abbott, "The Latter-day Saints Tradition," in *Religious Beliefs and Health Care*.

756   Shah, *Transcultural Aspects of Perinatal Health Care*, 248.

757   D. Harris-Abbott, "The Latter-day Saints Tradition," in *Religious Beliefs and Health Care*.

758-759   Shah, *Transcultural Aspects of Perinatal Health Care*, 249.

760   Ibid., 252.

761-762   Ibid., 254.

763   Ibid., 250.

764   Ibid., 249.

765   Ibid., 250.

766   "Abortion," LDS.net, accessed December 12, 2011, http://mormon.lds.net/abortion.

767   Shah, *Transcultural Aspects of Perinatal Health Care*, 252.

768   P.C. Nelson, *Bible Doctrines*, (Springfield, MO: Gospel Publishing House, 1998), 67–73, 96–98, 123.

769-771   Mead et al., "Pentecostal Churches" in *Handbook of Denominations*.

772   Nelson, *Bible Doctrines,* 52, 85.

773   "Pentecostals/Healing Service," AllExperts.com, accessed December 14, 2011, http://en.allexperts.com/q/Pentecostals-2256/Healing-Service.htm.

774   M.M. Poloma and J.C. Green, *The Assemblies of God* (New York: New York University Press, 2010), 31.

775   Ibid., 32.

776 "Religious Diversity: Practical Points for Health Care," Penn Medicine Pastoral Care and Education, accessed December 14, 2011, http://www.uphs.upenn.edu/pastoral/resed/diversity_points.html.

777 Poloma and Green, The Assemblies of God, 93.

778 "Heaven, Hell, and Judgment," Assemblies of God USA, accessed December 14, 2011, http://ag.org/top/Beliefs/gendoct_14_heaven_hell.cfm.

779 "Medical: Organ Donation," Assemblies of God USA, accessed December 14, 2011, http://ag.org/top/Beliefs/topics/contempissues_19_organ_donation.cfm.

780 "Fasting," Assemblies of God USA, accessed December 14, 2011, http://ag.org/top/beliefs/gendoct_04_fasting.cfm.

781 "Religious Diversity: Practical Points for Health Care," Penn Medicine Pastoral Care and Education, accessed December 14, 2011, http://www.uphs.upenn.edu/pastoral/resed/diversity_points.html.

782 "Medical: Euthanasia and Extraordinary Support to Sustain Life," Assemblies of God USA, accessed December 14, 2011, http://ag.org/top/Beliefs/topics/contempissues_18_euthanasia.cfm.

783 "Finding Faith, Hope, and Love," J. McClure, last updated February 27, 2011, http://rss.ag.org/articles/detail.cfm?RSS_RSSContentID=18592&RSS_OriginatingChannelID=global&RSS_OriginatingRSSFeedID=global&RSS_Source=search.

784 "Death and Dying," Assemblies of God USA, accessed December 14, 2011, http://ag.org/top/Beliefs/topics/gendoct_18_death.cfm.

785 "Defining Truths of the Assemblies of God: Divine Healing," T.E. Track, iValue, accessed January 31, 2012, http://agchurches.org/Sitefiles/Default/RSS/IValue/Resources/Divine%20Healing/Articles/Defining_DivineHealing.pdf.

786-787 "Medical: Euthanasia," http://ag.org/top/Beliefs/topics/contempissues_18_euthanasia.cfm.

788 J. Gillman, "Religious Perspectives on Organ Donation," Critical Care Nursing Quarterly 22, no.3 (1999): 26.

789 "Medical: Euthanasia," http://ag.org/top/Beliefs/topics/contempissues_18_euthanasia.cfm.

790 "Infant Baptism, Age of Accountability, Dedication of Children," Assemblies of God USA, accessed December 14, 2011, http://ag.org/top/Beliefs/topics/gendoct_11_accountability.cfm.

791 "Assemblies of God Fundamental Truths," Assemblies of God USA, last updated March 1, 2010, http://ag.org/top/Beliefs/Statement_of_Fundamental_Truths/sft_short.cfm.

792 Nelson, Bible Doctrines, 42–45.

793 "Do Assembly of God Men Get Circumcised?" Yahoo!Answers, accessed December 14, 2011, http://ph.answers.yahoo.com/question/index?qid=20100725030235AATDMXU.

794 "Medical: Birth Control," Assemblies of God USA, accessed December 14, 2011, http://ag.org/top/Beliefs/topics/relations_17_birth_control.cfm.

795-796 "Infertility," Assemblies of God USA, accessed December 14, 2011, http://ag.org/top/Beliefs/topics/relations_16_infertility.cfm.

797 "Abortion," Assemblies of God USA, accessed December 14, 2011, http://ag.org/top/Beliefs/topics/contempissues_01_abortion.cfm

798 S. Matlins and A. Magida, eds., "Presbyterian" in How to Be a Perfect Stranger: A Guide to Etiquette in Other People's Religions (Woodstock, VT: Skylight Paths Publishing, 2011).

799 "Presbyterian Practices," ReligionFacts, accessed December 14, 2011, http://www.religionfacts.com/christianity/denominations/presbyterian/practices.htm.

800 The Office of the Stated Clerk of the General Assembly of the Presbyterian Church in America, The Book of Church Order of the Presbyterian Church in America, 5th ed. (2010), chapter 56.

801 Nelson, Bible Doctrines, 95–96.

802 J. Roger, Presbyterian Creeds: A Guide to the Book of Confessions (Louisville, KY: Louisville John Knox Press, 1991), 262.

803 Ibid., 24.

804 Ibid., 115.

805 Ibid., 132.

806 "Blood and Organ Donation," New York-Presbyterian Morgan Stanley Children's Hospital, accessed December 14, 2011, http://childrensnyp.org/mschony/patients/blood-organ-donation.html.

807 "Food for Thought," New York Presbyterian Hospital, accessed December 14, 2011, http://nyp.org/nutrition/resources/index.html.

808 Office of General Assembly, *Book of Church Order*, chapter 60.

809 Roger, *Presbyterian Creeds*, 128.

810 "Who We Are," Presbyterian Elders in Prayer, accessed December 14, 2011, http://presbypray.org/.

811 "Office of External Relations," New York-Presbyterian Hospital, accessed December 14, 2011, http://nyp.org/oer/.

812 "Presbyterian: Advance Directives," Presbyterian Healthcare Decisions, accessed December 14, 2011, http://www.phs.org/PHS/Chaplaincy/Patient_Education/Advance/index.htm.

813 S. Gellar, "Religious Attitudes and the Autopsy," *Archives of Pathology & Laboratory Medicine* 108 (1984): 494.

814 "Religion and Spirituality," Death with Dignity National Center, accessed December 14, 2011, http://www.deathwithdignity.org/historyfacts/religion/.

815 "After Death: Religious Needs of Patients in Sickness, Dying, and Death," SWAHS Pastoral Care and Chaplaincy Services, accessed December 26, 2011, http://www.wsahs.nsw.gov.au/services/pastoralcare/relneeds.htm.

816 "Prayer for the Sick," Riverwood Presbyterian Church blog, August 26, 2006, http://www.riverwoodchurch.org/blog/2006/08/26/prayer-for-the-sick/.

817 "Things To Do Before You Die—Christianity," Find Your Fate, accessed December 14, 2011, http://death.findyourfate.com/christianity.html.

818 Matlins and Magida, eds., "Presbyterian" in *How to Be a Perfect Stranger*.

819 "What Do Presbyterians Believe About Life After Death?" Presbyterian Church USA, accessed December 14, 2011, http://gamc.pcusa.org/ministries/today/life-after-death/.

820 J. Gillman, "Religious Perspectives on Organ Donation," *Critical Care Nursing Quarterly* 22, no.3 (1999): 26.

821-822 "Religion and Spirituality," Death with Dignity, http://www.deathwithdignity.org/historyfacts/religion/.

823 "How to Decide When a Baby Should Be Baptized," eHow.com, accessed December 14, 2011, http://www.ehow.com/how_2214669_decide-baby-should-be-baptized.html.

824 "How to Be Baptized in the Presbyterian Church," eHow.com, accessed December 14, 2011, http://www.ehow.com/how_2214836_be-baptized-presbyterian-church.html.

825 "Circumcision," New York Presbyterian Hospital, accessed December 14, 2011, http://nyp.org/health/pediatrics_circumcision.html.

826 "Contraception/Birth Control," New York Presbyterian Hospital, accessed December 14, 2011, http://nyp.org/health/women-contra.html.

827 "Fetal Personhood Law Has Radical Implications For Freedom of Religion Says Religious Coalition," FreeRepublic.com, April 1, 2004, http://www.freerepublic.com/focus/f-news/1109601/posts.

828 D. Harris-Abbott, "The Presbyterian Tradition," in *Religious Beliefs and Health Care*.

829 "Ten Thousand Dreams Come True Through New York-Presbyterian/Weill Cornell's IVF Program," New York-Presbyterian Hospital, accessed December 14, 2011, http://nyp.org/news/hospital/crmi-ivf-milestone.html.

830 On this issue, Presbyterians differ widely, from extremely conservative totally anti-abortion stances to the perspective described in the following article: "Presbyterian Denomination Reaffirms Support for Abortion," *Columbus Dispatch*, Pro-Life Infonet, June 22, 2002, http://www.euthanasia.com/pres.html.

831   Mead et al., "Catholic Churches" in *Handbook of Denominations*.

832   "The Catholic Worship Service," Dummies.com, accessed December 15, 2011, http://www.dummies.com/how-to/content/the-catholic-worship-service-the-mass.html.

833-835   Mead et al., "Catholic Churches" in *Handbook of Denominations*.

836   "Faith Traditions and Health Care," Pennsylvania Medicine Pastoral Care and Education, revised June 2003, http://www.uphs.upenn.edu/pastoral/pubs/traditions.html.

837   "Healing Prayers," Our Catholic Faith, accessed December 15, 2011, http://www.ourcatholicfaith.org/prayer/p-healing.html.

838   "Visit the Sick," CatholoCity, accessed December 15, 2011, http://www.catholicity.com/commentary/shea/08249.html.

839   "Faith Traditions and Health Care," http://www.uphs.upenn.edu/pastoral/pubs/traditions.html.

840   "The Sin of Gluttony," Catholic Bible 101, accessed December 15, 2011, http://www.catholicbible101.com/overcominggluttony.htm.

841-842   "Faith Traditions and Health Care," http://www.uphs.upenn.edu/pastoral/pubs/traditions.html.

843   "Catholic Scriptures That Inspire, Comfort, and Celebrate," CatholicScripture.org, accessed December 15, 2011, http://www.catholicscripture.org/.

844   "Faith Traditions and Health Care," http://www.uphs.upenn.edu/pastoral/pubs/traditions.html.

845   "The Catholic Way of Dying," Fisheaters.com, accessed January 18, 2012, http://fisheaters.com/dying.html.

846   "Favorite Catholic Prayers," Daily Word of Life, accessed December 15, 2011, http://www.daily-word-of-life.com/catholic_prayers.htm.

847   R.P. Hamel, ed., "The Roman Catholic Tradition," in *Religious Beliefs and Health Care*.

848   B.M. Ashley, J. Deblois, K.D. O'Rourke, *Health Care Ethics: A Catholic Theological Analysis* (Washington, D.C.: Georgetown University Press, 2006), 199.

849   "Advance Care Planning—Catholic Perspective," Supportive Care Coalition, accessed December 15, 2011, http://www.supportivecarecoalition.org/AdvanceCarePlanning/Advance+Care+Planning+-+Catholics+Perspective.php.

850   Ashley et al., *Health Care Ethics*, 192.

851   S. Gellar, "Religious Attitudes and the Autopsy," *Archives of Pathology & Laboratory Medicine* 108 (1984): 494.

852   Ashley et al., *Health Care Ethics*, 184.

853   "What Leaves the Body at Death?" EnsignMessage.com, accessed December 15, 2011, http://www.ensignmessage.com/archives/leavesbody.html.

854   "Faith Traditions and Health Care," http://www.uphs.upenn.edu/pastoral/pubs/traditions.html.

855-856   A. Clarfield, M. Gordon, H. Markwell, and S. Alibhai, "Ethical Issues in End-of-Life Geriatric Care: The Approach of Three Monotheistic Religions—Judaism, Catholicism, and Islam," *Journal of American Geriatric Society* 51, no.8 (2003): 1151.

857   Ashley et al., *Health Care Ethics*, 184.

858-859   "Faith Traditions and Health Care," http://www.uphs.upenn.edu/pastoral/pubs/traditions.html.

860   Ashley et al., *Health Care Ethics*, 184.

861   "Faith Traditions and Health Care," http://www.uphs.upenn.edu/pastoral/pubs/traditions.html.

862   Clarfield et al., "Ethical Issues," *Journal of American Geriatric Society*, 1151.

863   Mead et al., "Catholic Churches" in *Handbook of Denominations*.

864   "Circumcision," Catholic Online, accessed December 15, 2011, http://www.catholic.org/encyclopedia/view.php?id=2977.

865   Mead et al., "Catholic Churches" in *Handbook of Denominations*.

866   "Contraception and Sterilization," Catholic Answers, accessed December 15, 2011, http://www.catholic.com/tracts/contraception-and-sterilization.

867   J.G. Lipson, S. Dibble, and P.A. Minarik, eds., *Culture and Nursing Care: A Pocket Guide* (San Francisco, CA: UCSF Nursing Press, 1996), B-8.

868   R.P. Hamel, "The Roman Catholic Tradition," in *Religious Beliefs and Health Care*.

869-870   "Faith Traditions and Health Care," http://www.uphs.upenn.edu/pastoral/pubs/traditions.html.

871-872   "History of Sikhism," ReligionFacts, accessed December 15, 2011, http://www.religionfacts.com/sikhism/history.htm.

873-874   "Sikhism, Its Beliefs, Practices, Symbol, and Names," Religious Tolerance.org, accessed December 15, 2011, http://www.religioustolerance.org/sikhism2.htm.

875   "Amrit the Sikh Baptism Ceremony," About.com, accessed December 15, 2011, http://sikhism.about.com/od/initiation/a/Amrit.htm.

876   "Beliefs and Doctrines of Sikhism," ReligionFacts, accessed December 15, 2011, http://www.religionfacts.com/sikhism/beliefs.htm.

877   R. Gatrad, S.S. Panesar, E. Brown, H. Notta, and A. Sheikh, "Palliative care for Sikhs," *International Journal of Palliative Nursing* 9, no.11 (2003): 496.

878   J.S. Mayell, *Universality of the Sikh Religion* (Columbia, MO: Mayell Publishers, 2006), 123.

879   S.S. Kohli, *The Sikh and Sikhism* (New Delhi: Atlantic Publishers & Distributors, 1993), 41–44.

880   M. Fowler, S. Reimer-Kirkham, R. Sawatzky, and E.J. Taylor, *Religion, Religious Ethics, and Nursing* (New York: Springer Publishing Company, 2012), 258–259.

881   "Health Care Providers' Handbook on Sikh Patients—Section 2, Sikh Beliefs Affecting Health Care," Queensland Government, accessed December 15, 2011, http://www.health.qld.gov.au/multicultural/health_workers/hbook-sikh.asp.

882   "Sikhism Fact Sheet," Culture and Religion, accessed December 15, 2011, http://www.omi.wa.gov.au/resources/publications/cr_diversity/sikh.pdf

883-884   "Health Care Providers' Handbook on Sikh Patients—Section 1, Guidelines for Health Services," Queensland Government, accessed December 15, 2011, http://www.health.qld.gov.au/multicultural/health_workers/hbook-sikh.asp.

885   Mayell, *Universality of the Sikh Religion*, 269–270.

886   Gatrad et al., "Palliative care for Sikhs," *International Journal of Palliative Nursing*, 497.

887   R. Gatrad, J. Jhutti-Johal, P.S. Gill, and A. Sheikh, "Sikh birth customs," *Archives of Disease in Childhood* 90, no. 6 (June 2005): 561.

888-889   B.K. Gill, "Nursing with Dignity: Part 6: Sikhism," *Nursing Times* 98, no. 14 (April 2002): 41.

890   "Health Care Providers' Handbook on Sikh Patients—Section 2, http://www.health.qld.gov.au/multicultural/health_workers/hbook-sikh.asp.

891   B.K. Gill, "Nursing with Dignity," *Nursing Times*, 40.

892-893   Mayell, *Universality of the Sikh Religion*, 331.

894   "Health Care Providers' Handbook on Sikh Patients—Section 1, http://www.health.qld.gov.au/multicultural/health_workers/hbook-sikh.asp.

895-896   Gatrad et al., "Palliative care for Sikhs," *International Journal of Palliative Nursing*, 497.

897   B.K. Gill, "Nursing with Dignity," *Nursing Times*, 41.

898   Gatrad et al., "Palliative care for Sikhs," *International Journal of Palliative Nursing*, 497.

899   B.K. Gill, "Nursing with Dignity," *Nursing Times*, 41.

900-901   "Health Care Providers' Handbook on Sikh Patients—Section 1, http://www.health.qld.gov.au/multicultural/
          health_workers/hbook-sikh.asp.

902   Gatrad et al., "Palliative care for Sikhs," *International Journal of Palliative Nursing*, 497.

903   "Health Care Providers' Handbook on Sikh Patients—Section 1, Guidelines for Health Services," Queensland
          Government, accessed December 15, 2011, http://www.health.qld.gov.au/multicultural/health_workers/hbook-
          sikh.asp.

904   Gatrad et al., "Palliative care for Sikhs," *International Journal of Palliative Nursing*, 498.

905   "Sikhs: Death and the Dead," Ethnicity Online, accessed December 15, 2011, http://www.ethnicityonline.net/
          sikh_death.htm.

906   Gatrad et al., "Palliative care for Sikhs," *International Journal of Palliative Nursing*, 498.

907   "Your Role as a Sikh Minister at the Time of Death," Sikhism, accessed December 15, 2011, http://fateh.sikhnet.
          com/sikhnet/sikhism.nsf/d22e910786b2d7a98725658f0002790d/b9334fece71488a0872565b7007b339b!OpenDocument.

908   B.K. Gill, "Nursing with Dignity," *Nursing Times*, 41.

909   "Sikhism Fact Sheet," Culture and Religion.

910   Gatrad et al., "Palliative care for Sikhs," *International Journal of Palliative Nursing*, 498.

911   "Health Care Providers' Handbook on Sikh Patients—Section 2, http://www.health.qld.gov.au/multicultural/
          health_workers/hbook-sikh.asp.

912   "Health Care Providers' Handbook on Sikh Patients—Section 1, http://www.health.qld.gov.au/multicultural/
          health_workers/hbook-sikh.asp.

913-915   B.K. Gill, "Nursing with Dignity," *Nursing Times*, 41.

916   Gatrad et al., "Palliative care for Sikhs," *International Journal of Palliative Nursing*, 497.

917   B.K. Gill, "Nursing with Dignity," *Nursing Times*, 41.

918   Gatrad et al., "Palliative care for Sikhs," *International Journal of Palliative Nursing*, 498.

919   "Sikh Ceremonies," Info About Sikhs, accessed December 15, 2011, http://www.infoaboutsikhs.com/sikh_
          ceremonies.htm.

920   B.K. Gill, "Nursing with Dignity," *Nursing Times*, 41.

921   "Health Care Providers' Handbook on Sikh Patients—Section 1, http://www.health.qld.gov.au/multicultural/
          health_workers/hbook-sikh.asp.

922-923   "Health Care Providers' Handbook on Sikh Patients—Section 2, http://www.health.qld.gov.au/multicultural/
          health_workers/hbook-sikh.asp.

924   B.K. Gill, "Nursing with Dignity," *Nursing Times*, 40.

925-928   Gatrad et al., "Sikh birth customs," *Archives of Disease in Childhood*, 561.

929   "Five Articles of Faith," Real Sikhism, accessed January 31, 2012, http://www.realsikhism.com/index.php?subacti
          on=showfull&id=1193703788&ucat=5.

930   Gatrad et al., "Sikh birth customs," *Archives of Disease in Childhood*, 562.

931   "Talk: Sikhism and Circumcision," Sikhi Wiki, accessed December 15, 2011, http://www.sikhiwiki.org/index.php/
          Talk:Sikhism_and_Circumcision.

932   B.K. Gill, "Nursing with Dignity," *Nursing Times*, 41.

933   Gatrad et al., "Sikh birth customs," *Archives of Disease in Childhood*, 561.

934   Gatrad et al., "Palliative care for Sikhs," *International Journal of Palliative Nursing*, 498.

935   "Sikhs: Birth, Babies, and Motherhood," Ethnicity Online, accessed December 15, 2011, http://www. ethnicityonline.net/sikh_birth.htm.

936   B.K. Gill, "Nursing with Dignity," *Nursing Times*, 41.

937-938 Gatrad et al., "Sikh birth customs," *Archives of Disease in Childhood*, 561.

939   "Health Care Providers' Handbook on Sikh Patients—Section 2, http://www.health.qld.gov.au/multicultural/ health_workers/hbook-sikh.asp.

940-941 Gatrad et al., "Sikh birth customs," *Archives of Disease in Childhood*, 561.

942-943 B.K. Gill, "Nursing with Dignity," *Nursing Times*, 41.

944   "Our Unitarian Universalist Principles," Unitarian Universalist Association of Congregations, accessed December 16, 2011, http://www.uua.org/beliefs/principles/.

945   "Membership," Unitarian Universalist Association of Congregations, accessed December 16, 2011, http://www. uua.org/beliefs/congregationallife/7004.shtml.

946   "Holidays," Unitarian Universalist Association of Congregations, accessed December 16, 2011, http://www.uua. org/beliefs/worship/holidays/index.shtml.

947   "What Good is Baptism?" From the Minister's Study, updated March 26, 1999, http://archive.uua.org/CONG/ column75.html.

948   "Sermons—How Shall We Be Healed?" Unitarian Universalist Association of Congregations, accessed December 16, 2011, http://www.uua.org/worship/words/sermons/submissions/183464.shtml.

949   "Chalice," Unitarian Universalist Association of Congregations, accessed December 16, 2011, http://www.uua. org/worship/words/chalice/submissions/151521.shtml.

950   "Governance and Management of the Unitarian Universalist Association," Unitarian Universalist Association of Congregations, accessed December 16, 2011, http://www.uua.org/uuagovernance/.

951   "Worship," Unitarian Universalist Association of Congregations, accessed December 16, 2011, http://www.uua. org/beliefs/worship/index.shtml.

952   "Our Unitarian Universalist Principles," Unitarian Universalist Association of Congregations, accessed December 16, 2011, http://www.uua.org/beliefs/principles/.

953   "Beliefs About Life and Death in Unitarian Universalism," Unitarian Universalist Association of Congregations, accessed December 16, 2011, http://www.uua.org/beliefs/welcome/183025.shtml.

954   "Sermons—Getting Serious About Unitarian Universalism," Unitarian Universalist Association of Congregations, accessed December 16, 2011, http://www.uua.org/worship/words/sermons/submissions/183412.shtml.

955   "Chalice," Unitarian Universalist Association of Congregations, accessed December 16, 2011, http://www.uua. org/worship/words/chalice/submissions/151521.shtml.

956   "Visiting the Ill or Hospitalized," Unitarian Universalist Association of Congregations, accessed December 16, 2011, http://www.uua.org/care/team/104543.shtml.

957   "A Guide for Nurses: Teaching Healthcare Effectively to Patients," Health Careers Journal, accessed December 16, 2011, http://www.healthcareersjournal.com/a-guide-for-nurses-teaching-healthcare-effectively-to-patients/.

958-959 "Unitarian Universalist Policy," http://www.uua.org/economic/healthcare/41672.shtml.

960   "Faith without a Creed: Asking Questions as a Unitarian Universalist," Unitarian Universalist Association of Congregations, accessed December 16, 2011, www.uuabookstore.org/client/client_pages/3089.pdf.

961   "Religion and Organ and Tissue Donation," The Gift of a Lifetime, accessed December 16, 2011, http://www. organtransplants.org/understanding/religion/.

962   "Faith without a Creed," www.uuabookstore.org/client/client_pages/3089.pdf.

963   P. Sewell, "Respecting a Patient's Care Needs After Death," *Nursing Times.net* 98, no. 39 (September 24, 2002), 36.

964   J.G. Haas, "Final Goodbye Isn't as Hard as You Might Think," *The Orange County Register*, June 11, 2007, http://www.ocregister.com/articles/people-36253-dying-death.html.

965-967   "Unitarian Universalist Policy," http://www.uua.org/economic/healthcare/41672.shtml.

968   J. Gillman, "Religious Perspectives on Organ Donation," *Critical Care Nursing Quarterly* 22, no.3 (1999): 19–29.

969   "Religion and Organ and Tissue Donation," The Gift of a Lifetime, accessed December 16, 2011, http://www.organtransplants.org/understanding/religion/.

970   "Religion and Spirituality," Death with Dignity, http://www.deathwithdignity.org/historyfacts/religion/.

971   "Baptism/Child Dedication," Unitarian Universalist Association of Congregations, accessed December 16, 2011, http://www.uua.org/beliefs/worship/ceremonies/6976.shtml.

972   "Faith without a Creed," www.uuabookstore.org/client/client_pages/3089.pdf.

973   "Unitarian Universalist Policy," http://www.uua.org/economic/healthcare/41672.shtml.

974   "Sermons—The Spiritual Imperative of Choice," Unitarian Universalist Association of Congregations, accessed December 16, http://www.uua.org/worship/words/sermons/submissions/8788.shtml.

975   "Religions Ponder the Stem Cell Issue," UUs and the News, updated August 27, 2001, http://archive.uua.org/news/010827.html.

976   "Abortion: Right to Choose," Unitarian Universalist Association of Congregations, accessed December 16, 2011, http://www.uua.org/statements/statements/20271.shtml.

CULTURES

977   J. Lipson and S. Dibble, eds. *Culture and Clinical Care* (San Francisco, CA: UCSF Nursing Press, 2005), xiii.

978   "State & County QuickFacts," U.S. Census Bureau, accessed January 18, 2012, http://quickfacts.census.gov/qfd/states/00000.html.

979   "Pakistani Migration to the US: An Economic Perspective," Institute of Developing Economies, accessed January 18, 2012, http://ir.ide.go.jp/dspace/bitstream/2344/839/1/196_oda.pdf.

980   "Communicating With and About People with Disabilities," U.S. Department of Labor, accessed January 18, 2012, http://www.dol.gov/odep/pubs/fact/comucate.htm.

981   National Institute on Aging, *A Clinician's Handbook: Talking with Your Older Patient* (Bethesda, MD: National Institutes of Health, Department of Health and Human Services, 2008).

982   W. Thompson and J. Hickey, *Society in Focus* (Boston: Pearson, 2005).

983-986   W.C. Rucker, *The River Flows On: Black Resistance, Culture, and Identity Formation in Early America* (Baton Rouge, LA: LSU Press, 2006).

987-989   "American Fact Finder," U.S. Census Bureau, accessed January 30, 2012, http://factfinder2.census.gov /faces/nav/jsf/pages/searchresults.xhtml?refresh=t.

990-993   K.R. Humes, N.A. Jones, and R.R. Ramirez, "Overview of Race and Hispanic Origin: 2010; 2010 Census Briefs," issued March 2011, http://www.census.gov/prod/cen2010/briefs/c2010br-02.pdf.

994-996   A. Sutherland, *Gypsies, The Hidden Americans* (Prospect Heights, IL: Waveland Press, Inc., 1975).

997-998   "A Cultural Identity," R. Rodriguez, Pacific News Service, June 18, 1997, http://www.pbs.org /newshour/essays/june97/rodriguez_6-18.html.

999   "The World Fact Book," Central Intelligence Agency, last updated January 4, 2012, https://www.cia.gov/library/publications/the-world-factbook/geos/us.html.

1000-1001   "Profiles of General Demographic Characteristics 2000 Census of Population and Housing," U.S. Department of Commerce, issued May 2001, http://www.census.gov/prod/cen2000/dp1/2kh00.pdf.

1002   "American Fact Finder," U.S. Census Bureau, accessed January 30, 2012, http://factfinder2.census.gov/faces/nav/jsf/pages/searchresults.xhtml?refresh=t.

1003   "Learning About America ...Through US Census Data," Slice and Dice Data.com, accessed January 30, 2012, http://www.sliceanddicedata.com/detfil16.htm.

1004   S.L. Engerman, "A Population History of the Caribbean," in *A Population History of North America*, ed. M.R. Haines and R.H. Steckel, 483–528 (New York: Cambridge University Press, 2000).

1005   J.G. Lipson, S. Dibble, and P.A. Minarik, eds., *Culture and Nursing Care: A Pocket Guide* (San Francisco, CA: UCSF Nursing Press, 1996), 41.

1006   M.A. Shah, *Transcultural Aspects of Perinatal Health Care: A Resource Guide* (Tampa, FL: National Perinatal Association, 2004), 27.

1007   L.D. Purnell and B.J. Paulanka, *Guide to Culturally Competent Health Care* (Philadelphia, PA: F. A. Davis Company, 2009), 32.

1008   J.N. Giger and R.E. Davidhizar, *Transcultural Nursing, Assessment and Intervention* (St. Louis, MO: Elsevier Mosby, 2008), 13, 203–207.

1009   Ibid., 203.

1010   Purnell and Paulanka, *Guide to Culturally Competent Health Care*, 33.

1011   Purnell and Paulanka, *Guide to Culturally Competent Health Care*, 32.

1012   G.A. Galanti, *Caring for Patients From Different Cultures,* 4th ed. (Philadelphia, PA: University of Pennsylvania Press, 2008), 197.

1013   S.M. Lassiter, *Multicultural Clients: A Professional Handbook for Health Care Providers and Social Workers* (Westport, CT: Greenwood Publishing Group, 1995), 9–10.

1014   Giger and Davidhizar, *Transcultural Nursing*, 13.

1015   Lipson et al., *Culture and Nursing Care*, 40.

1016   Giger and Davidhizar, *Transcultural Nursing*, 197.

1017   Ibid., 247.

1018-1019   E. Randall-David, *Strategies for Working with Culturally Diverse Communities and Clients* (Washington, DC: Association for the Care of Children's Health, 1989), 40.

1020   Giger and Davidhizar, *Transcultural Nursing*, 201.

1021   J. Lipson and S. Dibble, eds. *Culture and Clinical Care* (San Francisco, CA: UCSF Nursing Press, 2005), 16.

1022   Purnell and Paulanka, *Guide to Culturally Competent Health Care*, 22.

1023   Ibid., 28.

1024   Lipson and Dibble, eds., *Culture and Clinical Care*, 19.

1025   Giger and Davidhizar, *Transcultural Nursing*, 13, 214.

1026   Ibid., 249.

1027   Ibid., 200.

1028   Purnell and Paulanka, *Guide to Culturally Competent Health Care*, 34.

1029   L.A. Ritter and N.A. Hoffman, *Multicultural Health* (Sudbury, MA: Jones and Bartlett Publishers, 2010), 266–268.

1030   Purnell and Paulanka, *Guide to Culturally Competent Health Care*, 34.

1031   Lipson et al., *Culture and Nursing Care*, 39.

1032   Lipson and Dibble, eds., *Culture and Clinical Care*, 19.

1033   Giger and Davidhizar, *Transcultural Nursing*, 203.

1034   E.J. Phipps, G. True, and G.F. Murray, "Community Perspectives on Advance Care Planning: Report from the Community Ethics Program" *Journal of Cultural Diversity* 10, no.4 (Winter 2003): 118–23.

1035   Purnell and Paulanka, *Guide to Culturally Competent Health Care*, 31.

1036   Lipson and Dibble, eds., *Culture and Clinical Care*, 26.

1037   Lipson et al., *Culture and Nursing Care*, 40.

1038   B.R. Ferrell and N. Coyle, eds., *Oxford Textbook of Palliative Nursing* (New York: Oxford University Press, 2010), 599.

1039   "Death and Burial," Michael C. Carlos Museum of Emory University, Odyssey Online Africa, accessed December 28, 2011, http://www.carlos.emory.edu/ODYSSEY/AFRICA/AF_death.html.

1040   Lipson and Dibble, eds., *Culture and Clinical Care*, 25.

1041   Lipson et al., *Culture and Nursing Care*, 40.

1042   E.H. Hamilton, *The Health and Wellness Ministry in the African American Church* (n.p.: Xulon Press, 2004), 55–56.

1043   J. Klessig, "Cross-Cultural Medicine a Decade Later: The Effect of Values and Culture on Life-Support Decisions," *Western Journal of Medicine* 157, no. 3 (September 1992): 316.

1044   P. Jevon, *Advanced Cardiac Life Support: A Guide For Nurses* (Oxford, UK: Wiley-Blackwell, 2010), 276.

1045   R.H. Blum, *The Management of the Doctor-Patient Relationship* (n.p.: McGraw-Hill, Blakiston Division, 1960), 6.

1046   Lipson and Dibble, eds., *Culture and Clinical Care*, 24.

1047   J. Gillman, "Religious Perspectives on Organ Donation," *Critical Care Nursing Quarterly* 22, no.3 (1999): 22.

1048-1049   Purnell and Paulanka, *Guide to Culturally Competent Health Care*, 31.

1050   Shah, *Transcultural Aspects of Perinatal Health Care*, 15.

1051   Ibid., 13.

1052   Ibid., 25.

1053   Lipson and Dibble, eds., *Culture and Clinical Care*, 21.

1054   Lipson et al., *Culture and Nursing Care*, 40.

1055-1056   Lipson and Dibble, eds., *Culture and Clinical Care*, 21.

1057   Shah, *Transcultural Aspects of Perinatal Health Care*, 17.

1058   Ibid., 26.

1059   Lipson and Dibble, eds., *Culture and Clinical Care*, 21.

1060   Shah, *Transcultural Aspects of Perinatal Health Care*, 26.

1061   Ibid., 21.

1062   Purnell and Paulanka, *Guide to Culturally Competent Health Care*, 32.

1063   Shah, *Transcultural Aspects of Perinatal Health Care*, 19.

1064   Purnell and Paulanka, *Guide to Culturally Competent Health Care*, 30.

1065   Shah, *Transcultural Aspects of Perinatal Health Care*, 8.

1066   Ibid., 9.

1067   Ibid., 21.

1068   Ibid., 22.

1069   Ibid., 17.

1070-1071   Purnell and Paulanka, *Guide to Culturally Competent Health Care*, 30.

1072   Shah, *Transcultural Aspects of Perinatal Health Care*, 14.

1073   Ibid., 7.

1074   Lipson et al., *Culture and Nursing Care*, 40.

1075   J. Gates-Williams, M.N. Jackson, V. Jenkins-Monroe, and L.R. Williams, "The Business of Preventing African-American Infant Mortality," *Western Journal of Medicine* 157, no.3 (1992): 350.

1076   Purnell and Paulanka, *Guide to Culturally Competent Health Care*, 29.

1077   Shah, *Transcultural Aspects of Perinatal Health Care*, 11.

1078   Purnell and Paulanka, *Guide to Culturally Competent Health Care*, 29.

1079   Lipson and Dibble, eds., *Culture and Clinical Care*, 21.

1080   Shah, *Transcultural Aspects of Perinatal Health Care*, 22.

1081   Purnell and Paulanka, *Guide to Culturally Competent Health Care*, 124.

1082   Lipson and Dibble, eds., *Culture and Clinical Care*, 193.

1083   Ibid., 277.

1084   Ibid., 290.

1085   Purnell and Paulanka, *Guide to Culturally Competent Health Care*, 125.

1086   Ibid., 125.

1087   Ibid., 119.

1088   Ibid., 127.

1089-1090   Ibid., 118.

1091   Lipson and Dibble, eds., *Culture and Clinical Care*, 195, 279, 292.

1092   Purnell and Paulanka, *Guide to Culturally Competent Health Care*, 118.

1093   Ibid., 144.

1094   Lipson and Dibble, eds., *Culture and Clinical Care*, 196, 280, 293.

1095   Purnell and Paulanka, *Guide to Culturally Competent Health Care*, 144.

1096   C. Storti, *Americans at Work: A Guide to the Can-Do People* (Yarmouth, ME: Intercultural Press, Inc., 2004), 176.

1097   Purnell and Paulanka, *Guide to Culturally Competent Health Care*, 118.

1098   Ibid., 121.

1099   Ibid., 122.

1100   Lipson and Dibble, eds., *Culture and Clinical Care*, 197.

1101   Ibid., 281.

1102   Ibid., 294–95.

1103   Purnell and Paulanka, *Guide to Culturally Competent Health Care*, 126.

1104   Ibid., 127.

1105   Lipson and Dibble, eds., *Culture and Clinical Care*, 201.

1106   Ibid., 295.

1107   Ibid., 298.

1108   Purnell and Paulanka, *Guide to Culturally Competent Health Care*, 126.

1109   Lipson and Dibble, eds., *Culture and Clinical Care*, 198, 282, 295.

1110   Purnell and Paulanka, *Guide to Culturally Competent Health Care*, 125.

1111   Lipson and Dibble, eds., *Culture and Clinical Care*, 206.

1112   Ibid., 289.

1113   Ibid., 302.

1114   Ibid., 205, 288–89, 301.

1115   Purnell and Paulanka, *Guide to Culturally Competent Health Care*, 124.

1116   Lipson and Dibble, eds., *Culture and Clinical Care*, 205.

1117   Ibid., 288.

1118   Ibid., 301.

1119-1120   Purnell and Paulanka, *Guide to Culturally Competent Health Care*, 123.

1121   Lipson and Dibble, eds., *Culture and Clinical Care*, 205.

1122   Ibid., 288, 301.

1123   Ibid., 195.

1124   Ibid., 279.

1125   Ibid., 292.

1126   Purnell and Paulanka, *Guide to Culturally Competent Health Care*, 127.

1127   Ibid., 123–24.

1128   Lipson and Dibble, eds., *Culture and Clinical Care*, 199.

1129   Ibid., 283.

1130   Ibid., 297.

1131   Purnell and Paulanka, *Guide to Culturally Competent Health Care*, 123.

1132   Ibid., 124.

1133   Lipson and Dibble, eds., *Culture and Clinical Care*, 199.

1134   Ibid., 283.

1135   Ibid., 297.

1136   Ibid., 199.

1137   Ibid., 284

1138   Ibid., 297.

1139   Purnell and Paulanka, *Guide to Culturally Competent Health Care*, 123.

1140   Lipson and Dibble, eds., *Culture and Clinical Care*, 200.

1141   Ibid., 284.

1142   Ibid., 297.

1143   Purnell and Paulanka, *Guide to Culturally Competent Health Care*, 123.

1144   Lipson and Dibble, eds., *Culture and Clinical Care*, 199.

1145   Ibid., 283.

1146   Ibid., 297.

1147   Purnell and Paulanka, *Guide to Culturally Competent Health Care*, 124.

1148   Lipson and Dibble, eds., *Culture and Clinical Care*, 203.

1149   Ibid., 286, 299.

1150   Purnell and Paulanka, *Guide to Culturally Competent Health Care*, 124.

1151   Lipson and Dibble, eds., *Culture and Clinical Care*, 284.

1152-1153   Purnell and Paulanka, *Guide to Culturally Competent Health Care*, 123–24.

1154   Lipson and Dibble, eds., *Culture and Clinical Care*, 199.

1155   Ibid., 297.

1156   Ibid., 199.

1157   Ibid., 283.

1158   Ibid., 297.

1159   Purnell and Paulanka, *Guide to Culturally Competent Health Care*, 123.

1160   Ibid., 123–24.

1161   Ibid., 123.

1162   "Cultural Aspects of Healthcare," College of St. Scholastica Athens Project, accessed December 30, 2011, http://www.css.edu/Academics/ATHENS-Project/Help-Page/Cultural-Aspects-of-Healthcare.html#American%20Indians.

1163   "Teachers; Apprenticeships," The Heart of the Healer Foundation, accessed December 30, 2011, http://www.heartofthehealer.org/apprenticeships/Teachers.

1164   "Native American Spirituality, Beliefs of Native Americans from the Arctic to the Southwest," Religious Tolerance.org, accessed December 30, 2011, http://www.religioustolerance.org/nataspir3.htm.

1165   A. Peelman, *Christ is a Native American* (Toronto, Ontario, Canada, Novalis-Saint Paul University, 1995), 41.

1166   "A Native American Approach to Teaching and Learning," L. Wakau-Villagomez, Critical Multicultural Pavilion Research Room, last updated September 2003, http://www.edchange.org/multicultural/papers/medicinewheel.html.

1167   "Cultural Aspects of Healthcare," http://www.css.edu/Academics/ATHENS-Project/Help-Page/Cultural-Aspects-of-Healthcare.html#American%20Indians..

1168-1169   B.J. Kramer, "Health and Aging of Urban American Indians," *Western Journal of Medicine* 157, no. 3 (1992): 281–283.

1170   T.L. Crofoot Graham, "Using Reasons for Living to Connect to American Indian Healing Traditions," *Journal of Sociology and Social Welfare* 29, no.1 (March 2002): 55.

1171-1172   M.A. Shah, *Transcultural Aspects of Perinatal Health Care: A Resource Guide* (Tampa, FL: National Perinatal Association, 2004), 258.

1173   M.M. Andrews and J.S. Boyle, *Transcultural Concepts in Nursing Care*, 2nd ed. (New York: Lippincott, 1995), 94.

1174   Kramer, "Health and Aging of Urban American Indians," *Western Journal of Medicine*, 284.

1175   Giger and Davidhizar, *Transcultural Nursing*, 285.

1176   Ibid., 276–299.

1177   G.O. Gabbard, L.W. Roberts, H. Crisp-Han, V. Ball, G. Hobday, and F. Rachal, *Professionalism in Psychiatry* (Arlington, VA: American Psychiatric Publishing, 2012), 94.

1178-1179   L. Araba-Owoyele, R. Littaua, M. Hughes, and J. Berecochea, "Determinants of Voluntary Blood Donation Among California's Racial/Ethnic Minorities," in *Minority Health Issues for an Emerging Majority* (Washington, DC: 4th National Forum on Cardiovascular Health, Pulmonary Disorders, and Blood Resources, June 26–27, 1992), 123.

1180   "Cultural Aspects of Healthcare," http://www.css.edu/Academics/ATHENS-Project/Help-Page/Cultural-Aspects-of-Healthcare.html#American%20Indians.

1181   Kramer, "Health and Aging of American Indians," *Western Journal of Medicine*, 282.

1182   Giger and Davidhizar, *Transcultural Nursing*, 281.

1183   Kramer, "Health and Aging of Urban American Indians," *Western Journal of Medicine*, 283.

1184-1187   "Cultural Aspects of Healthcare," http://www.css.edu/Academics/ATHENS-Project/Help-Page/Cultural-Aspects-of-Healthcare.html#American%20Indians.

1188   Giger and Davidhizar, *Transcultural Nursing,* 292.

1189   Ibid., 169.

1190   "Lactose Intolerance," PubMed Health, last updated July 7, 2010, http://www.ncbi.nlm.nih.gov/pubmedhealth/PMH0001321/.

1191   Andrews and Boyle, *Transcultural Concepts in Nursing Care*, 289.

1192   Andrews and Boyle, *Transcultural Concepts in Nursing Care*, 290.

1193   K. Cohen, *Honoring the Medicine: The Essential Guide to Native American Healing*, (New York: Ballantine Books, 2006), 43.

1194   Andrews and Boyle, *Transcultural Concepts in Nursing Care*, 23.

1195   J.G. Lipson, S. Dibble, and P.A. Minarik, eds., *Culture and Nursing Care: A Pocket Guide* (San Francisco, CA: UCSF Nursing Press, 1996), 17.

1196   "Patient Gender Preferences for Medical Care," J. Sherman, MedPage Today's KevinMD.com, accessed December 30, 2011, http://www.kevinmd.com/blog/2010/11/patient-gender-preferences-medical-care.html.

1197   Lipson et al., *Culture and Nursing Care*, 14.

1198   "Cultural Aspects of Healthcare," http://www.css.edu/Academics/ATHENS-Project/Help-Page/Cultural-Aspects-of-Healthcare.html#American%20Indians.

1199   Giger and Davidhizar, *Transcultural Nursing*, 276–299.

1200   Andrews and Boyle, *Transcultural Concepts in Nursing Care*, 459–60.

1201   "Cultural Aspects of Healthcare," http://www.css.edu/Academics/ATHENS-Project/Help-Page/Cultural-Aspects-of-Healthcare.html#American%20Indians.

1202   G.A. Galanti, *Caring for Patients From Different Cultures,* 4th ed. (Philadelphia, PA: University of Pennsylvania Press, 2008), 240.

1203-1207   "Cultural Aspects of Healthcare," http://www.css.edu/Academics/ATHENS-Project/Help-Page/Cultural-Aspects-of-Healthcare.html#American%20Indians.

1208   Giger and Davidhizar, *Transcultural Nursing*, 276–299.

1209-1211   Lipson et al., *Culture and Nursing Care*, 17.

1212   Ibid., 13–19.

1213   Lipson and Dibble, eds., *Culture and Clinical Care*, 29.

1214   Ibid., 39.

1215   Lipson et al., *Culture and Nursing Care*, 18.

1216   K.L. Braun, J.H. Pietsch, and P.L. Blanchette, eds., "End-of-Life Decision Making in American Indian and Alaska Native Cultures," in *Cultural Issues in End-of-Life Decision Making* (Thousand Oaks, CA: Sage Publications, Inc., 2000), 127–144.

1217   Shah, *Transcultural Aspects of Perinatal Health Care*, 265.

1218   S.J. Crawford and D.F. Kelley, *American Indian Religious Traditions* (Santa Barbara, CA: ABC-CLIO, Inc., 2005), 107.

1219-1220   Shah, *Transcultural Aspects of Perinatal Health Care*, 261.

1221   Ibid., 264.

1222   Lipson et al., *Culture and Nursing Care*, 13–16.

1223   Andrews and Boyle, *Transcultural Concepts*, 458.

1224   Giger and Davidhizar, *Transcultural Nursing*, 282.

1225   Shah, *Transcultural Aspects of Perinatal Health Care*, 263.

1226   Ibid., 265.

1227   Lipson et al., *Culture and Nursing Care*, 16.

1228   C.P. Nelson, R. Dunn, J. Wan, and J. Wei, "The Increasing Incidence of Newborn Circumcision: Data from the Nationwide Inpatient Sample," *Journal of Urology* 173, no.3 (March 2005): 978–981.

1229   Shah, *Transcultural Aspects of Perinatal Health Care*, 262.

1230   Ibid., 266.

1231   Lipson and Dibble, eds., *Culture and Clinical Care*, 35.

1232   Shah, *Transcultural Aspects of Perinatal Health Care*, 261.

1233   Lipson et al., *Culture and Nursing Care*, 13–16.

1234-1235   "Southern Paiute—Religion and Expressive Culture," Countries and Their Cultures, accessed December 30, 2011, http://www.everyculture.com/North-America/Southern-Paiute-and-Chemehuevi-Religion-and-Expressive-Culture.html.

1236   Lipson et al., *Culture and Nursing Care*, 16.

1237   R.L. Coles, *Race and Family: A Structural Approach* (Thousand Oaks, CA: Sage Publications, Inc., 2006), 129.

1238-1239   Shah, *Transcultural Aspects of Perinatal Health Care*, 262.

1240-1241   Ibid., 259, 265.

1242-1243   Lipson and Dibble, eds., *Culture and Clinical Care*, 35.

1244   Giger and Davidhizar, *Transcultural Nursing*, 280.

1245   Shah, *Transcultural Aspects of Perinatal Health Care*, 262.

1246   Ibid., 264.

1247   Lipson and Dibble, eds., *Culture and Clinical Care*, 35.

1248-1249   Shah, *Transcultural Aspects of Perinatal Health Care*, 260.

1250-1251   Ibid., 263.

1252-1253   Lipson et al., *Culture and Nursing Care*, 13–16.

1254   ICTMN Staff, "New Bill Would Authorize Federally Funded Abortions for Servicewomen," *Indian Country Today Media Network*, June 7, 2011.

1255   Giger and Davidhizar, *Transcultural Nursing*, 450–54.

1256   Giger and Davidhizar, *Transcultural Nursing*, 13, 450–54.

1257   Shah, *Transcultural Aspects of Perinatal Health Care*, 64.

1258   Giger and Davidhizar, *Transcultural Nursing*, 452.

1259   C. D'Avanzo, *Pocket Guide to Cultural Health Assessment* (St. Louis, MO: Elsevier Mosby, 2008), 158–164.

1260   Ibid., 159.

1261   Ibid., 158–64.

1262   A. Ong and N.N. Chen, eds., *Asian Biotech: Ethics and Communities of Fate* (Durham, NC: Duke University Press, 2010), 170–71.

1263   Giger and Davidhizar, *Transcultural Nursing*, 29.

1264   D'Avanzo, *Pocket Guide to Cultural Health Assessment* (2008), 161.

1265   Giger and Davidhizar, *Transcultural Nursing*, 445.

1266   Lipson et al., *Culture and Nursing Care*, 75.

1267   D'Avanzo, *Pocket Guide to Cultural Health Assessment* (2008), 161.

1268   Giger and Davidhizar, *Transcultural Nursing*, 15.

1269   Lipson et al., *Culture and Nursing Care*, 74

1270   Lipson et al., *Culture and Nursing Care*, 75.

1271   D'Avanzo, *Pocket Guide to Cultural Health Assessment* (2008), 162.

1272   G.C. White, *Believers and Beliefs: A Practical Guide to Religious Etiquette for Business and Social Occasions* (New York: Berkley Publishing Group, 1997), 122.

1273   Giger and Davidhizar, *Transcultural Nursing*, 451–52.

1274   Lipson et al., *Culture and Nursing Care*, 76.

1275-1276   Ibid., 75.

1277   Giger and Davidhizar, *Transcultural Nursing*, 454.

1278   J.H. Muller and B. Desmond, "Ethical Dilemmas in a Cross-Cultural Context. A Chinese Example" *Western Journal of Medicine* 157, no.3 (September 1992): 325–26.

1279   Giger and Davidhizar, *Transcultural Nursing*, 454.

1280   Lipson et al., *Culture and Nursing Care*, 75.

1281   Giger and Davidhizar, *Transcultural Nursing*, 454.

1282   Giger and Davidhizar, *Transcultural Nursing*, 452.

1283   C.D. Bryant and D.L. Peck, eds., *Encyclopedia of Death and the Human Experience* (Thousand Oaks, CA: Sage Publications, 2009), 191.

1284   A. Thompson, *Feng Shui* (New York: St. Martin's Press, 1996), 75, 103.

1285   N. Dresser, *Multicultural Manners: Essential Rules of Etiquette for the 21st Century* (Hoboken, NJ: John Wiley and Sons, Inc., 1996), 64.

1286   D'Avanzo, *Pocket Guide to Cultural Health Assessment* (2008), 158–64.

1287   Andrews and Boyle, *Transcultural Concepts in Nursing Care*, 318.

1288   Giger and Davidhizar, *Transcultural Nursing*, 445.

1289   Lipson et al., *Culture and Nursing Care*, 77.

1290   D'Avanzo, *Pocket Guide to Cultural Health Assessment* (2008), 162.

1291-1293	Lipson et al., *Culture and Nursing Care*, 78.
1294	Andrews and Boyle, *Transcultural Concepts in Nursing Care*, 368.
1295	Lipson et al., *Culture and Nursing Care*, 78.
1296	C.L.W. Chan and A.Y.M. Chow, eds., *Death, Dying, and Bereavement: A Hong Kong Chinese Experience* (Aberdeen, Hong Kong: Hong Kong University Press, 2006), 188.
1297	G.C. White, *Believers and Beliefs*, 124.
1298	D'Avanzo, *Pocket Guide to Cultural Health Assessment* (2008), 162.
1299-1300	Muller and Desmond, "Ethical Dilemmas. A Chinese Example" *Western Journal of Medicine*, 318, 325.
1301	Ibid., 325–26.
1302	D'Avanzo, *Pocket Guide to Cultural Health Assessment* (2008), 162.
1303	Giger and Davidhizar, *Transcultural Nursing,* 454.
1304	J. Klessig, "Cross-Cultural Medicine a Decade Later: The Effect of Values and Culture on Life-Support Decisions," *Western Journal of Medicine* 157, no. 3 (September 1992): 318.
1305	Muller and Desmond, "Ethical Dilemmas. A Chinese Example" *Western Journal of Medicine*, 325–26.
1306	Lipson et al., *Culture and Nursing Care*, 78.
1307	D'Avanzo, *Pocket Guide to Cultural Health Assessment* (2008), 162.
1308	G.A. Galanti, *Caring for Patients From Different Cultures*, 4th ed. (Philadelphia, PA: University of Pennsylvania Press, 2008), 165–66.
1309	H. Selin and P.K. Stone, *Childbirth Across Cultures: Ideas and Practices of Pregnancy, Childbirth, and the Postpartum* (New York: Springer, 2009), 74.
1310	G.C. White, *Believers and Beliefs*, 123.
1311	H. Donaldson, J. Kratzer, S. Okoturo-Ketter, and P. Tung, "Breastfeeding Among Chinese Immigrants in the United States," *Journal of Midwifery and Women's Health* 55, no. 3 (2010), 277–81.
1312	Shah, *Transcultural Aspects of Perinatal Health Care*, 72.
1313	Lipson et al., *Culture and Nursing Care*, 78.
1314-1315	Shah, *Transcultural Aspects of Perinatal Health Care*, 74.
1316	Ibid., 71.
1317	D'Avanzo, *Pocket Guide to Cultural Health Assessment* (2008), 162.
1318	Lipson et al., *Culture and Nursing Care*, 77.
1319	Shah, *Transcultural Aspects of Perinatal Health Care*, 68.
1320	Galanti, *Caring for Patients From Different Cultures*, 198.
1321	Shah, *Transcultural Aspects of Perinatal Health Care*, 77.
1322	L.D. Purnell and B.J. Paulanka, *Guide to Culturally Competent Health Care* (Philadelphia, PA: F. A. Davis Company, 2009), 94.
1323	Shah, *Transcultural Aspects of Perinatal Health Care*, 72.
1324	Ibid., 73.
1325-1326	Ibid., 75.
1327	Ibid., 68.
1328	Purnell and Paulanka, *Guide to Culturally Competent Health Care*, 92.

1329   Lipson et al., *Culture and Nursing Care*, 77.

1330   Shah, *Transcultural Aspects of Perinatal Health Care*, 70.

1331   "Abortion Confusion," Act Now.com, updated November 4, 2008, http://www.actnow.com.au /Issues/Abortion_ confusion.aspx.

1332   N.L. Potts and B.L. Mandleco, *Pediatric Nursing: Caring for Children and Their Families* (Clifton Park, NY: Delmar Publishing, 2012), 1185.

1333   Muller and Desmond, "Ethical Dilemmas. A Chinese Example" *Western Journal of Medicine*, 325–26.

1334   Shah, *Transcultural Aspects of Perinatal Health Care*, 77.

1335   S. Salimbene, *What Language Does Your Patient Hurt In?,* 2nd ed. (Amherst, MA: Diversity Resources, Inc., 2005), 96.

1336   Lipson and Dibble, eds., *Culture and Clinical Care*, 147.

1337   Ibid., 158.

1338   Salimbene, *What Language Does Your Patient Hurt In?,* 98.

1339   Lipson and Dibble, eds., *Culture and Clinical Care*, 159.

1340-1341   Ibid., 148.

1342   Salimbene, *What Language Does Your Patient Hurt In?,* 96.

1343   Lipson and Dibble, eds., *Culture and Clinical Care*, 149–50.

1344   Ibid., 150.

1345   Ibid., 148.

1346   Salimbene, *What Language Does Your Patient Hurt In?,* 97.

1347   Lipson and Dibble, eds., *Culture and Clinical Care*, 152.

1348   Salimbene, *What Language Does Your Patient Hurt In?,* 98.

1349   Ibid., 97.

1350   Lipson and Dibble, eds., *Culture and Clinical Care*, 152.

1351   Ibid., 158.

1352   Ibid., 149.

1353   Ibid., 157.

1354   Salimbene, *What Language Does Your Patient Hurt In?,* 96.

1355   Lipson and Dibble, eds., *Culture and Clinical Care,* 149.

1356   Ibid., 148–49.

1357   Salimbene, *What Language Does Your Patient Hurt In?,* 97.

1358   Lipson and Dibble, eds., *Culture and Clinical Care*, 151.

1359   Ibid., 150.

1360   Ibid., 159.

1361-1362   Ibid., 151.

1363   Ibid., 150.

1364   Ibid., 160.

1365   Ibid., 153.

1366   Editors of Hinduism Today Magazine, What is Hinduism? Modern Adventures Into a Profound Global Faith, (Kapaa, HI: Himalayan Academy, 2007), 351.

1367   A. Clarfield, M. Gordon, H. Markwell, and S. Alibhai, "Ethical Issues in End-of-Life Geriatric Care: The Approach of Three Monotheistic Religions—Judaism, Catholicism, and Islam," Journal of American Geriatric Society 51, no.8 (2003): 1152.

1368   "Health Care Providers' Handbook on Sikh Patients—Section 1, Guidelines for Health Services," Queensland Government, accessed December 15, 2011, http://www.health.qld.gov.au/multicultural/health_workers/hbook-sikh.asp.

1368   Lipson and Dibble, eds., Culture and Clinical Care, 161.

1369-1371   Ibid., 161.

1372   Ibid., 160.

1373-1375   Ibid., 161.

1376   S. Thrane, "Hindu End of Life," Journal of Hospice and Palliative Nursing, 337.

1377-1379   N. Sarhill, S. LeGrand, R. Islambouli, M.P. Davis, and D. Walsh, "The Terminally Ill Muslim: Death and Dying from the Muslim Perspective," American Journal of Hospice & Palliative Medicine 18, no. 4 (July/August, 2001): 251–53.

1380   B.K. Gill, "Nursing with Dignity: Part 6: Sikhism," Nursing Times 98, no. 14 (April 2002): 41.

1381   Lipson and Dibble, eds., Culture and Clinical Care, 149.

1382-1383   Ibid., 157.

1384   Salimbene, What Language Does Your Patient Hurt In?, 96.

1385-1387   Ibid., 159.

1388   M. Crawshaw and M. Balen, eds., Adopting After Infertility (Philadelphia, PA: Jessica Kingsley Publishers, 2010), 112.

1389   Lipson and Dibble, eds., Culture and Clinical Care, 155.

1390   Ibid., 154.

1391-1393   Ibid., 155.

1394   Ibid., 157.

1395-1396   Salimbene, What Language Does Your Patient Hurt In?, 98.

1397   Lipson and Dibble, eds., Culture and Clinical Care, 156.

1398   Lipson and Dibble, eds., Culture and Clinical Care, 155.

1399   Andrews and Boyle, Transcultural Concepts in Nursing Care, 49.

1400   Ibid., 159.

1401   Lipson and Dibble, eds., Culture and Clinical Care, 156.

1402-1405   Ibid., 155.

1406   Ibid., 154.

1407   Salimbene, What Language Does Your Patient Hurt In?, 98.

1408-1409   Lipson and Dibble, eds., *Culture and Clinical Care*, 156.

1410   J.J. Paris and A. Bell, "Ethical Issues in Perinatology: Guarantee My Child Will Be 'Normal' or Stop All Treatment" *Journal of Perinatology* 13, no.6 (1993), 469.

1411   Giger and Davidhizar, *Transcultural Nursing,* 477.

1412   Ibid., 480.

1413   Purnell and Paulanka, *Guide to Culturally Competent Health Care*, 141.

1414   D'Avanzo, *Pocket Guide to Cultural Health Assessment* (2008), 53.

1415   Purnell and Paulanka, *Guide to Culturally Competent Health Care*, 140.

1416   Lipson et al., *Culture and Nursing Care*, 122.

1417   Giger and Davidhizar, *Transcultural Nursing,* 481.

14181419   Lipson et al., *Culture and Nursing Care*, 120–23.

1420   Ibid., 116.

1421   Giger and Davidhizar, *Transcultural Nursing,* 473, 476.

1422   Giger and Davidhizar, *Transcultural Nursing,* 473.

1423   Purnell and Paulanka, *Guide to Culturally Competent Health Care*, 136.

1424   Giger and Davidhizar, *Transcultural Nursing,* 473.

1425   Ibid., 485.

1426   Ibid., 485, 487.

1427   Purnell and Paulanka, *Guide to Culturally Competent Health Care*, 135.

1428   N. Dresser, *Multicultural Manners: Essential Rules of Etiquette for the 21st Century* (Hoboken, NJ: John Wiley and Sons, Inc., 2005), 74.

1429-1430   Purnell and Paulanka, *Guide to Culturally Competent Health Care*, 140.

1431   Andrews and Boyle, *Transcultural Concepts in Nursing Care*, 308.

1432   Galanti, *Caring for Patients From Different Cultures*, 56.

1433   Purnell and Paulanka, *Guide to Culturally Competent Health Care*, 139.

1434-1436   Lipson et al., *Culture and Nursing Care*, 121.

1437   Ibid., 117–20.

1438   Purnell and Paulanka, *Guide to Culturally Competent Health Care*, 139.

1439   M.R. Leming and G.E. Dickinson, *Understanding Dying, Death, and Bereavement* (Belmont, CA: Wadsworth, 2011), 499–505.

1440   Lipson et al., *Culture and Nursing Care*, 120–23.

1441   Purnell and Paulanka, *Guide to Culturally Competent Health Care*, 138.

1442   Galanti, *Caring for Patients From Different Cultures*, 169.

1443   Lipson et al., *Culture and Nursing Care*, 121.

1444   J. Klessig, "Cross-Cultural Medicine a Decade Later: The Effect of Values and Culture on Life-Support Decisions," *Western Journal of Medicine* 157, no. 3 (September 1992): 320.

1445   Purnell and Paulanka, *Guide to Culturally Competent Health Care*, 140.

1446   "Filipino Culture Paper; Nursing Culture Class," Nurses Neighborhood, accessed January 6, 2012, http://www.nurses-neighborhood.com/filipino-culture.html.

1447   Purnell and Paulanka, *Guide to Culturally Competent Health Care*, 138.

1448   Lipson et al., *Culture and Nursing Care*, 120.

1449-1450   R.T. Francoeur and R.J. Noonan, eds., *The Continuum Complete International Encyclopedia of Sexuality* (New York: Continuum International Publishing Group, Inc., 2004), 839.

1451   Lipson et al., *Culture and Nursing Care*, 119.

1452   M.L. Murray and G.M. Huelsmann, *Labor and Delivery Nursing: A Guide to Evidence-Based Practice* (New York: Springer Publishing Company, Inc., 2009), 201.

1453   Purnell and Paulanka, *Guide to Culturally Competent Health Care*, 141.

1454   Ibid., 140.

1455   Lipson et al., *Culture and Nursing Care*, 120.

1456   Giger and Davidhizar, *Transcultural Nursing*, 482.

1457   Ibid., 480.

1458-1459   Lipson et al., *Culture and Nursing Care*, 120.

1460   Ibid., 119.

1461   Purnell and Paulanka, *Guide to Culturally Competent Health Care*, 137.

1462   Ibid., 136.

1463   Ibid., 136.

1464   Giger and Davidhizar, *Transcultural Nursing*, 371.

1465   D'Avanzo, *Pocket Guide to Cultural Health Assessment* (2008), 371.

1466   Shah, *Transcultural Aspects of Perinatal Health Care*, 174.

1467   Lipson and Dibble, eds., *Culture and Clinical Care*, 314.

1468   Giger and Davidhizar, *Transcultural Nursing*, 366.

1469   D'Avanzo, *Pocket Guide to Cultural Health Assessment* (2008), 367.

1470   Giger and Davidhizar, *Transcultural Nursing*, 372.

1471   Ibid., 367.

1472   Ibid., 373, 380.

1473   Shah, *Transcultural Aspects of Perinatal Health Care*, 168.

1474   Giger and Davidhizar, *Transcultural Nursing*, 380.

1475   D'Avanzo, *Pocket Guide to Cultural Health Assessment* (2008), 363.

1476   G.A. Galanti, *Caring for Patients From Different Cultures*, 4th ed. (Philadelphia, PA: University of Pennsylvania Press, 2008), 181–82.

1477   D'Avanzo, *Pocket Guide to Cultural Health Assessment* (2008), 361.

1478   S. Matsumura, S. Bito, H. Liu, K. Kahn, S. Fukuhara, M. Kagawa-Singer, and N. M. Wenger, "Acculturation of Attitudes Toward End-of-Life Care: A Cross-Cultural Survey of Japanese Americans and Japanese" *Journal of General Internal Medicine* 17, no. 7 (July 2002), 531-539.

1479   D'Avanzo, *Pocket Guide to Cultural Health Assessment* (2008), 372.

1480   Giger and Davidhizar, *Transcultural Nursing*, 371.

1481   Ibid., 368.

1482   Andrews and Boyle, *Transcultural Concepts*, 308.

1483   Giger and Davidhizar, *Transcultural Nursing*, 365.

1484   Lipson et al., *Culture and Nursing Care*, 183.

1485-1486   S. Matsumura et al., "Acculturation of Attitudes Toward End-of-Life Care," *Journal of General Internal Medicine*, 531-539.

1487-1488   Lipson et al., *Culture and Nursing Care*, 186.

1489   W.E. Finkbeiner, P.C. Ursell, and R.L. Davis, *Autopsy Pathology: A Manual and Atlas* (Philadelphia, PA: Saunders Elsevier, 2009), 22.

1490   Lipson and Dibble, eds., *Culture and Clinical Care*, 315.

1491   Lipson et al., *Culture and Nursing Care*, 186.

1492   White, *Believers and Beliefs*, 104.

1493   D'Avanzo, *Pocket Guide to Cultural Health Assessment* (2008), 362.

1494   S. Matsumura et al., "Acculturation of Attitudes Toward End-of-Life Care," *Journal of General Internal Medicine*, 537.

1495   Purnell and Paulanka, *Guide to Culturally Competent Health Care*, 252–64.

1496   S. Matsumura et al., "Acculturation of Attitudes Toward End-of-Life Care," *Journal of General Internal Medicine*, 537.

1497   Purnell and Paulanka, *Guide to Culturally Competent Health Care*, 260.

1498   S. Matsumura et al., "Acculturation of Attitudes Toward End-of-Life Care," *Journal of General Internal Medicine*, 534.

1499   J. Gillman, "Religious Perspectives on Organ Donation," *Critical Care Nursing Quarterly* 22, no.3 (1999): 22.

1500   Lipson et al., *Culture and Nursing Care*, 186.

1501   Gillman, "Religious Perspectives on Organ Donation," *Critical Care Nursing Quarterly*, 24.

1502   Purnell and Paulanka, *Guide to Culturally Competent Health Care*, 252–64.

1503   S. Matsumura et al., "Acculturation of Attitudes Toward End-of-Life Care," *Journal of General Internal Medicine*, 537.

1504   Purnell and Paulanka, *Guide to Culturally Competent Health Care*, 261.

1505   Shah, *Transcultural Aspects of Perinatal Health Care*, 169.

1506   M. Kriegman-Chin, "A Japanese Birth" *Midwifery Today* 26 (1993), 32–3, 40.

1507   Shah, *Transcultural Aspects of Perinatal Health Care*, 171.

1508   J. Riordan, *Breastfeeding and Human Lactation* (Sudbury, MA: Jones and Bartlett Publishers, 2005), 719.

1509   Kriegman-Chin, "A Japanese Birth" *Midwifery Today*, 32–3, 40.

1510   Shah, *Transcultural Aspects of Perinatal Health Care*, 172.

1511   Lipson et al., *Culture and Nursing Care*, 183.

1512   Ibid., 184.

1513   Shah, *Transcultural Aspects of Perinatal Health Care*, 170.

1514   Ibid., 176.

1515   Lipson et al., *Culture and Nursing Care*, 188.

1516   Ibid., 185.

1517   Purnell and Paulanka, *Guide to Culturally Competent Health Care*, 261–62.

1518   Lipson and Dibble, eds., *Culture and Clinical Care*, 311.

1519   Shah, *Transcultural Aspects of Perinatal Health Care*, 173.

1520   D'Avanzo, *Pocket Guide to Cultural Health Assessment* (2008), 362.

1521	Kriegman-Chin, "A Japanese Birth" *Midwifery Today*, 33.
1522	Lipson and Dibble, eds., *Culture and Clinical Care*, 310.
1523	Kriegman-Chin, "A Japanese Birth" *Midwifery Today*, 32–3, 40.
1524	E.M. Hetherington, R.D. Parke, and V.O Locke, *Child Psychology: A Contemporary Viewpoint* (Boston, MA: McGraw-Hill, 2003), 112.
1525-1526	Shah, *Transcultural Aspects of Perinatal Health Care*, 166.
1527	Kriegman-Chin, "A Japanese Birth" *Midwifery Today*, 33.
1528	Shah, *Transcultural Aspects of Perinatal Health Care*, 168.
1529	Kriegman-Chin, "A Japanese Birth" *Midwifery Today*, 32.
1530-1531	Purnell and Paulanka, *Guide to Culturally Competent Health Care*, 259.
1532	Shah, *Transcultural Aspects of Perinatal Health Care*, 167.
1533	Giger and Davidhizar, *Transcultural Nursing,* 627.
1534	Ibid., 619–641.
1535	D'Avanzo, *Pocket Guide to Cultural Health Assessment* (2008), 388.
1536	Lipson et al., *Culture and Nursing Care*, 200.
1537	C.M. Roberson, "ASNA Independent Study Activity – Cultural Assessment of Koreans," *Alabama Nurse* 30, no. 3 (Sep–Nov 2003): 13–16.
1538-1539	J.D. Andrews, *Cultural, Religious, Ethnic: Reference Manual for Healthcare Providers* (Winston-Salem, NC: Jamarda Resources, 1995), 34–35.
1540	D'Avanzo, *Pocket Guide to Cultural Health Assessment* (2008), 389.
1541	Giger and Davidhizar, *Transcultural Nursing,* 625.
1542	Ibid., 635.
1543	Dresser, *Multicultural Manners* (2005), 74.
1544	Giger and Davidhizar, *Transcultural Nursing,* 633.
1545	D'Avanzo, *Pocket Guide to Cultural Health Assessment* (2008), 361.
1546	S. Salimbene, *What Language Does Your Patient Hurt In?,* 2nd ed. (Amherst, MA: Diversity Resources, Inc., 2005), 80.
1547	Galanti, *Caring for Patients From Different Cultures*, 181–82.
1548	Dresser, *Multicultural Manners* (2005), 64.
1549-1550	Roberson, "Cultural Assessment of Koreans," *Alabama Nurse*, 13–16.
1551	D'Avanzo, *Pocket Guide to Cultural Health Assessment* (2008), 389.
1552	Roberson, "Cultural Assessment of Koreans," *Alabama Nurse*, 13–16.
1553	E.J. Phipps, G. True, and G.F. Murray, "Community Perspectives on Advance Care Planning: Report from the Community Ethics Program" *Journal of Cultural Diversity* 10, no.4 (Winter 2003): 118–23.
1554	Roberson, "Cultural Assessment of Koreans," *Alabama Nurse*, 13–16.
1555	Lipson et al., *Culture and Nursing Care*, 198.
1556	Roberson, "Cultural Assessment of Koreans," *Alabama Nurse*, 13–16.
1557	Lipson et al., *Culture and Nursing Care*, 198.
1558	Shah, *Transcultural Aspects of Perinatal Health Care*, 216.

1559	Purnell and Paulanka, *Guide to Culturally Competent Health Care*, 289.
1560	J. Klessig, "Cross-Cultural Medicine," *Western Journal of Medicine*, 318.
1561	J.R. Kim, D. Elliott, and C. Hyde, "The Influence of Sociocultural Factors on Organ Donation and Transplantation in Korea: Findings From Key Informant Interviews" *Journal of Transcultural Nursing* 15, no. 2 (April 2004): 147.
1562	Purnell and Paulanka, *Guide to Culturally Competent Health Care*, 289.
1563	Lipson et al., *Culture and Nursing Care*, 199.
1564	Ibid., 194.
1565	J. Gillman, "Religious Perspectives on Organ Donation," *Critical Care Nursing Quarterly* 22, no.3 (1999): 22.
1566	Kim et al., "The Influence of Sociocultural Factors on Organ Donation and Transplantation in Korea," *Journal of Transcultural Nursing*, 147.
1567-1568	J. Klessig, "Cross-Cultural Medicine," *Western Journal of Medicine*, 318.
1569	Purnell and Paulanka, *Guide to Culturally Competent Health Care*, 289.
1570-1571	Shah, *Transcultural Aspects of Perinatal Health Care*, 214.
1572	Roberson, "Cultural Assessment of Koreans," *Alabama Nurse*, 13–16.
1573	Purnell and Paulanka, *Guide to Culturally Competent Health Care*, 288.
1574	S.H. Kim, W.K. Kim, K.A. Lee, Y.S. Song, S.Y. Oh, "Breastfeeding in Korea," *World Review of Nutrition and Dietetics* 78 (1995): 114–27.
1575	Roberson, "Cultural Assessment of Koreans," *Alabama Nurse*, 13–16.
1576	Shah, *Transcultural Aspects of Perinatal Health Care*, 215.
1577	Andrews and Boyle, *Transcultural Concepts in Nursing Care*, 113–16.
1578	Shah, *Transcultural Aspects of Perinatal Health Care*, 216.
1579	Giger and Davidhizar, *Transcultural Nursing,* 630.
1580	Shah, *Transcultural Aspects of Perinatal Health Care,* 215.
1581	Ibid., 216.
1582	Lipson et al., *Culture and Nursing Care*, 197–98.
1583	Roberson, "Cultural Assessment of Koreans," *Alabama Nurse*, 13–16.
1584-1585	Shah, *Transcultural Aspects of Perinatal Health Care,* 215.
1586	Lipson et al., *Culture and Nursing Care*, 197.
1587-1589	Shah, *Transcultural Aspects of Perinatal Health Care*, 214.
1590	Ibid., 213.
1591	Ibid., 214.
1592-1593	Roberson, "Cultural Assessment of Koreans," *Alabama Nurse*, 13–16.
1594	Andrews and Boyle, *Transcultural Concepts in Nursing Care*, 103.
1595-1596	Shah, *Transcultural Aspects of Perinatal Health Care*, 213.
1597	Purnell and Paulanka, *Guide to Culturally Competent Health Care*, 288.
1598	Ibid., 216.
1599-1600	Lipson et al., *Culture and Nursing Care*, 201.
1601-1610	Lipson and Dibble, eds., *Culture and Clinical Care*, 361.

1611	"Blood Transfusion Service," Pakistan Red Crescent Society, accessed January 7, 2012, http://prcs.org.pk/blood.asp.
1612	Lipson and Dibble, eds., *Culture and Clinical Care*, 372.
1613-1615	Ibid., 361.
1616-1617	Ibid., 362.
1618	Ibid., 361.
1619-1621	Ibid., 362.
1622	Ibid., 362–63.
1623-1624	Ibid., 363.
1625-1638	Ibid., 365.
1639-1641	Ibid., 362.
1642-1645	Ibid., 363.
1646-1651	Ibid., 364.
1652	Ibid., 367.
1653	Ibid., 371.
1654-1660	Ibid., 372
1661-1666	Ibid., 373.
1667	Ibid., 372.
1668	Ibid., 373.
1669-1670	Ibid., 372.
1671-1672	Ibid., 368.
1673-1683	Ibid., 367.
1684-1687	Ibid., 368.
1688	Ibid., 369.
1689	Ibid., 368.
1690-1691	Ibid., 367.
1692	Ibid., 368.
1693-1694	Ibid., 371.
1695-1704	Ibid., 368.
1705	Ibid., 364.
1706-1708	Ibid., 367.
1709-1710	Ibid., 369.
1711-1712	Andrews and Boyle, *Transcultural Concepts in Nursing Care*, 513–15
1713	Lipson and Dibble, eds., *Culture and Clinical Care*, 370.
1714	Giger and Davidhizar, *Transcultural Nursing,* 505.
1715	Ibid., 509, 513.
1716	Ibid., 508–09.
1717	Ibid., 499.

1718   Ibid., 527.

1719   D.S. Mull, N. Nguyen, and J.D. Mull, "Vietnamese Diabetic Patients and Their Physicians: What Ethnography Can Teach Us," *Western Journal of Medicine* 175, no. 5 (November 2001): 308.

1720   Giger and Davidhizar, *Transcultural Nursing,* 512.

1721-1722   J.D. Andrews, *Cultural, Religious, Ethnic: Reference Manual for Healthcare Providers* (Winston-Salem, NC: Jamarda Resources, 1995), 34–35.

1723   Giger and Davidhizar, *Transcultural Nursing,* 512.

1724   Roberson, "Cultural Assessment of Koreans," *Alabama Nurse*, 13–16.

1725   Giger and Davidhizar, *Transcultural Nursing,* 498.

1726   Giger and Davidhizar, *Transcultural Nursing,* 499.

1727   Ibid., 499.

1728   Giger and Davidhizar, *Transcultural Nursing,* 499.

1729   Lipson and Dibble, eds., *Culture and Clinical Care*, 448.

1730   Giger and Davidhizar, *Transcultural Nursing,* 520.

1731   Mull et al., "Vietnamese Diabetic Patients and Their Physicians," *Western Journal of Medicine*, 307.

1732   Lipson et al., *Culture and Nursing Care*, 283.

1733   Giger and Davidhizar, *Transcultural Nursing,* 521.

1734   Ibid., 512.

1735   Lipson et al., *Culture and Nursing Care*, 193.

1736   Lipson and Dibble, eds., *Culture and Clinical Care*, 456.

1737   Mull et al., "Vietnamese Diabetic Patients and Their Physicians," *Western Journal of Medicine*, 308.

1738   Ibid., 309.

1739-1740   Lipson and Dibble, eds., *Culture and Clinical Care*, 448.

1741   Giger and Davidhizar, *Transcultural Nursing,* 502.

1742   Ibid., 502.

1743   Ibid., 525.

1744   Lipson and Dibble, eds., *Culture and Clinical Care*, 455.

1745   Ibid., 457.

1746   Dresser, *Multicultural Manners* (2005), 160.

1747   Giger and Davidhizar, *Transcultural Nursing,* 506.

1740   Lipson et al., *Culture and Nursing Care*, 203.

1749   Lipson and Dibble, eds., *Culture and Clinical Care*, 459.

1750   Andrews and Boyle, *Transcultural Concepts in Nursing Care*, 369.

1751   Lipson et al., *Culture and Nursing Care*, 286.

1752   Ibid., 282.

1753   D'Avanzo, *Pocket Guide to Cultural Health Assessment* (2008), 777.

1754   Lipson and Dibble, eds., *Culture and Clinical Care*, 459.

1755   Giger and Davidhizar, *Transcultural Nursing,* 499.

1756   Lipson and Dibble, eds., *Culture and Clinical Care*, 459.

1757   Lipson et al., *Culture and Nursing Care*, 286.

1758   Giger and Davidhizar, *Transcultural Nursing,* 512.

1759   Ibid., 512.

1760   Galanti, *Caring for Patients From Different Cultures*, 175.

1761   Lipson and Dibble, eds., *Culture and Clinical Care*, 459.

1762   M.A. Calhoun, "The Vietnamese Woman: Health/Illness Attitudes and Behaviors," special issue "Women, Health, and Culture" in *Health Care for Women International* 6, no. 1–3 (1985): 61–72.

1763   D'Avanzo, *Pocket Guide to Cultural Health Assessment* (2008), 776.

1764   Lipson et al., *Culture and Nursing Care*, 285.

1765   Dresser, *Multicultural Manners* (2005), 87–89, 106–07, 138.

1766   Galanti, *Caring for Patients From Different Cultures*, 157.

1767   D'Avanzo, *Pocket Guide to Cultural Health Assessment* (2008), 777.

1768   Lipson and Dibble, eds., *Culture and Clinical Care*, 454.

1769   Ibid., 453.

1770   Ibid., 457.

1771   Ibid., 454.

1772-1773   Ibid., 453.

1774   Giger and Davidhizar, *Transcultural Nursing,* 501.

1775   Lipson et al., *Culture and Nursing Care*, 284.

1776-1777   Lipson and Dibble, eds., *Culture and Clinical Care*, 454.

1778   Lipson et al., *Culture and Nursing Care*, 135–36.

1779-1780   A. Sutherland, "Gypsies and Health Care," *Western Journal of Medicine* 157, no. 3 (September 1992): 276–80.

1781   J.P. Liégeois, *Roma, Gypsies, Travellers* (The Netherlands: Council of Europe, 1994), 83.

1782-1783   S.J. Danis, "The Gypsy Culture in South Florida," *Florida Nurse* 44, no. 7 (August 1996): 17.

1784   Lipson et al., *Culture and Nursing Care*, 136.

1785   D. Honer and P. Hoppie, "The Enigma of the Gypsy Patient," *Modern Medicine* (August 1, 2004), http://www.modernmedicine.com/modernmedicine/article/articleDetail.jsp?id=114152.

1786   A. Sutherland, "Gypsies and Health Care," *Western Journal of Medicine* 157, no. 3 (September 1992): 276–78.

1787   Honer and Hoppie, "The Enigma of the Gypsy Patient," *Modern Medicine*.

1788-1791   Sutherland, "Gypsies and Health Care," *Western Journal of Medicine*, 276–78.

1792   Ibid., 277–79.

1793   Ibid., 276–77.

1794   Ibid., 276–78.

1795   Honer and Hoppie, "The Enigma of the Gypsy Patient," *Modern Medicine*.

1796   Lipson et al., *Culture and Nursing Care*, 126–29.

1797   Honer and Hoppie, "The Enigma of the Gypsy Patient," *Modern Medicine*.

1798   Sutherland, "Gypsies and Health Care," *Western Journal of Medicine*, 276–78.

1799   Lipson et al., *Culture and Nursing Care*, 136.

1800   Ibid., 128.

1801   Sutherland, "Gypsies and Health Care," *Western Journal of Medicine*, 277–79.

1802   Lipson et al., *Culture and Nursing Care*, 126–29.

1803   Sutherland, "Gypsies and Health Care," *Western Journal of Medicine*, 276–78.

1804   Lipson et al., *Culture and Nursing Care*, 126–32.

1805   C. Vivian and L. Dundes, "The Crossroads of Culture and Health Among the Roma (Gypsies)" *Journal of Nursing Scholarship* 36, no.1 (March 2004): 86–91.

1806   Lipson et al., *Culture and Nursing Care*, 132.

1807   "Gypsy Death Rituals and Customs," Gypsy Vodou, accessed January 9, 2012, http://gypsyvodou.com/gypsies/875/.

1808   Sutherland, "Gypsies and Health Care," *Western Journal of Medicine*, 280.

1809   Galanti, *Caring for Patients From Different Cultures*, 268.

1810   Lipson et al., *Culture and Nursing Care*, 132.

1811   "Religion and Donation," LifeCenter Northwest, accessed January 31, 2012, http://www.lcnw.org/understanding-donation/religion-and-donation/.

1812   "Religious Views," Ochsner, accessed January 9, 2012, http://www.ochsner.org/services/multi_organ_transplant/transplant_organ_donation_religious_views/#GYP.

1813   Sutherland, "Gypsies and Health Care," *Western Journal of Medicine*, 278.

1814   Ibid., 276–78.

1815-1816   Lipson et al., *Culture and Care*, 131.

1817   Ibid., 136.

1818-1821   Sutherland, "Gypsies and Health Care," *Western Journal of Medicine*, 278.

1822   Lipson et al., *Culture and Nursing Care*, 126–32.

1823   Ibid., 131.

1824   Sutherland, "Gypsies and Health Care," *Western Journal of Medicine*, 278.

1825-1827   "The Roma: Their Beliefs and Practices," Religious Tolerance.org, accessed January 9, 2012, http://www.religioustolerance.org/roma2.htm.

1828   Vivian and Dundes, "Crossroads of Culture and Health," *Journal of Nursing Scholarship*, 90

1829-1833   Lipson and Dibble, eds., *Culture and Clinical Care*, 59.

1834   Ibid., 59–60.

1835-1836   Lipson et al., *Culture and Nursing Care*, 52.

1837   Lipson and Dibble, eds., *Culture and Clinical Care*, 70.

1838   Lipson et al., *Culture and Nursing Care*, 45.

1839-1840   Lipson and Dibble, eds., *Culture and Clinical Care*, 60.

1841-1844   Ibid., 61.

1845-1849   Ibid., 62.

1850   Ibid., 63.

1851   Purnell and Paulanka, *Guide to Culturally Competent Health Care*, 88.

1852   Lipson et al., *Culture and Nursing Care*, 45.

1853-1854   Ibid., 46.

1855   Ibid., 51.

1856   Ibid., 47.

1857-1865   Lipson and Dibble, eds., *Culture and Clinical Care*, 64.

1866   Lipson et al., *Culture and Nursing Care*, 53.

1867-1868   Ibid., 46.

1869-1872   Ibid., 47.

1873-1874   Ibid., 53.

1875   Ibid., 51.

1876-1877   Ibid., 48.

1878   Lipson and Dibble, eds., *Culture and Clinical Care*, 65.

1879   Ibid., 64.

1880   Lipson et al., *Culture and Nursing Care*, 48.

1881   Ibid., 53.

1882   Lipson and Dibble, eds., *Culture and Clinical Care*, 64, 70.

1883   Lipson et al., *Culture and Nursing Care*, 50.

1884-1889   Lipson and Dibble, eds., *Culture and Clinical Care*, 71.

1890   Lipson et al., *Culture and Nursing Care*, 93.

1891   Lipson and Dibble, eds., *Culture and Clinical Care*, 61.

1892-1893   F.C. Barcellos, C.L. Araujo, and J. Dias da Costa, "Organ Donation: A Population-Based Study" *Clinical Transplantation* 19, no. 1 (February 2005), 33.

1894   Lipson et al., *Culture and Nursing Care*, 93.

1895-1896   "The Sacraments: Baptism," American Catholic.org, accessed January 9, 2012, http://www.americancatholic.org/features/special/default.aspx?id=30.

1897   Lipson et al., *Culture and Nursing Care*, 48–49.

1898-1866   Lipson and Dibble, eds., *Culture and Clinical Care*, 66.

1900   Purnell and Paulanka, *Guide to Culturally Competent Health Care*, 94.

1901   Lipson et al., *Culture and Nursing Care*, 50.

1902-1904   Lipson and Dibble, eds., *Culture and Clinical Care*, 67.

1905   Lipson et al., *Culture and Nursing Care*, 49.

1906   Lipson and Dibble, eds., *Culture and Clinical Care*, 66.

1907   Lipson et al., *Culture and Nursing Care*, 50.

1908   Ibid., 52.

1909   Lipson and Dibble, eds., *Culture and Clinical Care*, 66.

1910	Purnell and Paulanka, *Guide to Culturally Competent Health Care*, 95.
1911	"The Sacraments: Baptism," American Catholic.org, accessed January 9, 2012, http://www.americancatholic.org/features/special/default.aspx?id=30.
1912	Lipson et al., *Culture and Nursing Care*, 49.
1913	Lipson and Dibble, eds., *Culture and Clinical Care*, 66.
1914-1915	Lipson et al., *Culture and Nursing Care*, 49.
1916	Lipson and Dibble, eds., *Culture and Clinical Care*, 65.
1917	Purnell and Paulanka, *Guide to Culturally Competent Health Care*, 94.
1918-1919	Lipson and Dibble, eds., *Culture and Clinical Care*, 67.
1920	Purnell and Paulanka, *Guide to Culturally Competent Health Care*, 94.
1921	Lipson and Dibble, eds., *Culture and Clinical Care*, 109.
1922-1923	Lipson et al., *Culture and Nursing Care*, 89.
1924	Ibid., 90.
1925	Ibid., 87.
1926-1928	Ibid., 88.
1929	Ibid., 87.
1930	Lipson and Dibble, eds., *Culture and Clinical Care*, 118.
1931	Ibid., 109.
1932	Lipson et al., *Culture and Nursing Care*, 82.
1933-1934	Lipson and Dibble, eds., *Culture and Clinical Care*, 111.
1935-1937	Lipson et al., *Culture and Nursing Care*, 83.
1938	Ibid., 83–84.
1939-1940	Lipson and Dibble, eds., *Culture and Clinical Care*, 111.
1941	Ibid., 112–13.
1942	Ibid., 113.
1943	Ibid., 112.
1944	Ibid., 113.
1945-1946	Lipson et al., *Culture and Nursing Care*, 84.
1947	Lipson and Dibble, eds., *Culture and Clinical Care*, 113.
1948	Lipson et al., *Culture and Nursing Care*, 84.
1949	Lipson and Dibble, eds., *Culture and Clinical Care*, 118–19.
1950	Ibid., 109–10.
1951	Ibid., 114.
1952-1955	Ibid., 112.
1956-1959	Ibid., 113.
1960	Ibid., 112.
1961	Ibid., 120.

1962	Ibid., 119.
1963-1964	Ibid., 119–20.
1965-1969	Ibid., 119.
1970	Ibid., 109.
1971	Ibid., 119.
1972	Ibid., 120.
1973	F.S. Mead, S.S. Hill, C.D. Atwood, "Roman Catholic Church" in *Handbook of Denominations in the United States*, 13th ed., (Nashville, TN: Abingdon Press, 2010).
1974	Lipson and Dibble, eds., *Culture and Clinical Care*, 114.
1975-1977	Lipson et al., *Culture and Nursing Care*, 86.
1978	Lipson and Dibble, eds., *Culture and Clinical Care*, 114–15.
1979-1981	Ibid., 115.
1982	C. Browner, "The Management of Early Pregnancy: Colombian Folk Concepts of Fertility Control," *Social Science Medicine. Part B: Medical Anthropology* 14, no.1 (Feb. 1980): 25.
1983	W.H. Baldwin and T.R. Ford, "Modernism and Contraceptive Use in Colombia," *Studies in Family Planning* 7, no. 3 (March 1976), 75–79.
1984	Lipson and Dibble, eds., *Culture and Clinical Care*, 115.
1985	Lipson et al., *Culture and Nursing Care*, 89.
1986	D.K. Fina, "The Spiritual Needs of Pediatric Patients and Their Families," *AORN* 62, no. 4 (October 1995): 556–58, 560, 562, 564.
1987	Lipson et al., *Culture and Nursing Care*, 86.
1988-1989	Browner, "Colombian Folk Concepts of Fertility Control," *Social Science Medicine*, 27.
1990	Lipson and Dibble, eds., *Culture and Clinical Care*, 115.
1991	Browner, "Colombian Folk Concepts of Fertility Control," *Social Science Medicine*, 27.
1992-1994	Lipson and Dibble, eds., *Culture and Clinical Care*, 115.
1995-1996	Ibid., 114.
1997	Browner, "Colombian Folk Concepts of Fertility Control," *Social Science Medicine*, 25–32.
1998	Lipson and Dibble, eds., *Culture and Clinical Care*, 116.
1999	Browner, "Colombian Folk Concepts of Fertility Control," Social Science Medicine, 25.
2000-2001	Purnell and Paulanka, *Guide to Culturally Competent Health Care*, 111.
2002	Ibid., 112.
2003	Shah, *Transcultural Aspects of Perinatal Health Care*, 115.
2004	Lipson et al., *Culture and Nursing Care*, 98–99.
2005	Ibid., 98.
2006	D'Avanzo, *Pocket Guide to Cultural Health Assessment* (2008), 193.
2007-2008	Lipson et al., *Culture and Nursing Care*, 99.
2009	Shah, *Transcultural Aspects of Perinatal Health Care*, 92.
2010	Lipson et al., *Culture and Nursing Care*, 99.

2011	Purnell and Paulanka, *Guide to Culturally Competent Health Care*, 116.
2012	Lipson et al., *Culture and Nursing Care*, 92.
2013	Purnell and Paulanka, *Guide to Culturally Competent Health Care*, 103.
2014	Ibid., 102–03.
2015-2017	Ibid., 103.
2018-2019	Ibid., 104.
2020-2023	Lipson et al., *Culture and Nursing Care*, 92.
2024	Ibid., 93.
2025	C. D'Avanzo, *Pocket Guide to Cultural Health Assessment* (St. Louis, MO: Elsevier Mosby, 1996), 238.
2026	Lipson et al., *Culture and Nursing Care*, 93.
2027	Lipson et al., *Culture and Nursing Care*, 94.
2028	D'Avanzo, *Pocket Guide to Cultural Health Assessment* (2008), 196.
2029-2032	Purnell and Paulanka, *Guide to Culturally Competent Health Care*, 107.
2033	Lipson et al., *Culture and Nursing Care*, 94.
2034	Purnell and Paulanka, *Guide to Culturally Competent Health Care*, 107.
2035-2036	Lipson et al., *Culture and Nursing Care*, 94.
2037	Ibid., 97.
2038	Ibid., 93–94.
2039-2042	Ibid., 94.
2043	Purnell and Paulanka, *Guide to Culturally Competent Health Care*, 114.
2044	Ibid., 113–14, 116.
2045	Ibid., 115–16.
2046	Ibid., 114.
2047	Lipson et al., Culture and Nursing Care, 99.
2048	Ibid., 97.
2049	Ibid., 98.
2050	Shah, *Transcultural Aspects of Perinatal Health Care*, 86.
2051	Lipson et al., *Culture and Nursing Care*, 97.
2052	Purnell and Paulanka, *Guide to Culturally Competent Health Care*, 112.
2053	Lipson et al., *Culture and Nursing Care*, 97.
2054	Ibid., 94–95
2055	Ibid., 94.
2056-2057	Ibid., 95.
2058-2059	Ibid., 97.
2060	Purnell and Paulanka, *Guide to Culturally Competent Health Care*, 111.
2061	Ibid., 110-11.
2062	Ibid., 110.

2063-2065   Ibid., 110.

2066-2067   Ibid., 111.

2068   Lipson et al., *Culture and Nursing Care*, 93.

2069   Shah, *Transcultural Aspects of Perinatal Health Care*, 91–100.

2070-2071   Lipson et al., *Culture and Nursing Care*, 96.

2072-2073   Ibid., 97.

2074   Ibid., 93, 97.

2075   Giger and Davidhizar, "Cuban Americans" in *Transcultural Nursing*.

2076   Purnell and Paulanka, *Guide to Culturally Competent Health Care*, 110.

2077-2078   Lipson et al., *Culture and Nursing Care*, 96.

2079   Shah, *Transcultural Aspects of Perinatal Health Care*, 105.

2080   Ibid., 107.

2081   Lipson et al., *Culture and Nursing Care*, 96.

2082-2083   Purnell and Paulanka, *Guide to Culturally Competent Health Care*, 110.

2084   Lipson et al., *Culture and Nursing Care*, 96.

2085   Lipson and Dibble, eds., *Culture and Clinical Care*, 127.

2086   Shah, *Transcultural Aspects of Perinatal Health Care*, 108.

2087   Lipson et al., *Culture and Nursing Care*, 96.

2088   Shah, *Transcultural Aspects of Perinatal Health Care*, 101.

2089   Ibid., 115.

2090   Ibid., 109.

2091   Lipson et al., *Culture and Nursing Care*, 96.

2092   Shah, *Transcultural Aspects of Perinatal Health Care*, 105.

2093   Ibid., 109.

2094   Ibid., 110.

2095   D.K. Fina, "The Spiritual Needs of Pediatric Patients," *AORN*, 556–58, 560, 562, 564.

2096   Shah, *Transcultural Aspects of Perinatal Health Care*, 110.

2097   Ibid., 114.

2098   Ibid., 106.

2099   Purnell and Paulanka, *Guide to Culturally Competent Health Care*, 110.

2100-2101   Shah, *Transcultural Aspects of Perinatal Health Care*, 106.

2102   Purnell and Paulanka, *Guide to Culturally Competent Health Care*, 109.

2103-2104   Lipson et al., *Culture and Nursing Care*, 96.

2105   Ibid., 95.

2106   Shah, *Transcultural Aspects of Perinatal Health Care*, 101.

2107   Ibid., 111.

2108   Ibid., 87, 92.

2109   Ibid., 112.

2110   Ibid., 97.

2111   Ibid., 101.

2112-2113   Lipson and Dibble, eds., *Culture and Clinical Care*, 126.

2114   Ibid., 127.

2115-2120   Lipson and Dibble, eds., *Culture and Clinical Care*, 133.

2121   Ibid., 142–43.

2122   Ibid., 143.

2123   Ibid., 140.

2124   Ibid., 141.

2125   Ibid., 143.

2126-2134   Ibid., 134.

2135-2141   Ibid., 135.

2142   Ibid., 135–36.

2143   Ibid., 141.

2144-2152   Ibid., 137.

2153-2159   Ibid., 136.

2160-2161   Ibid., 138.

2162-2163   Ibid., 142.

2164-2165   Ibid., 137.

2166-2169   Ibid., 138.

2170-2171   Ibid., 145.

2172-2176   Ibid., 144.

2177-2178   Ibid., 145.

2179   "The Sacraments: Baptism," American Catholic.org, accessed January 9, 2012, http://www.americancatholic.org/features/special/default.aspx?id=30.

2180   Lipson and Dibble, eds., *Culture and Clinical Care*, 137.

2181-2186   Ibid., 139.

2100-2100   Ihid., 140.

2189-2190   Ibld., 139.

2191   Ibid., 143.

2192-2193   Ibid., 139.

2194   "The Sacraments: Baptism," American Catholic.org, accessed January 9, 2012, http://www.americancatholic.org/features/special/default.aspx?id=30.

2195-2196   Lipson and Dibble, eds., *Culture and Clinical Care*, 139.

2197   Ibid., 136.

2198-2201   Ibid., 139.

2202   Ibid., 138.

2203   Ibid., 140.

2204   Ibid., 144.

2205   Giger and Davidhizar, *Transcultural Nursing,* 257–58.

2206   H. Dominguez-Ruvalcaba and I. Corona, eds., *Gender Violence at the U.S.–Mexico Border* (Arizona: University of Arizona Press, 2010), 79.

2207   D.A. Prentice and D.T. Miller, eds., *Cultural Divides: Understanding and Overcoming Group Conflict* (New York: Russell Sage Foundation, 1999), 323.

2208   Giger and Davidhizar, *Transcultural Nursing,* 254.

2209   Ibid., 256.

2210   E.R. Calvillo, and J.H. Flaskerud, "Review of Literature on Culture and Pain of Adults with Focus on Mexican-Americans" *Journal of Transcultural Nursing* 2, no. 2 (Winter 1991), 19.

2211   M.J. Dummer Clark, *Community Health Nursing: Caring for Populations* (Upper Saddle River, NJ: Prentice Hall, 2003), 121.

2212   Dresser, *Multicultural Manners* (2005), 136.

2213   Ibid., 87–88.

2214   Lipson and Dibble, eds., *Culture and Clinical Care,* 334.

2215   Giger and Davidhizar, *Transcultural Nursing,* 248–49, 251..

2216   Lipson and Dibble, eds., *Culture and Clinical Care,* 337.

2217   Ibid., 348.

2218   Shah, *Transcultural Aspects of Perinatal Health Care,* 229.

2219-2220   Lipson and Dibble, eds., *Culture and Clinical Care,* 331.

2221-2222   Ibid., 332.

2223   Ibid., 332–34.

2224-2225   Ibid., 331.

2226   Ibid., 331–32.

2227-2228   Ibid., 332.

2229-2230   Ibid., 333.

2231   J. Klessig, "Cross-Cultural Medicine a Decade Later: The Effect of Values and Culture on Life-Support Decisions," *Western Journal of Medicine* 157, no. 3 (September 1992): 321.

2232-2234   Lipson and Dibble, eds., *Culture and Clinical Care,* 333.

2235-2236   Ibid., 332.

2237   Ibid., 334.

2238   Purnell and Paulanka, *Guide to Culturally Competent Health Care,* 295.

2239   Galanti, *Caring for Patients From Different Cultures,* 238.

2240   Lipson and Dibble, eds., *Culture and Clinical Care,* 334.

2241   Purnell and Paulanka, *Guide to Culturally Competent Health Care,* 295.

2242-2245   Lipson and Dibble, eds., *Culture and Clinical Care,* 334.

2246-2247	Ibid., 333.
2248-2251	Ibid., 334.
2252	Ibid., 339.
2253	Andrews and Boyle, *Transcultural Concepts in Nursing Care*, 212.
2254	Ibid., 222.
2255	Prentice and Miller, *Cultural Divides*, 323.
2256	N. Dresser, *Multicultural Manners* (1996), 247.
2257	J. Klessig, "Cross-Cultural Medicine," *Western Journal of Medicine*, 321.
2258	Giger and Davidhizar, *Transcultural Nursing,* 258.
2259	D'Avanzo, *Pocket Guide to Cultural Health Assessment* (1994), 154.
2260	Giger and Davidhizar, *Transcultural Nursing,* 253.
2261	Calvillo and Flaskerud, "Review of Literature on Culture and Pain," *Journal of Transcultural Nursing*, 19.
2262-2263	Lipson and Dibble, eds., *Culture and Clinical Care*, 335.
2264	Ibid., 342.
2265-2270	Ibid., 341.
2271-2273	Purnell and Paulanka, *Guide to Culturally Competent Health Care*, 298.
2274	N. Williams, *The Mexican American Family: Tradition and Change* (Walnut Creek, CA: AltaMira Press, 2003), 75.
2275	J. Klessig, "Cross-Cultural Medicine," *Western Journal of Medicine*, 321.
2276-2277	Lipson and Dibble, eds., *Culture and Clinical Care*, 341.
2278	Lipson et al., *Culture and Nursing Care*, 213.
2279	Giger and Davidhizar, *Transcultural Nursing,* 258.
2280	Ibid., 248.
2281-2282	Shah, *Transcultural Aspects of Perinatal Health Care*, 230.
2283	Lipson and Dibble, eds., *Culture and Clinical Care*, 336.
2284	Giger and Davidhizar, *Transcultural Nursing*, 34, 262.
2285	Lipson and Dibble, eds., *Culture and Clinical Care*, 337.
2286-2287	Shah, *Transcultural Aspects of Perinatal Health Care*, 234.
2288	Lipson and Dibble, eds., *Culture and Clinical Care*, 337.
2289	Shah, *Transcultural Aspects of Perinatal Health Care*, 231.
2290	Purnell and Paulanka, *Guide to Culturally Competent Health Care*, 297.
2291	Lipson and Dibble, eds., *Culture and Clinical Care*, 336.
2292	Shah, *Transcultural Aspects of Perinatal Health Care*, 232.
2293	Ibid., 235.
2294	Lipson and Dibble, eds., *Culture and Clinical Care*, 340.
2295	Shah, *Transcultural Aspects of Perinatal Health Care*, 228.
2296-2298	Lipson and Dibble, eds., *Culture and Clinical Care*, 337.

2299   "The Sacraments: Baptism," American Catholic.org, accessed January 9, 2012, http://www.americancatholic.org/features/special/default.aspx?id=30.

2300   Shah, *Transcultural Aspects of Perinatal Health Care*, 235.

2301-2302   Purnell and Paulanka, *Guide to Culturally Competent Health Care*, 297.

2303   Lipson and Dibble, eds., *Culture and Clinical Care*, 336.

2304   Shah, *Transcultural Aspects of Perinatal Health Care*, 232.

2305   Ibid., 233.

2306   Ibid., 234.

2307   Giger and Davidhizar, *Transcultural Nursing,* 245, 259.

2308   Lipson and Dibble, eds., *Culture and Clinical Care*, 336.

2309   Shah, *Transcultural Aspects of Perinatal Health Care*, 232.

2310   Lipson and Dibble, eds., *Culture and Clinical Care*, 336.

2311   Purnell and Paulanka, *Guide to Culturally Competent Health Care*, 297.

2312   Shah, *Transcultural Aspects of Perinatal Health Care*, 232.

2313   Purnell and Paulanka, *Guide to Culturally Competent Health Care*, 297.

2314   Shah, *Transcultural Aspects of Perinatal Health Care*, 232.

2315   Ibid., 227–28.

2316   Andrews and Boyle, *Transcultural Concepts in Nursing Care*, 342.

2317   Shah, *Transcultural Aspects of Perinatal Health Care*, 228–29.

2318   Ibid., 228.

2319   Ibid., 230.

2320   Ibid., 227.

2321   G.A. Galanti, *Caring for Patients From Different Cultures*, 3rd ed. (Philadelphia, PA: University of Pennsylvania Press, 2004), 125.

2322-2323   Shah, *Transcultural Aspects of Perinatal Health Care*, 230.

2324   Purnell and Paulanka, *Guide to Culturally Competent Health Care*, 297.

2325   Lipson and Dibble, eds., *Culture and Clinical Care*, 337.

2326   Shah, *Transcultural Aspects of Perinatal Health Care*, 229.

2327   Lipson and Dibble, eds., Culture and Clinical Care, 336.

2328   J.L. Bonkowsky, J.K. Frazer, K.F. Buchi, and C.L. Byington, "Metamizole Use by Latino Immigrants: A Common and Potentially Harmful Home Remedy" *Pediatrics* 109, no. 6 (June 1, 2002).

2329   Lipson and Dibble, eds., *Culture and Clinical Care*, 331.

2330   Giger and Davidhizar, *Transcultural Nursing*, 259.

2331-2334   Lipson et al., Culture and Nursing Care, 235.

2335   Dresser, Multicultural Manners (2005), 87–88.

2336   Purnell and Paulanka, Guide to Culturally Competent Health Care, 338.

2337   Ibid., 339–40.

2338   Ibid., 325.

2339	Ibid., 341.
2340-2343	Lipson et al., Culture and Nursing Care, 223.
2344-2345	Ibid., 224.
2346-2347	Purnell and Paulanka, Guide to Culturally Competent Health Care, 322.
2348	Lipson and Dibble, eds., Culture and Clinical Care, 339.
2349	Purnell and Paulanka, Guide to Culturally Competent Health Care, 322, 325.
2350	Purnell and Paulanka, Guide to Culturally Competent Health Care, 323.
2351	Ibid., 322.
2352	Ibid., 322, 326.
2353-2354	Lipson et al., Culture and Nursing Care, 225.
2355	Lipson et al., Culture and Nursing Care, 227.
2356-2357	Purnell and Paulanka, Guide to Culturally Competent Health Care, 328.
2358-2364	Lipson et al., Culture and Nursing Care, 228.
2365	Ibid., 228.
2366	Purnell and Paulanka, Guide to Culturally Competent Health Care, 338.
2367	Lipson et al., Culture and Nursing Care, 233.
2368	Ibid., 229–30.
2369	Ibid., 233.
2370	Ibid., 234.
2371	Ibid., 233–34.
2372	Purnell and Paulanka, Guide to Culturally Competent Health Care, 338.
2373	Lipson et al., Culture and Nursing Care, 234.
2374-2376	Lipson et al., Culture and Nursing Care, 228.
2377	Ibid., 229–30.
2378	Purnell and Paulanka, Guide to Culturally Competent Health Care, 340.
2379	Ibid., 232.
2380	Purnell and Paulanka, Guide to Culturally Competent Health Care, 337.
2381	Lipson et al., Culture and Nursing Care, 231–32.
2382	Ibid., 232.
2383	Ibid., 231–32.
2384	Ibid., 231.
2385	Andrews and Boyle, Transcultural Concepts in Nursing Care, 367.
2386	Ibid., 226.
2387	"The Sacraments: Baptism," American Catholic.org, accessed January 9, 2012, http://www.americancatholic.org/features/special/default.aspx?id=30.
2388	Lipson et al., Culture and Nursing Care, 230.
2389	C.B. Rosdahl, M.T. Kowalski, Textbook of Basic Nursing (Philadelphia, PA: Lippincott Williams & Wilkins, 2008), 909.

2390   Purnell and Paulanka, Guide to Culturally Competent Health Care, 336.

2391   Lipson et al., *Culture and Nursing Care*, 230.

2392   Purnell and Paulanka, *Guide to Culturally Competent Health Care*, 336.

2393   Ibid., 328, 336.

2394   Ibid., 336.

2395   Lipson et al., *Culture and Nursing Care*, 231.

2396   Purnell and Paulanka, *Guide to Culturally Competent Health Care*, 335.

2397   Ibid., 327.

2398   Lipson et al., *Culture and Nursing Care*, 230.

2399   Ibid., 231.

2400   Ibid., 236.

2401   Ibid., 231.

2402   "The Sacraments: Baptism," American Catholic.org, accessed January 9, 2012, http://www.americancatholic.org/features/special/default.aspx?id=30.

2403   Lipson and Dibble, eds., *Culture and Clinical Care*, 397.

2404   Lipson et al., *Culture and Nursing Care*, 231.

2405   Ibid., 231.

2406-2407   Purnell and Paulanka, *Guide to Culturally Competent Health Care*, 335.

2408-2409   Lipson et al., *Culture and Nursing Care*, 230.

2410   Purnell and Paulanka, *Guide to Culturally Competent Health Care*, 335.

2411   "Abortion: What the Church Teaches," American Catholic.org, accessed January 13, 2012, http://www.americancatholic.org/Newsletters/CU/ac0898.asp.

2412-2413   Lipson et al., *Culture and Nursing Care*, 227.

2414   "Cultural Aspects of Healthcare," College of St. Scholastica Athens Project, accessed December 30, 2011, http://www.css.edu/Academics/ATHENS-Project/Help-Page/Cultural-Aspects-of-Healthcare.html.

2415   Purnell and Paulanka, *Guide to Culturally Competent Health Care*, 75.

2416   "Islam and Health," Boston University School of Medicine, Boston Healing Landscape Project, accessed January 14, 2012, http://www.bu.edu/bhlp/Resources/Islam/index.html.

2417   Purnell and Paulanka, *Guide to Culturally Competent Health Care*, 72.

2418   Lipson and Dibble, eds., *Culture and Clinical Care*, 44–45.

2419   Ibid., 43–45.

2420   Ibid., 45.

2421-2422   Ibid., 47.

2423   "Cultural Aspects of Healthcare," http://www.css.edu/Academics/ATHENS-Project/Help-Page/Cultural-Aspects-of-Healthcare.html.

2424   "Cultural Aspects of Healthcare," http://www.css.edu/Academics/ATHENS-Project/Help-Page/Cultural-Aspects-of-Healthcare.html.

2425   Lipson and Dibble, eds., *Culture and Clinical Care*, 46.

2426   "Cultural Aspects of Healthcare," http://www.css.edu/Academics/ATHENS-Project/Help-Page/Cultural-Aspects-of-Healthcare.html.

2427   Lipson and Dibble, eds., *Culture and Clinical Care*, 46.

2428   L.A. Abushaikha, "Methods of Coping with Labor Pain Used by Jordanian Women," *Journal of Transcultural Nursing* 18, no. 1 (January 2007): 39.

2429   "Cultural Aspects of Healthcare," http://www.css.edu/Academics/ATHENS-Project/Help-Page/Cultural-Aspects-of-Healthcare.html.

2430   Lipson and Dibble, eds., *Culture and Clinical Care*, 48.

2431   "Cultural Aspects of Healthcare," http://www.css.edu/Academics/ATHENS-Project/Help-Page/Cultural-Aspects-of-Healthcare.html.

2432   Lipson and Dibble, eds., *Culture and Clinical Care*, 47.

2433   N. Sarhill, S. LeGrand, R. Islambouli, M.P. Davis, and D. Walsh, "The Terminally Ill Muslim: Death and Dying from the Muslim Perspective," *American Journal of Hospice & Palliative Medicine* 18, no. 4 (July/August, 2001): 253.

2434   Andrews and Boyle, *Transcultural Concepts in Nursing Care*, 393.

2435   "Cultural Aspects of Healthcare," http://www.css.edu/Academics/ATHENS-Project/Help-Page/Cultural-Aspects-of-Healthcare.html.

2436   "Cultural Aspects of Healthcare," http://www.css.edu/Academics/ATHENS-Project/Help-Page/Cultural-Aspects-of-Healthcare.html.

2437-2438   Lipson and Dibble, eds., *Culture and Clinical Care*, 56.

2439   Sarhill et al., "The Terminally Ill Muslim," *American Journal of Hospice & Palliative Medicine*, 252.

2440   Lipson and Dibble, eds., *Culture and Clinical Care*, 55.

2441   Ibid., 56.

2442   Ibid., 44.

2443   Ibid., 56.

2444   M. Crawshaw and M. Balen, eds., *Adopting After Infertility* (Philadelphia, PA: Jessica Kingsley Publishers, 2010), 112.

2445   Lipson and Dibble, eds., *Culture and Clinical Care*, 50.

2446   M.M. Leininger and M.R. McFarland, *Culture Care Diversity and Universality: A Worldwide Nursing Theory* (Sudbury, MA: Jones and Bartlett Publishers, 2006), 173.

2447   "Cultural Aspects of Healthcare," http://www.css.edu/Academics/ATHENS-Project/Help-Page/Cultural-Aspects-of-Healthcare.html.

2448   Abushaikha, "Methods of Coping with Labor Pain," *Journal of Transcultural Nursing*, 39.

2449   Ibid., 38–39.

2450   K.L. Mauk and N.K. Schmidt, *Spiritual Care in Nursing Practice* (Philadelphia, PA: Lippincott Williams & Wilkins, 2004), 105.

2451   Lipson and Dibble, eds., *Culture and Clinical Care*, 50.

2452   Ibid., 51.

2453   M.M. Hammoud, C.B. White, and M.D. Fetters, "Opening Cultural Doors: Providing Culturally Sensitive Healthcare to Arab American and American Muslim Patients," *American Journal of Obstetrics & Gynecology* 193, no. 4 (October 2005): 1310.

2454-2455   Lipson and Dibble, eds., *Culture and Clinical Care*, 50.

2456   Hammoud et al., "Opening Cultural Doors," *American Journal of Obstetrics & Gynecology*, 1311.

2457   Lipson and Dibble, eds., *Culture and Clinical Care*, 50.

2458   Ibid., 46.

2459   Ibid., 50.

2460-2461   Ibid., 49.

2462   Ibid., 51.

2463   Hammoud et al., "Opening Cultural Doors," *American Journal of Obstetrics & Gynecology*, 1311.

2464   Lipson et al., *Culture and Nursing Care*, 146–51.

2465-2466   Andrews and Boyle, *Transcultural Concepts in Nursing Care*, 195–97.

2467   Giger and Davidhizar, *Transcultural Nursing*, 578.

2468   Ibid., 575–77, 583.

2469   D'Avanzo, *Pocket Guide to Cultural Health Assessment* (2008), 304.

2470   Giger and Davidhizar, *Transcultural Nursing*, 573.

2471   J. Reier, *McGraw-Hill's GED Language Arts, Reading* (New York: McGraw-Hill, 2003), 2.

2472   Purnell and Paulanka, *Guide to Culturally Competent Health Care*, 184.

2473   Giger and Davidhizar, *Transcultural Nursing*, 569–70.

2474-2476   Purnell and Paulanka, *Guide to Culturally Competent Health Care*, 170, 174.

2477   D'Avanzo, *Pocket Guide to Cultural Health Assessment* (2008), 307.

2478   Lipson et al., *Culture and Nursing Care*, 144.

2479   Andrews and Boyle, *Transcultural Concepts in Nursing Care*, 196.

2480   Ibid., 192–99.

2481   D'Avanzo, *Pocket Guide to Cultural Health Assessment* (2008), 304–08.

2482   Giger and Davidhizar, *Transcultural Nursing*, 568, 573, 576.

2483   Lipson et al., *Culture and Nursing Care*, 147.

2484   Purnell and Paulanka, *Guide to Culturally Competent Health Care*, 187.

2485   Andrews and Boyle, *Transcultural Concepts in Nursing Care*, 196.

2486   Purnell and Paulanka, *Guide to Culturally Competent Health Care*, 170, 183.

2487   Lipson et al., *Culture and Nursing Care*, 145–47.

2488   Ibid., 145–47.

2489   Ibid., 150.

2490-2491   Ibid., 142–50.

2492   D'Avanzo, *Pocket Guide to Cultural Health Assessment* (2008), 306.

2493   Ibid., 306.

2494   Ibid., 150.

2495   Purnell and Paulanka, *Guide to Culturally Competent Health Care*, 184.

2496   Giger and Davidhizar, *Transcultural Nursing*, 576–77.

2497   D'Avanzo, *Pocket Guide to Cultural Health Assessment* (2008), 306.

2498   Purnell and Paulanka, *Guide to Culturally Competent Health Care*, 169–85.

2499   Lipson et al., *Culture and Nursing Care*, 145–47.

2500   Giger and Davidhizar, *Transcultural Nursing,* 582.

2501   Lipson et al., *Culture and Nursing Care*, 148–49.

2502   Andrews and Boyle, *Transcultural Concepts in Nursing Care*, 199.

2503   Purnell and Paulanka, *Guide to Culturally Competent Health Care*, 173.

2504   Ibid., 179.

2505   Giger and Davidhizar, *Transcultural Nursing,* , 576.

2506   Ibid., 577.

2507   Andrews and Boyle, *Transcultural Concepts in Nursing Care*, 196.

2508   Giger and Davidhizar, *Transcultural Nursing*, 576.

2509   Ibid., 576–77.

2510   D'Avanzo, *Pocket Guide to Cultural Health Assessment* (2008), 307.

2511   Ibid., 306.

2512   Purnell and Paulanka, *Guide to Culturally Competent Health Care*, 177.

2513   "Religion in Jamaica," Jamaica-Guide.info, accessed January 14, 2012, http://jamaica-guide.info/past.and.present/religion/.

2514   "Jamaica—Religion," Countries and their Cultures, accessed January 14, 2012, http://www.everyculture.com/Ja-Ma/Jamaica.html.

2515   Shah, *Transcultural Aspects of Perinatal Health Care*, 148.

2516   D'Avanzo, *Pocket Guide to Cultural Health Assessment* (2008), 356.

2517   "Jamaica—Marriage, Family, and Kinship," Countries and their Cultures, accessed January 14, 2012, http://www.everyculture.com/Ja-Ma/Jamaica.html.

2518   D'Avanzo, *Pocket Guide to Cultural Health Assessment* (2008), 359.

2519-2520   Shah, *Transcultural Aspects of Perinatal Health Care*, 142.

2521   Lipson et al., *Culture and Nursing Care*, 302.

2522   "Culture of Jamaica," Jamaica-Guide.info, accessed January 14, 2012, http://jamaica-guide.info/past.and.present/culture/.

2523-2524   Lipson et al., *Culture and Nursing Care*, 292.

2525   Ibid., 293.

2526   Lipson and Dibble, eds., *Culture and Clinical Care*, 463–65.

2527   Lipson et al., *Culture and Nursing Care*, 293.

2528   Shah, *Transcultural Aspects of Perinatal Health Care*, 139.

2529   Lipson et al., *Culture and Nursing Care*, 295.

2530   "Culture of Jamaica," Jamaica-Guide.info, accessed January 14, 2012, http://jamaica-guide.info/past.and.present/culture/.

2531   Lipson and Dibble, eds., *Culture and Clinical Care*, 465–67.

2532   Shah, *Transcultural Aspects of Perinatal Health Care*, 139.

2533   Lipson and Dibble, eds., *Culture and Clinical Care*, 465–67.

2534   Shah, *Transcultural Aspects of Perinatal Health Care*, 136.

2535   "Jamaica—Medicine and Health Care," Countries and their Cultures, accessed January 14, 2012, http://www.everyculture.com/Ja-Ma/Jamaica.html.

2536-2538   Shah, *Transcultural Aspects of Perinatal Health Care*, 134.

2539   Lipson and Dibble, eds., *Culture and Clinical Care*, 463.

2540   Lipson et al., *Culture and Nursing Care*, 298.

2541   Ibid., 296.

2542-2543   Ibid., 299.

2544   Lipson and Dibble, eds., *Culture and Clinical Care*, 472.

2545   Lipson et al., *Culture and Nursing Care*, 299.

2546   "Jamaica—Religion," Countries and their Cultures, accessed January 14, 2012, http://www.everyculture.com/Ja-Ma/Jamaica.html.

2547   Lipson et al., *Culture and Nursing Care*, 293.

2548   J. Gillman, "Religious Perspectives on Organ Donation," *Critical Care Nursing Quarterly* 22, no.3 (1999): 22.

2549   "Jamaica—Socialization," Countries and their Cultures, accessed January 14, 2012, http://www.everyculture.com/Ja-Ma/Jamaica.html.

2550-2551   Lipson et al., *Culture and Nursing Care*, 298.

2552   Shah, *Transcultural Aspects of Perinatal Health Care*, 144.

2553   D'Avanzo, *Pocket Guide to Cultural Health Assessment* (2008), 359.

2554   Shah, *Transcultural Aspects of Perinatal Health Care*, 145.

2555   Ibid., 146.

2556   Lipson et al., *Culture and Nursing Care*, 298.

2557   Lipson and Dibble, eds., *Culture and Clinical Care*, 467–68.

2558   Shah, *Transcultural Aspects of Perinatal Health Care*, 147.

2559   Ibid., 149.

2560   Lipson et al., *Culture and Nursing Care*, 297.

2561   Ibid., 302.

2562   Shah, *Transcultural Aspects of Perinatal Health Care*, 142.

2563   Lipson et al., *Culture and Nursing Care*, 298.

2564   "Jamaica—Socialization," Countries and their Cultures, accessed January 14, 2012, http://www.everyculture.com/Ja-Ma/Jamaica.html.

2565   Dresser, *Multicultural Manners* (1996), 18.

2566   Shah, *Transcultural Aspects of Perinatal Health Care*, 146.

2567   Lipson and Dibble, eds., *Culture and Clinical Care*, 465–67.

2568   Shah, *Transcultural Aspects of Perinatal Health Care*, 151.

2569   Lipson et al., *Culture and Nursing Care*, 293–94.

2570   Shah, *Transcultural Aspects of Perinatal Health Care*, 139–41.

2571   Ibid., 142.

2572   "Jamaica—Socialization," Countries and their Cultures, accessed January 14, 2012, http://www.everyculture.com/Ja-Ma/Jamaica.html.

2573   Lipson and Dibble, eds., *Culture and Clinical Care*, 467–68.

2574   Lipson et al., *Culture and Nursing Care*, 297.

2575-2576   Shah, *Transcultural Aspects of Perinatal Health Care*, 143.

2577   Ibid., 146.

DISABILITIES

2578   "Americans with Disabilities: 2005," M.W. Brault, US Census Bureau, updated December 2008), http://www.census.gov/prod/2008pubs/p70-117.pdf.

2579   L.I. Iezzoni, R.B. Davis, J. Soukup, and B. O'Day, "Satisfaction with Quality and Access to Health Care Among People with Disabling Conditions," *International Journal for Quality in Health Care* 14, no. 5 (2002), 369–81.

2580-2581   Institute of Medicine, Committee on Quality of Health Care in America, *Crossing the Quality Chasm: A New Health System for the 21st Century* (Washington, DC: National Academy Press, 2001).

2582   "Left Out in the Cold: Healthcare Experiences of Adults with Intellectual and Developmental Disabilities in Massachusetts," A.D. Nichols, R.L. Ward, R.I. Freedman, and L.V. Sarkissian , The Boston Foundation, updated December 2008), http://www.arcmass.org/Portals/0/TheArcofMassHealthCareFullReport_12.08.pdf.

2583   "Categories of Disability Under IDEA," National Dissemination Center for Children with Disabilities, updated April 2009, http://nichcy.org/disability/categories/.

2584-2585   "Communicating With and About People with Disabilities," U.S. Department of Labor, accessed January 18, 2012, http://www.dol.gov/odep/pubs/fact/comucate.htm.

2586-2587   "Advance Health Care Directives and Health Care Decision-making for Incompetent Patients: A Guide to Act 169 of 2006 for Physicians and Other Health Care Professionals," Pennsylvania Medical Society, accessed January 18, 2012, http://www.pcacc.org/advance_health_directives.pdf.

2588-2591   E.M. Carty, Disability and Childbirth: Meeting the Challenges, *Canadian Medical Association Journal* 159, no. 4 (Aug. 1998): 363–69, http://www.canadianmedicaljournal.ca/content/159/4/363.full.pdf

2592-2593   "Gynecologic and Obstetric Issues Confronting Women with Disabilities," S. Welner and C. Hammond, Global Library of Women's Medicine, last updated August 2009, http://www.glowm.com/index.html?p=glowm.cml/section_view&articleid=76.

2594-2597   "Communicating With and About People with Disabilities," U.S. Department of Labor, accessed January 18, 2012, http://www.dol.gov/odep/pubs/fact/comucate.htm.

2598   "Health Care Reform: What Does it Mean for the Autism Community?" Autism Speaks Official Blog, posted March 23, 2010, http://blog.autismspeaks.org/2010/03/23/health-care-reform/.

2599-2601   J.G. Goepp, "Autism: A Nutraceutical Approach, *Life Extension Magazine* (December 2007), 53–60.

2002   R. Ray Mihm, "Autism: Part 1 Deficits, Prevalence, Symptoms, and Environmental Factors" *Journal of Continuing Education in Nursing* 39, no. 2 (February 2008): 55–56.

2603-2605   "Autism," University of Virginia Children's Hospital, accessed January 15, 2012, http://uvahealth.com/services/childrens-hospital/conditions-treatments/12028/?searchterm=autism.

2606   Goepp, "Autism: A Nutraceutical Approach," *Life Extension Magazine* (December 2007), 53–60.

2607   "Autism," University of Virginia, http://uvahealth.com/services/childrens-hospital/conditions-treatments/12028/?searchterm=autism.

2608-2611   D. Nelson and K. Amplo, "Care of the Autistic Patient in the Perioperative Area" *AORN Journal* 89, no. 2 (February 2009): 391–397.

2612-2613   *Goepp, "Autism," Life Extension Magazine,* 53–60.

2614-2618   Nelson and Amplo, "Care of the Autistic Patient in the Perioperative Area" *AORN Journal,* 391–397.

2619-2620   M. Beard-Pfeuffer, "Understanding the World of Children with Autism" *RN* 71, no. 2 (February 2008): 40–46.

2621-2623   Nelson and Amplo, "Care of the Autistic Patient in the Perioperative Area" *AORN Journal,* 391–397.

2624   M. Beard-Pfeuffer, "Understanding the World," *RN,* 40–46.

2625   Nelson and Amplo, "Care of the Autistic Patient in the Perioperative Area" *AORN Journal,* 391–397.

2626   M. Beard-Pfeuffer, "Understanding the World," *RN,* 40–46.

2627-2629   Nelson and Amplo, "Care of the Autistic Patient in the Perioperative Area" *AORN Journal,* 391–397.

2630   D.D. Dell, M. Feleccia, L. Hicks, E. Longstreth-Papsun, S. Politsky, and C. Trommer, "Care of Patients with Autism Spectrum Disorder Undergoing Surgery for Cancer," *Oncology Nursing Forum* 35, no. 2 (March 2008): 177–182.

2631-2633   B.L. Handen and M. Lubetsky, "Pharmacotherapy in Autism and Related Disorders" *School Psychology Quarterly* 20, no. 2 (2005): 155–171.

2634   E. Hollander, R. Dolgoff-Kaspar, C. Cartwright, R. Rawitt, and S. Novotny, "An Open Trial of Divalproex Sodium in Autism Spectrum Disorders," *Journal of Clinical Psychiatry* 62, no. 7 (July 2001): 530–534.

2635   J. Komoto, S. Usui, and J. Hirata, "Infantile Autism and Affective Disorder," *Journal of Autism and Developmental Disorders* 14, no. 1 (1984), 81–84.

2636   T.A. Rugino and T.C. Samsock, "Levetiracetam in Autistic Children: An Open-Label Study," *Journal of Developmental & Behavioral Pediatrics* 23, no. 4 (August 2002): 225–230.

2637   B.L. Handen, C.R. Johnson, and M. Lubetsky, "Efficacy of Methylphenidate Among Children with Autism and Symptoms of Attention-Deficit Hyperactivity Disorder," *Journal of Autism and Developmental Disorders* 30, no. 3 (2000), 245–255.

2638   R. Antochi, C. Stavrakaki, and P.C. Emery, "Psychopharmacological Treatments in Persons with Dual Diagnosis of Psychiatric Disorders and Developmental Disabilities," *Postgraduate Medical Journal* 79, no. 929 (2003): 139–46.

2639   M. Campbell, B. Fish, R. David, T. Shapiro, P. Collins, and C. Koh, "Response to Triiodothyronine and Dextroamphetamine: A Study of Preschool Schizophrenic Children," *Journal of Autism and Developmental Disorders* 2, no. 4, 343–358.

2640   A. Di Martino, G. Melis, C. Cianchetti, and A. Zuddas, "Methylphenidate for Pervasive Developmental Disorders: Safety and Efficacy of Acute Single Dose Test and Ongoing Therapy: An Open-Pilot Study," *Journal of Child and Adolescent Psychopharmacology* 14, no. 2 (Aug. 25, 2004): 207–218.

2641   K. Bock and C. Stauth, *Healing the New Childhood Epidemics: Autism, ADHD, Asthma, and Allergies* (New York: Ballantine Books, 2007), 340.

2642   Handen et al.,"Efficacy of Methylphenidate," *Journal of Autism and Developmental Disorders,* 245–255.

2643-2645   D.J. Lee, B.L. Lam, S. Arora, K.L. Arheart, K.E. McCollister, D.D. Zheng, S.L. Christ, and E.P. Davila, "Reported Eye Care Utilization and Health Insurance Status Among US Adults," *Archives of Ophthalmology* 127, no. 3 (March 2009): 303–310.

2646   T.L. Carter, "Age-related Vision Changes: A Primary Care Guide," *Geriatrics* 49, no. 9 (1994): 37–42, 45.

2647   D.C. Fletcher, "Low Vision: The Physician's Role in Rehabilitation and Referral," *Geriatrics* 49, no. 5 (May 1994): 50–53.

2648   E.A. Rosenberg and L.C. Sperazza, "The Visually Impaired Patient," *American Family Physician* 77, no. 10 (2008): 1431–1436, 1437–38. Available from www.aafp.org/afp.

2649   Carter, "Age-related Vision Changes," *Geriatrics,* 37–42, 45.

2650   T.D. Castor and T.L. Carter, "Low Vision: Physician Screening Helps to Improve Patient Function," *Geriatrics* 50, no. 12 (Dec. 1995): 51–52, 55–57.

2651-2652   U.S. Equal Employment Opportunity Commission, *Communicating and Interacting with People Who Have Disabilities* (Upland, PA: DIANE Publishing Company, n.d.): 5–6.

2653   U.S. EEOC, *Communicating and Interacting with People Who Have Disabilities*, 5–6.

2654   L.A. Samovar, R.E. Porter, and E.R. McDaniel, *Intercultural Communication: A Reader*, 13ᵗʰ ed. (Boston, MA: Wadsworth, 2012), 250.

2655-2657   U.S. EEOC, *Communicating and Interacting with People Who Have Disabilities*, 5–6.

2658   "Guidelines for Medical Professionals," Earle Baum Center, updated April 2004, http://earlebaum.org/guidelines-and-information/guidelies-for-medical-professionals/.

2659   "The Blind Child in the Elementary Classroom," C. Castellano, accessed January 15, 2012, http://www.blindchildren.org/textonly/to_edu_dev/3_5_5.html.

2660   "Guidelines for Medical Professionals," Earle Baum Center, updated April 2004, http://earlebaum.org/guidelines-and-information/guidelies-for-medical-professionals/.

2661   "Guidelines for Medical Professionals," Earle Baum Center, updated April 2004, http://earlebaum.org/guidelines-and-information/guidelies-for-medical-professionals/.

2662   H.R. Taylor, "Fred Hollows Lecture: Eye Care for the Community," *Clinical and Experimental Ophthalmology* 30, no. 3 (June 2002): 151–154.

2663   M. Scheiman, M. Scheiman, and S.G. Whittaker, *Low Vision Rehabilitation: A Practical Guide for Occupational Therapists* (Thorofare, NJ: Slack Incorporated, 2007), 62.

2664-2665   M.C. Bilyk, J.M. Sontrop, G.E. Chapman, S.I. Barr, and L. Mamer, "Food Experiences and Eating Patterns of Visually Impaired and Blind People," *Canadian Journal of Dietetic Practice and Research* 70, no. 1 (Spring 2009): 13–18.

2666   "Diabetes Diet: Create Your Healthy-Eating Plan," Mayo Clinic.org, accessed January 15, 2012, http://www.mayoclinic.com/health/diabetes-diet/DA00027.

2667   U.S. EEOC, *Communicating and Interacting with People Who Have Disabilities*, 5–6.

2668   U.S. EEOC, *Communicating and Interacting with People Who Have Disabilities*, 5–6.

2669   "Guidelines for Medical Professionals," Earle Baum Center, updated April 2004, http://earlebaum.org/guidelines-and-information/guidelies-for-medical-professionals/.

2670-2671   "How to Care for a Blind Person," eHow.com Health, updated March 7, 2011, http://www.ehow.com/how_2040980_care-blind-person.html.

2672-2674   U.S. EEOC, *Communicating and Interacting with People Who Have Disabilities*, 5–6.

2675-2676   "Guidelines for Medical Professionals," Earle Baum Center, updated April 2004, http://earlebaum.org/guidelines-and-information/guidelies-for-medical-professionals/.

2677   Rosenberg and Sperazza, "The Visually Impaired Patient," *American Family Physician*, 1431–1436, 1437–38.

2678   Carter, "Age-related Vision Changes," *Geriatrics*, 37–42, 45.

2679   Rosenberg and Sperazza, "The Visually Impaired Patient," *American Family Physician*, 1431–1436, 1437–38.

2680   J. Seale and M. Nind, eds., *Understanding and Promoting Access for People with Learning Disabilities* (New York: Routledge, 2010), 145.

2681   M. Brown, J. MacArthur, and S. Gibbs, "Emergency Care for People with Learning Disabilities: What All Nurses and Midwives Need to Know," *Accident and Emergency Nursing* 13, no. 4 (Oct. 2005): 224–231.

2682   J. Nunn, R. Freeman, E. Anderson, L.C. Carneiro, M.S.A. Carneiro, and A. Formicola et al., "Inequalities in Access to Education and Healthcare," special issue "Global Congress on Dental Education" in *European Journal of Dental Education* 12 (Feb. 2008), 30–39.

2683   J. Brylewski and I. Duggan, "Antipsychotic Medication for Challenging Behaviour in People with Learning Disability," *Cochrane Database of Systematic Reviews* 3 (2004), http://onlinelibrary.wiley.com/doi/10.1002/14651858.CD000377.pub2/abstract.

2684   N. Davies, "Learning Disabilities," *Nursing Standard* 20, no. 44 (July 2006): 67.

2685   Seale and Nind, *Understanding and Promoting Access for People with Learning Disabilities*, 75.

2686   Ibid., 146.

2687-2688 Brown et al., "Emergency Care," *Accident and Emergency Nursing*, 224–231.

2689   "Intellectual Disability Fact Sheet," Centers for Disease Control, accessed January 16, 2012, http://www.cdc.gov/ncbddd/dd/ddmr.htm.

2690-2691 H.M. Van Schrojenstein Lantman-De Valk, J.F. Metsemakers, J.M. Haveman, and H.F.J.M. Crebolder, "Health Problems in People with Intellectual Disability in General Practice: A Comparative Study," *Family Practice* 17, no. 5 (2000), 405–7.

2692   S. Cumella, N. Ransford, J. Lyons, and H. Burnham, "Needs for Oral Care Among People with Intellectual Disability Not in Contact with Community Dental Services," *Journal of Intellectual Disability Research* 44, no. 1 (Feb. 2000): 45–52.

2693   M. Sowney, M. Brown, and O. Barr, "Caring for People with Learning Disabilities in Emergency Care," *Emergency Nurse* 14, no. 2 (May 2006): 23–30.

2694   S.A. Cooper, E. Smiley, J. Morrison, A. Williamson, and L. Allan, "Mental Ill-Health in Adults with Intellectual Disabilities: Prevalence and Associated Factors" *British Journal of Psychiatry* 190 (2007), 27–35.

2695-2698 Sowney et al., "Caring for People," *Emergency Nurse*, 23–30.

2699   S.A. Cooper, E. Smiley, J. Morrison, L. Allan, A. Williamson, and J. Finlayson et al., "Psychosis and Adults with Intellectual Disabilities: Prevalence, Incidence, and Related Factors," *Social Psychiatry and Psychiatric Epidemiology* 42, no. 7 (2007): 530–36.

2700   A. Strydom, G. Livingston, M. King, and A. Hassiotis, "Prevalence of Dementia in Intellectual Disability Using Different Diagnostic Criteria," *British Journal of Psychiatry* 191 (2007): 150–57.

2701   C.J.M. Böhmer, E.C. Klinkenberg-Knol, M.C. Niezen-de Boer, and S.G.M. Meuwissen, "Gastroesophageal Reflux Disease in Intellectually Disabled Individuals: How Often, How Serious, How Manageable?" *American Journal of Gastroenterology* 94 (1999): 804–10.

2702   K. Patja, P. Eero, and M. Iivanlainen, "Cancer Incidence Among People with Intellectual Disability" *Journal of Intellectual Disability Research* 45, no. 4 (Aug. 2001): 300–07.

2703-2704 C.A. Melville, J. Morrison, L. Allan, E. Smiley, and A. Williamson, "The Prevalence and Determinants of Obesity in Adults with Intellectual Disabilities," *Journal of Applied Research in Intellectual Disabilities* 21, no. 5 (Sept. 2008): 425–37.

2705   R. Ferris-Taylor, "Communication," in *Learning Disabilities: Toward Inclusion*, 5th ed., edited by B. Gates, (Oxford, UK: Churchill Livingstone, 2003).

2706   "Checklist for Learning Disabilities," Milestones, accessed January 16, 2012, http://www.advancingmilestones.com/PDFs/m_resources_LD-checklist.pdf

2707   H. Van Schrojenstein Lantman-de Valk, C. Linehan, M. Kerr, P. Noonan-Walsh, "Developing Health Indicators for People with Intellectual Disabilities. The Method of the Pomona Project," *Journal of Intellectual Disability Research* 51, no. 6 (June 2007): 427–34.

2708   D.C. Harper and J.S. Wadsworth, "Improving Health Care Communication for Persons with Mental Retardation," *Public Health Reports* 107, no. 3 (1992): 297–302.

2709   C.K. Sigelman, *Communicating with Mentally Retarded Persons: Asking Questions and Getting Answers* (Lubbock, TX: Texas Tech University, 1983).

2710   H.A. Taub, G.E. Kline, and M.T. Baker, "The Elderly and Informed Consent: Effects of Vocabulary Level and Corrected Feedback," *Experimental Aging Research* 7, no. 2 (1981), 137–146.

2711   Sowney et al., "Caring for People," *Emergency Nurse*, 23–30.

2712   "Healthy Diet May Slow Alzheimer's Disease," American Academy of Anti-Aging Medicine, updated June 16, 2010, http://www.worldhealth.net/news/healthy-diet-may-slow-alzheimers-disease/.

2713-2719	Sowney et al., "Caring for People," *Emergency Nurse*, 23–30.
2720	Van Schrojenstein Lantman-de Valk et al., "Developing Health Indicators," *Journal of Intellectual Disability Research*, 427–34.
2721-2728	Sowney et al., "Caring for People," *Emergency Nurse*, 23–30.
2729-2730	E. Emerson, "Poverty and People with Intellectual Disabilities," *Mental Retardation and Developmental Disabilities Research Reviews* 13, no. 2 (2007), 107–13.
2731	J. Donovan, "Learning Disability Nurses' Experiences of Being with Clients Who May be in Pain" *Journal of Advanced Nursing* 38, no. 5 (June 2002): 458–466.
2732-2733	"For Teachers: Understanding Learning Disabilities and ADHD," Learning Disabilities Association of America, accessed January 16, 2012, http://www.ldanatl.org/aboutld/teachers/index.asp.
2734-2737	A.G. Steinberg, S. Barnett, H.E. Meador, E. Wiggins, and P. Zazove, "Health Care System Accessibility. Experiences and Perceptions of Deaf People," *Journal of General Internal Medicine* 21, no. 3 (March 2006), 260–66.
2738	C. Chong-hee Lieu, G.R. Sadler, J.T. Fullerton, and P.D. Stohlmann "Communication Strategies for Nurses Interacting with Patients Who are Deaf," *Dermatology Nursing* 19, no. 6 (2007): 541–44; 549–55.
2739	L.I. Iezzoni , B.L. O'Day, M. Killeen, and H. Harker, "Communicating About Health Care: Observations from Persons Who are Deaf or Hard of Hearing," *Annals of Internal Medicine* 140, no. 5 (March 2,2004): 356–362.
2740	C. Chong-hee Lieu et al., "Communication Strategies for Nurses," *Dermatology Nursing*, 541–44; 549–55.
2741	I.M. Munoz-Baell and M.T. Ruiz,"Empowering the Deaf. Let the Deaf be Deaf," *Journal of Epidemiology and Community Health* 54, no. 1 (2000): 40–44.
2742	A. Zaidman-Zait, "Everyday Problems and Stress Faced by Parents of Children with Cochlear Implants," *Rehabilitation Psychology* 53, no. 2 (May 2008): 139–152.
2743-2750	D. Jeffery, "Adapting De-escalation Techniques with Deaf Service Users," *Nursing Standard* 19, no. 49 (2005): 41–47.
2751-2758	"Health and Well-Being: Physical Health," Deaf Info.org, accessed January 16, 2012, http://www.deafinfo.org.uk/ wellbeing/physical.html .
2759	"Health and Well-Being," Deaf Info.org, accessed January 16, 2012, http://www.deafinfo.org.uk /wellbeing/ physical.html .
2760-2766	M. McAleer, "Communicating Effectively with Deaf Patients," *Nursing Standard* 20, no. 19 (2006): 51–54.
2767-2774	"Healthcare for People with Physical Disabilities: Access Issues," *Medscape General Medicine* 3, no. 2 (2001), http://www.medscape.com/viewarticle/408122_4.
2775	D. Deutsch Smith, "Physical Impairments and Special Health Care Needs," *IDEA Update. Introduction to Special Education: Teaching in an Age of Opportunity* (Boston, MA: Allyn and Bacon, 2004). http://www. csus.edu/indiv/l/lillyf/EDS100/smith%20physical%20and%20health%20issues.pdf.
2776-2781	S. Arthur and G. Zarb, "Measuring Disablement in Society: Working Paper 4. Barriers to Employment for Disabled People" (1995), http://www.leeds.ac.uk/disability-studies/archiveuk/Zarb/barriers%20to%20employment.pdf.
2782-2786	Deutsch Smith, "Physical Impairments and Special Health Care Needs," *IDEA Update*. http://www.csus.edu/ indiv/l/lillyf/EDS100/smith%20physical%20and%20health%20issues.pdf.
2787	"Physical Medicine/Pain Management," Midwest Orthopaedics at Rush, accessed January 16, 2012, http://www. rushortho.com/pain_management.cfm.
2788-2790	Deutsch Smith, "Physical Impairments and Special Health Care Needs," *IDEA Update*. http://www.csus.edu/ indiv/l/lillyf/EDS100/smith%20physical%20and%20health%20issues.pdf.
2791	"Education of Individuals with Speech and Language Impairment," Answers.com, accessed January 16, 2012, http://www.answers.com/topic/education-of-individuals-with-speech-and-language-impairment.
2792	"Knowledge and Skills Needed by Speech-Language Pathologists Providing Services to Individuals With Swallowing and/or Feeding Disorders," The American Speech-Language Hearing Association, accessed January 16, 2012, http://www.asha.org/docs/html/KS2002-00079.html#sec1.3.1.

2793-2794   "Swallowing Disorders (Dysphagia) in Adults," The American Speech-Language Hearing Association, accessed January 16, 2012, http://www.asha.org/public/speech/swallowing/SwallowingAdults.htm.

2795   "Helping Adolescents Who Stutter Focus on Fluency," The American Speech-Language Hearing Association, accessed January 16, 2012, http://www.asha.org/.../academic/curriculum/slp-flu/HelpAdolescentsWhoStutter.pdf.

2796   "Aphasia," The American Speech-Language Hearing Association, accessed January 16, 2012, http://www.asha.org/public/speech/disorders/Aphasia.htm.

2797   "Apraxia of Speech in Adults," The American Speech-Language Hearing Association, accessed January 16, 2012, http://www.asha.org/public/speech/disorders/ApraxiaAdults.htm.

2798   "Vocal Cord Nodules and Polyps," The American Speech-Language Hearing Association, accessed January 16, 2012, http://www.asha.org/public/speech/disorders/NodulesPolyps.htm.

2799   "Augmentative and Alternative Communication (AAC)," The American Speech-Language Hearing Association, accessed January 16, 2012, http://www.asha.org/public/speech/disorders/AAC/.

2800-2801   "Knowledge and Skills Needed by Speech-Language Pathologists Providing Services to Individuals With Swallowing and/or Feeding Disorders," The American Speech-Language Hearing Association, accessed January 16, 2012, http://www.asha.org/docs/html/KS2002-00079.html#sec1.3.1 .

2802   "Videofluoroscopic Swallowing Studies (VFSS)," The American Speech-Language Hearing Association, accessed January 16, 2012, http://www.asha.org/slp/clinical/dysphagia/VFSS.htm.

2803-2804   "Endoscopic Evaluation of Swallowing," The American Speech-Language Hearing Association, accessed January 16, 2012, http://www.asha.org/slp/clinical/dysphagia/endoscopy.htm.

2805   "Aphasia: Benefits of Speech-Language Pathology Services," The American Speech-Language Hearing Association, accessed January 16, 2012, http://www.asha.org/public/speech/disorders/AphasiaSLPBenefits.htm.

2806   "Orofacial Myofunctional Disorders (OMD)," The American Speech-Language Hearing Association, accessed January 16, 2012, http://www.asha.org/public/speech/disorders/OMD.htm.

2807-2808   "Feeding and Swallowing Disorders (Dysphagia) in Children," The American Speech-Language Hearing Association, accessed January 16, 2012, http://www.asha.org/public/speech/swallowing/FeedSwallowChildren.htm.

2809-2810   "Traumatic Brain Injury – The Medical Insurance Maze," Head and Brain Injuries, accessed January 16, 2012, http://www.headbraininjuries.com/brain-injury-medical-insurance.

2811-2812   "Why Immigrants Lack Adequate Access to Health Care and Health Insurance," Migration Policy Institute, updated September 2006, http://www.migrationinformation.org/Feature/display.cfm?ID=417.

2813-2821   "Cognitive and Communication Disorders," Centre for Neuro Skills, accessed January 16, 2012, http://www.neuroskills.com/brain-injury/cognitive-and-communication-disorders.php.

2822   "Balanced Diet Quadruples Survival Chances After Traumatic Brain Injury," Thaindian News, accessed January 16, 2012, http://www.thaindian.com/newsportal/lifestyle/balanced-diet-quadruples-survival-chances-after-traumatic-brain-injury_10066971.html.

2823   A. Wu, R. Molteni, Z. Ying, and F. Gomez-Pinilla, "A Saturated-Fat Diet Aggravates the Outcome of Traumatic Brain Injury on Hippocampal Plasticity and Cognitive Function by Reducing Brain-derived Neurotrophic Factor," *Neuroscience* 119, no. 2 (June 2003): 365–75.

2824   "Pecans May Help Protect Neuro Function," American Academy of Anti-aging Medicine, updated June 17, 2010, http://www.worldhealth.net/news/pecans-may-help-protect-neurological-function/.

2825-2831   "Cognitive and Communication Disorders," Centre for Neuro Skills, accessed January 16, 2012, http://www.neuroskills.com/brain-injury/cognitive-and-communication-disorders.php.

GENERATIONS

2032   "Population Estimate Data," Annual Estimates of the Resident Population by Sex and Five-year Age Groups for the United States: April 1, 2000 to July 1, 2008 (NC-EST2008-01), accessed January 17, 2012, http://www.census.gov/popest/data/national/asrh/pre-1980/PE-11.html.

2833   S. Phelan, "Generational Issues in the ob-gyn Workplace: 'Marcus Welby, MD' versus 'Scrubs,'" *Obstetrics and Gynecology* 116, no. 3 (Sept. 2010), 568–69.

2834-2839   "The Millennials: Confident. Connected. Open to Change.," Pew Research Center, accessed January 17, 2012, http://pewresearch.org/pubs/1501/millennials-new-survey-generational-personality-upbeat-open-new-ideas-technology-bound?src=prc-latest&proj=peoplepress.

2840   S. Phelan, "Generational Issues," *Obstetrics and Gynecology*, 568–69.

2841-2843   "The Millennials: Confident. Connected. Open to Change.," http://pewresearch.org/pubs/1501 /millennials-new-survey-generational-personality-upbeat-open-new-ideas-technology-bound?src=prc-latest&proj=peoplepress.

2844   S. Phelan, "Generational Issues," *Obstetrics and Gynecology*, 568–69.

2845-2847   "The Millennials: Confident. Connected. Open to Change.," http://pewresearch.org/pubs/1501 /millennials-new-survey-generational-personality-upbeat-open-new-ideas-technology-bound?src=prc-latest&proj=peoplepress.

2848   S. Phelan, "Generational Issues ," *Obstetrics and Gynecology*, 568–69.

2849-2851   "The Millennials: Confident. Connected. Open to Change.," http://pewresearch.org/pubs/1501/ millennials-new-survey-generational-personality-upbeat-open-new-ideas-technology-bound?src=prc-latest&proj=peoplepress.

2852   "Thomson Reuters Study Finds Baby Boomers and Generation X Face Healthcare Cost Hurdles," RedOrbit, updated June 22, 2009, http://www.redorbit.com/news/health/1708934/thomson_reuters_study _finds_baby_boomers_and_generation_x_face/.

2853-2863   "The Traditional Generation [Born 1922–1945]," Value Options, accessed January 16, 2012, http://www.valueoptions.com/spotlight_YIW/traditional.htm.

2864-2868   "Tips to Improve Communication Across Generations," National Oceanographic and Atmospheric Association Office of Diversity, accessed January 17, 2012, http://honolulu.hawaii.edu/intranet /committees/FacDevCom/ guidebk/teachtip/intergencomm.htm.

2869   L. Gravett and R. Throckmorton, *Bridging the Generation Gap: How to Get Radio Babies, Boomers, Gen Xers, and Gen Yers to Work Together and Achieve More* (Franklin Lakes, NJ: Career Press, Inc., 2007), 35.

2870-2871   Ibid., 36.

2872   R. Salkowitz, *Generation Blend: Managing Across the Technology Age Gap* (Hoboken, NJ: John Wiley & Sons, Inc., 2008), 66.

2873   Ibid., 65.

2874-2875   "Different Generations, Different Worlds," Sysco, accessed January 17, 2012, http://www.syscosf.com/about/ DECEMBER2009_GENERATION3.pdf .

2876-2883   "The Traditional Generation," http://www.valueoptions.com/spotlight_YIW/traditional.htm.

2884-2885   D.A. Monti and E.J.S. Kunkel, "Practical Geriatrics: Management of Chronic Pain Among Elderly Patients," *Psychiatric Services* 49, no. 12 (1998), 1537–1539.

2886   "The Traditional Generation," http://www.valueoptions.com/spotlight_YIW/traditional.htm.

2887   "Talking to a Loved One About Death," Caring.com, accessed January 17, 2012, http://www.caring.com/articles/ talking-to-a-dying-parent.

2888-2893   "Grandparents Raising Grandchildren," Dr. Kornhaber, accessed January 17, 2012, http://www.grandparenting. org/Grandparents_Raising_Grandchildren.htm.

2894-2897   "Societal Blind Spots as Barriers to Health Care Reform," J. Geyman, Physicians for a National Health Program, updated July 15, 2009, http://pnhp.org/blog/2009/07/15/societal-blind-spots-as-barriers-to-health-care-reform/ .

2898-2903   "The Baby Boomer Generation [Born 1946–1964]," Value Options, accessed January 17, 2012, http://www. eapexpress.com/spotlight_YIW/baby_boomers.htm.

2904-2907   "Tips to Improve Communication Across Generations," http://honolulu.hawaii.edu/intranet/committees/ FacDevCom/guidebk/teachtip/intergencomm.htm.

2908-2912   "The Baby Boomer Generation," http://www.eapexpress.com/spotlight_YIW/baby_boomers.htm.

2913-2915   "Different Generations, Different Worlds," http://www.syscosf.com/about /DECEMBER2009_GENERATIONS.pdf .

2916-2918   "As They Age, Baby Boomers Seek Spirituality," R. Ellis, NBC Nightly News, updated November 8, 2005, http://www.msnbc.msn.com/id/9971428/ns/nightly_news_with_brian_williams.

2919-2929   "The Baby Boomer Generation," http://www.eapexpress.com/spotlight_YIW/baby_boomers.htm.

2930-2934   "Multigenerational Households are Growing," S. O'Brien, About.Com., accessed January 17, 2012, http://seniorliving.about.com/od/boomerscaringforparents/a/multigeneration-household.htm.

2935   "The Baby Boomer Generation," http://www.eapexpress.com/spotlight_YIW/baby_boomers.htm.

2936-2947   "Generation X," Value Options, accessed January 17, 2012, http://www.valueoptions.com /spotlight_YIW/gen_x.htm.

2948-2952   "Tips to Improve Communication Across Generations," http://honolulu.hawaii.edu /intranet/committees/FacDevCom/guidebk/teachtip/intergencomm.htm.

2953-2957   "Generation X," http://www.valueoptions.com/spotlight_YIW/gen_x.htm.

2958-2960   "Different Generations, Different Worlds," http://www.syscosf.com/about /DECEMBER2009_GENERATIONS.pdf.

2961-2963   "Practical: Generation X and Discipleship—Some Simple Do's and Don'ts," G. Codrington, Youth Pastor.com, posted November 19, 1997, http://www.youthpastor.com/lessons/index.cfm/Practical-Generation_X_and_Discipleship_some_simple_Dos_and_Donts_148.htm.

2964-2968   "Generation X," http://www.valueoptions.com/spotlight_YIW/gen_x.htm.

2969-2979   "Generation Y [Born 1980-1994]," Value Options, accessed January 17, 2012, http://www.valueoptions.com/spotlight_YIW/gen_y.htm.

2980-2985   "Tips to Improve Communication Across Generations," http://honolulu.hawaii.edu /intranet/committees/FacDevCom/guidebk/teachtip/intergencomm.htm.

2986-2990   "Generation Y," http://www.valueoptions.com/spotlight_YIW/gen_y.htm.

2991-2993   "Different Generations, Different Worlds," http://www.syscosf.com/about /DECEMBER2009_GENERATIONS.pdf .

2994-2995   "Religious Composition of the U.S.—U.S. Religious Landscape Survey," Pew Forum on Religion & Public Life, accessed January 17, 2012, http://religions.pewforum.org/pdf/affiliations-all-traditions.pdf.

2996-3001   "Generation Y," http://www.valueoptions.com/spotlight_YIW/gen_y.htm.

Bibliography Of Works Consulted

About.com. "Amrit the Sikh Baptism Ceremony." Accessed December 15, 2011. http://sikhism.about.com /od/initiation/a/ Amrit.htm.

About.com. "Christianity Today - General Statistics and Facts of Christianity." Accessed January 17, 2012. http://christianity.about.com/od/denominations/p/christiantoday.htm.

About.com. "Latter-Day Saints." Accessed December 12, 2011. http://lds.about.com/od /basicsgospelprinciples/p/death.htm.

About.com Islam. "What is Ramadan?" Accessed December 6, 2011. http://islam.about.com/od/ramadan /f/ramadanintro.htm.

Abushaikha, L.A. "Methods of Coping with Labor Pain Used by Jordanian Women." *Journal of Transcultural Nursing* 18, no. 1 (January 2007): 35–40. DOI: 10.1177/1043659606294194.

Abyad, A. "The Role of Different Faiths and Their Attitudes Toward Death." *Healing Ministry* (Jan/Feb, 1996): 23.

Act Now.com. "Abortion Confusion." Updated November 4, 2008. http://www.actnow.com.au /Issues/Abortion_confusion.aspx.

Adherents.com. "Major Religions of the World Ranked by Number of Adherents." Accessed January 17, 2012. http://www.adherents.com/Religions_By_Adherents.html.

Adventure Travellers Club. "Culture and Customs of India." Accessed December 5, 2011. http://www.nepaltravellers.com/Culture_and_Customs.htm.

Aish.com. "Do We Own our Bodies, or are They Only on Loan?" Accessed December 8, 2011. http://www.aish.com/ci/sam/48960576.html.

Aish.com. "When and Why Do We Wear a Kippah?" Accessed December 8, 2011. http://www.aish.com/jl/m/pb/48949686.html.

All About Cults. "What is the Birth Practice in Christian Scientist?" Accessed December 26, 2011. http://www.allaboutcults.org/birth-practice-in-christian-scientist-faq.htm.

Alleman, H.C. and W.H. Dunbar. *Lutheran Teacher Training Series for the Sunday School, Volume 1*. Philadelphia, PA: Lutheran Publication Society, 1909.

AllExperts.com. "Jehovah's Witnesses." Updated August 20, 2006. http://en.allexperts.com/q/Jehovah-s-Witness-1617/Diet.htm.

AllExperts.com. "Jehovah's Witness—Rites of Passage." Updated June 5, 2005. http://en.allexperts.com/q/Jehovah-s-Witness-1617/Rites-Passage.htm.

AllExperts.com. "Pentecostals/Healing Service." Accessed December 14, 2011. http://en.allexperts.com/q/Pentecostals-2256/Healing-Service.htm.

AllExperts.com. "Seventh-day Adventists: Infant Circumcision." Updated April 28, 2009. http://en.allexperts.com/q/Seventh-Day-Adventists-2318/2009/4/infant-circumcision.htm.

Al-Munajjid, S.M.S. Islamic Q and A. "Basic Tenets of Faith." Accessed December 6, 2011. http://islamqa.com/en/ref/20207/amulets.

American Academy of Anti-Aging Medicine. "Healthy Diet May Slow Alzheimer's Disease." Updated June 16, 2010. http://www.worldhealth.net/news/healthy-diet-may-slow-alzheimers-disease/.

American Academy of Anti-aging Medicine. "Pecans May Help Protect Neuro Function." Updated June 17, 2010. http://www.worldhealth.net/news/pecans-may-help-protect-neurological-function/.

American Catholic.org. "Abortion: What the Church Teaches." Accessed January 13, 2012. http://www.americancatholic.org/Newsletters/CU/ac0898.asp.

American Catholic.org. "The Sacraments: Baptism." Accessed January 9, 2012. http://www.americancatholic.org/features/special/default.aspx?id=30.

The American Speech-Language Hearing Association. "Aphasia." Accessed January 16, 2012, http://www.asha.org/public/speech/disorders/Aphasia.htm.

The American Speech-Language Hearing Association. "Aphasia: Benefits of Speech-Language Pathology Services." Accessed January 16, 2012. http://www.asha.org/public/speech/disorders/AphasiaSLPBenefits.htm.

The American Speech-Language Hearing Association. "Apraxia of Speech in Adults." Accessed January 16, 2012. http://www.asha.org/public/speech/disorders/ApraxiaAdults.htm.

The American Speech-Language Hearing Association. "Augmentative and Alternative Communication (AAC)." Accessed January 16, 2012. http://www.asha.org/public/speech/disorders/AAC/.

The American Speech-Language Hearing Association. "Endoscopic Evaluation of Swallowing," Accessed January 16, 2012. http://www.asha.org/slp/clinical/dysphagia/endoscopy.htm.

The American Speech-Language Hearing Association. "Feeding and Swallowing Disorders (Dysphagia) in Children." Accessed January 16, 2012. http://www.asha.org/public/speech/swallowing/FeedSwallowChildren.htm.

The American Speech-Language Hearing Association. "Helping Adolescents Who Stutter Focus on Fluency." Accessed January 16, 2012. http://www.asha.org/.../academic/curriculum/slp-flu/HelpAdolescentsWhoStutter.pdf.

The American Speech-Language Hearing Association. "Knowledge and Skills Needed by Speech-Language Pathologists Providing Services to Individuals With Swallowing and/or Feeding Disorders." Accessed January 16, 2012. http://www.asha.org/docs/html/KS2002-00079.html#sec1.3.1 .

The American Speech-Language Hearing Association. "Orofacial Myofunctional Disorders (OMD)." Accessed January 16, 2012. http://www.asha.org/public/speech/disorders/OMD.htm.

The American Speech-Language Hearing Association. "Swallowing Disorders (Dysphagia) in Adults." Accessed January 16, 2012. http://www.asha.org/public/speech/swallowing/SwallowingAdults.htm.

The American Speech-Language Hearing Association. "Videofluoroscopic Swallowing Studies (VFSS)." Accessed January 16, 2012. http://www.asha.org/slp/clinical/dysphagia/VFSS.htm.

The American Speech-Language Hearing Association. "Vocal Cord Nodules and Polyps," Accessed January 16, 2012. http://www.asha.org/public/speech/disorders/NodulesPolyps.htm.

Amish America. "Do Amish Use Birth Control?" Accessed December 22, 2011. http://amishamerica.com/do-amish-use-birth-control/.

Andrews, J.D. Cultural, Ethic and Religious: Reference Manual for Health Care Providers. Winston-Salem, NC: Jamarda Resources, 1995.

Andrews, M.M. and J.S. Boyle. Transcultural Concepts in Nursing Care, 2nd ed. New York: Lippincott, 1995.

Annual Estimates of the Resident Population by Sex and Five-year Age Groups for the United States: April 1, 2000 to July 1, 2008 (NC-EST2008-01). "Population Estimate Data." Accessed January 17, 2012. http://www.census.gov/popest/data/national/asrh/pre-1980/PE-11.html.

Answers.com. "Education of Individuals with Speech and Language Impairment." Accessed January 16, 2012. http://www.answers.com/topic/education-of-individuals-with-speech-and-language-impairment.

Answers.com. "What are Jehovah's Witness Beliefs About Birth Control?" Accessed December 7, 2011. http://wiki.answers.com/Q/What_are_Jehovah%27s_witnesses_beliefs_about_birth_control.

Answers.com. "What Do Baptists Believe About Abortion?" Accessed December 26, 2011. http://wiki.answers.com/Q/What_do_Baptists_believe_about_abortion.

Antochi, R., C. Stavrakaki, and P.C. Emery. "Psychopharmacological Treatments in Persons with Dual Diagnosis of Psychiatric Disorders and Developmental Disabilities." Postgraduate Medical Journal 79, no. 929 (2003): 139–46. DOI:10.1136/pmj.79.929.139.

Araba-Owoyele, L., R. Littaua, M. Hughes, and J. Berecochea. Minority Health Issues for an Emerging Majority. Washington, DC: 4th National Forum on Cardiovascular Health, Pulmonary Disorders, and Blood Resources, June 26–27, 1992.

Arthur, S. and G. Zarb. "Measuring Disablement in Society: Working Paper 4. Barriers to Employment for Disabled People." (1995). http://www.leeds.ac.uk/disability-studies/archiveuk/Zarb /barriers%20to%20employment.pdf.

Ashley, B.M., J. Deblois, and K.D. O'Rourke. Health Care Ethics: A Catholic Theological Analysis. Washington, D.C.: Georgetown University Press, 2006.

Assemblies of God USA. "Abortion." Accessed December 14, 2011. http://ag.org/top/Beliefs/topics/contempissues_01_abortion.cfm.

Assemblies of God USA. "Assemblies of God Fundamental Truths." Last updated March 1, 2010. http://ag.org/top/Beliefs/Statement_of_Fundamental_Truths/sft_short.cfm.

Assemblies of God USA. "Death and Dying." Accessed December 14, 2011. http://ag.org/top/Beliefs /topics/gendoct_18_death.cfm.

Assemblies of God USA. "Fasting." Accessed December 14, 2011. http://ag.org/top/beliefs /gendoct_04_fasting.cfm.

Assemblies of God USA. "Heaven, Hell, and Judgment." Accessed December 14, 2011. http://ag.org/top/Beliefs/gendoct_14_heaven_hell.cfm.

Assemblies of God USA. "Infant Baptism, Age of Accountability, Dedication of Children." Accessed December 14, 2011. http://ag.org/top/Beliefs/topics/gendoct_11_accountability.cfm.

Assemblies of God USA. "Infertility." Accessed December 14, 2011. http://ag.org/top/Beliefs /topics/relations_16_infertility.cfm.

Assemblies of God USA. "Medical: Birth Control." Accessed December 14, 2011. http://ag.org/top /Beliefs/topics/relations_17_birth_control.cfm.

Assemblies of God USA. "Medical: Euthanasia and Extraordinary Support to Sustain Life." Accessed December 14, 2011. http://ag.org/top/Beliefs/topics/contempissues_18_euthanasia.cfm.

Assemblies of God USA. "Medical: Organ Donation." Accessed December 14, 2011. http://ag.org/top/Beliefs/topics/contempissues_19_organ_donation.cfm.

Autism Speaks Official Blog. "Health Care Reform: What Does it Mean for the Autism Community?" Posted March 23, 2010. http://blog.autismspeaks.org/2010/03/23/health-care-reform/.

Baldwin, W.H. and T.R. Ford. "Modernism and Contraceptive Use in Colombia." *Studies in Family Planning* 7, no. 3 (March 1976), 75–79. http://www.jstor.org/pss/1965038.

Baptist Health and Wellness Center."Blood Transfusions." Accessed December 26, 2011. http://community.e-baptisthealth.com/health-info/content/ped/eng/hematology/trans.html.

Baptist Hospital East. "Circumcision." Accessed December 26, 2011. http://baptisteast.adam.com /content.aspx?productId=14&pid=14&gid=000133.

Barcellos, F.C., C.L. Araujo, and J. Dias da Costa. "Organ Donation: A Population-Based Study." *Clinical Transplantation* 19, no. 1 (February 2005), 33–37. DOI: 10.1111/j.1399-0012.2005.00280.x.

BBC Religions. "Mormons and Organ Donation." Accessed December 12, 2011. http://www.bbc.co.uk/religion/religions/mormon/socialvalues/organ_donation.shtml.

Beachy, A., E. Hershberger, R. Davidhizar, G. Davidhizar, and J.N. Giger. "Cultural Implications for Nursing Care of the Amish." *Journal of Cultural Diversity* 4, no. 4 (1997). http://www.ncbi.nlm.nih.gov/pubmed/9555377.

Beard-Pfeuffer, M. "Understanding the World of Children with Autism." *RN* 71, no. 2 (February 2008): 40–46. http://www.ncbi.nlm.nih.gov/pubmed/18386443.

Biema, D. "Kingdom Come." *Time*. (August 4, 1997), 38–39.

The Bigview.com. "The Noble Eightfold Path." Accessed December 26, 2011. http://www.thebigview.com /buddhism/eightfoldpath.html.

Bilyk, M.C., J.M. Sontrop, G.E. Chapman, S.I. Barr, and L. Mamer. "Food Experiences and Eating Patterns of Visually Impaired and Blind People." *Canadian Journal of Dietetic Practice and Research* 70, no. 1 (Spring 2009): 13–18. DOI: 10.3148/70.1.2009.13.

Blevins, D., C. Lewis, Jr., F. Moore, R. Samples, and J. Stone, eds. *Manual Church of the Nazarene 2005–2009*. Kansas City, MO: Nazarene Publishing House,2005. http://sermons.logos.com/submissions /107737-Manual-Church-Of-The-Nazarene-2005-2009-manual2005-2009-Church-#content =/submissions/107737.

Blum, R.H. *The Management of the Doctor-Patient Relationship*. n.p.: McGraw-Hill, Blakiston Division, 1960.

Bock, K. and C. Stauth. *Healing the New Childhood Epidemics: Autism, ADHD, Asthma, and Allergies*. New York: Ballantine Books, 2007.

Böhmer, C.J.M., E.C. Klinkenberg-Knol, M.C. Niezen-de Boer, and S.G.M. Meuwissen. "Gastroesophageal Reflux Disease in Institutionalized Intellectually Disabled Individuals: How Often, How Serious, How Manageable?" *American Journal of Gastroenterology* 94 (1999): 804–10. DOI:10.1111/j.1572-0241.1999.00854.x.

Bonkowsky, J.L., J.K. Frazer, K.F. Buchi, and C.L. Byington. "Metamizole Use by Latino Immigrants: A Common and Potentially Harmful Home Remedy." *Pediatrics* 109, no. 6 (June 1, 2002). DOI: 10.1542 /peds.109.6.e98.

Boston University School of Medicine. Boston Healing Landscape Project. "General Guidelines." Accessed December 6, 2011. http://www.bu.edu/bhlp/Resources/Islam/health/guidelines.html.

Boston University School of Medicine. Boston Healing Landscape Project. "Islam and Health." Accessed January 14, 2012. http://www.bu.edu/bhlp/Resources/Islam/index.html.

Bratcher, D., ed. "Doctrinal and Ethical Positions, Church of the Nazarene." *CRI/Voice*. Last modified November 11, 2011. http://www.crivoice.org/creednazarene.html.

Brault, M.W., U.S. Census Bureau. "Americans with Disabilities: 2005." Updated December 2008. http://www.census.gov/prod/2008pubs/p70-117.pdf.

Braun, K., J.H. Pietsch, and P.L. Blanchette. *Cultural Issues in End-Of-Life Decisions*. Thousand Oaks, CA: Sage Publications, 2000.

Bregman, L. *Religion, Death, and Dying, Volume 3, Bereavement and Death Rituals*. Santa Barbara, CA: Greenwood Publishing Group, 2010.

Breitowitz, Y. Jewish Law Articles. "The Preembryo in Halacha." Accessed December 8, 2011. http://www.jlaw.com/Articles/preemb.html.

Brown, M., J. MacArthur, and S. Gibbs, "Emergency Care for People with Learning Disabilities: What All Nurses and Midwives Need to Know." *Accident and Emergency Nursing* 13, no. 4 (Oct. 2005): 224–231. http://dx.doi.org/10.1016/j.aaen.2005.06.001.

Browner, C. "The Management of Early Pregnancy: Colombian Folk Concepts of Fertility Control." *Social Science Medicine. Part B: Medical Anthropology* 14, no.1 (Feb. 1980): 25–32. http://dx.doi.org/10.1016/0160-7987(80)90037-X.

Bryant, C.D. and D.L. Peck, eds. *Encyclopedia of Death and the Human Experience*. Thousand Oaks, CA: Sage Publications, 2009.

Brylewski, J. and L. Duggan. "Antipsychotic Medication for Challenging Behaviour in People with Learning Disability." *Cochrane Database of Systematic Reviews* 3 (2004). http://onlinelibrary.wiley.com /doi/10.1002/14651858.CD000377.pub2/abstract.

Buchanan, E. *Parent/Teacher Handbook: Teaching Children Ages 10 to 12 Everything They Need to Know About Their Christian Heritage*. Nashville, TN: Broadman and Holman Publishers, 2006.

Burton, E.C., K.A. Collins, and S.A. Gurevitz. "Religions and the Autopsy." Medscape Reference. Accessed December 27, 2011. http://emedicine.medscape.com/article/1705993-overview#aw2aab6b7.

Calhoun, M.A. "The Vietnamese Woman: Health/Illness Attitudes and Behaviors." special issue "Women, Health, and Culture" in *Health Care for Women International* 6, no. 1–3 (1985): 61–72. DOI:10.1080/07399338509515683.

Calvillo, E.R. and J.H. Flaskerud. "Review of Literature on Culture and Pain of Adults with Focus on Mexican-Americans." *Journal of Transcultural Nursing* 2, no. 2 (Winter 1991), 16–23. DOI: 10.1177 /104365969100200203.

Campbell, M., B. Fish, R. David, T. Shapiro, P. Collins, and C. Koh. "Response to Triiodothyronine and Dextroamphetamine: A Study of Preschool Schizophrenic Children." *Journal of Autism and Developmental Disorders* 2, no. 4, 343–358. DOI: 10.1007/BF01538168.

Caring.com. "Talking to a Loved One About Death." Accessed January 17, 2012. http://www.caring.com/articles/talking-to-a-dying-parent

Carter, C., OhioLINK. "Food Intake, Dietary Practices, and Nutritional Supplement Use Among the Amish." Accessed December 21, 2011. http://drc.ohiolink.edu/handle/2374.OX/5155.

Carter, T.L. "Age-related Vision Changes: A Primary Care Guide." *Geriatrics* 49, no. 9 (1994): 37–42, 45. http://ukpmc.ac.uk/abstract/MED/8088558.

Carty, E.M. "Disability and Childbirth: Meeting the Challenges." *Canadian Medical Association Journal* 159, no. 4 (Aug. 1998): 363–69. http://www.canadianmedicaljournal.ca/content/159/4/363.full.pdf

Castellano, C. "The Blind Child in the Elementary Classroom." Accessed January 15, 2012. http://www.blindchildren.org/textonly/to_edu_dev/3_5_5.html.

Castor, T.D. and T.L. Carter. "Low Vision: Physician Screening Helps to Improve Patient Function." *Geriatrics* 50, no. 12 (Dec. 1995): 51–52, 55–57. http://www.ncbi.nlm.nih.gov/pubmed/7498801.

Catholic Answers. "Contraception and Sterilization." Accessed December 15, 2011. http://www.catholic.com/tracts/contraception-and-sterilization.

Catholic Bible 101. "The Sin of Gluttony." Accessed December 15, 2011. http://www.catholicbible101.com /overcominggluttony.htm.

CatholoCity. "Visit the Sick." Accessed December 15, 2011. http://www.catholicity.com /commentary/shea/08249.html.

Catholic Online. "Circumcision." Accessed December 15, 2011. http://www.catholic.org /encyclopedia/view.php?id=2977.

CatholicScripture.org. "Catholic Scriptures That Inspire, Comfort, and Celebrate." Accessed December 15, 2011. http://www.catholicscripture.org/.

Centers for Disease Control. "Intellectual Disability Fact Sheet." Accessed January 16, 2012. http://www.cdc.gov/ncbddd/dd/ddmr.htm.

Central Intelligence Agency. "The World Fact Book." Last updated January 4, 2012. https://www.cia.gov/library/publications/the-world-factbook/geos/us.html.

Centre for Neuro Skills. "Cognitive and Communication Disorders." Accessed January 16, 2012. http://www.neuroskills.com/brain-injury/cognitive-and-communication-disorders.php.

ChaCha. "Will Mormons Do Blood Transfusions?" Accessed December 12, 2011. http://www.chacha.com/question/will-mormons-do-blood-transfusions.

Chan, C.L.W. and A.Y.M. Chow, eds. *Death, Dying, and Bereavement: A Hong Kong Chinese Experience*. Aberdeen, Hong Kong: Hong Kong University Press, 2006.

Chesapeake Conference of Seventh-day Adventists ."Trust Services and Planned Giving." Accessed December 21, 2011. http://www.ccosda.org/article.php?id=48.

Chichester, M. "Multicultural Issues in Perinatal Loss." *Association of Women's Health, Obstetric, and Neonatal Nurses: Lifelines* 9, no. 4 (August 2005): 318. DOI: 10.1177/1091592305280875.

Chong-hee Lieu, C., G.R. Sadler, J.T. Fullerton, and P.D. Stohlmann. "Communication Strategies for Nurses Interacting with Patients Who are Deaf." *Dermatology Nursing* 19, no. 6 (2007): 541–44; 549–55. http://www.medscape.com/viewarticle/569802_1.

The Christian Post. "Lutheran Report Gives Biblical Response to Stem Cell, Cloning, In-Vitro Fertilization." December 6, 2005. http://www.christianpost.com/news/lutheran-report-gives-biblical-response-to-stem-cell-cloning-in-vitro-fertilization-3969/.

Christian Science.com. "Sunday Church Services and Wednesday Testimony Meetings." Accessed December 26, 2011. http://christianscience.com/church-of-christ-scientist/the-mother-church-in-boston-ma-usa/sunday-church-services-and-wednesday-testimony-meetings.

Circlist.com. "Circumcision in the United States of America." Accessed December 12, 2011. http://www.circlist.com/rites/usa.html.

Clarfield, A., M. Gordon, H. Markwell, and S. Alibhai. "Ethical Issues in End-of-Life Geriatric Care: The Approach of Three Monotheistic Religions—Judaism, Catholicism, and Islam." *Journal of American Geriatric Society* 51, no.8 (2003): 1149–54. DOI: 10.1046/j.1532-5415.2003.51364.x.

Codrington, G. "Practical: Generation X and Discipleship—Some Simple Do's and Don'ts." Youth Pastor.com. Posted November 19, 1997. http://www.youthpastor.com/lessons/index.cfm/Practical-Generation_X_and_Discipleship_some_simple_Dos_and_Donts_148.htm.

Cohen, K. *Honoring the Medicine: The Essential Guide to Native American Healing*. New York: Ballantine Books, 2006.

Coles, R.L. *Race and Family: A Structural Approach*. Thousand Oaks, CA: Sage Publications, Inc., 2006

College of St. Scholastica Athens Project. "Cultural Aspects of Healthcare." Accessed December 30, 2011. http://www.css.edu/Academics/ATHENS-Project/Help-Page/Cultural-Aspects-of-Healthcare.html#American%20Indians.

Columbus Dispatch. Pro-Life Infonet. "Presbyterian Denomination Reaffirms Support for Abortion." June 22, 2002. http://www.euthanasia.com/pres.html.

Cooper, S.A., E. Smiley, J. Morrison, L. Allan, A. Williamson, and J. Finlayson et al., "Psychosis and Adults with Intellectual Disabilities: Prevalence, Incidence, and Related Factors," *Social Psychiatry and Psychiatric Epidemiology* 42, no. 7 (2007): 530–38. DOI: 10.1007/s00127-007 0197-9.

Cooper, S.A., E. Smiley, J. Morrison, A. Williamson, and L. Allan. "Mental Ill-Health in Adults with Intellectual Disabilities: Prevalence and Associated Factors." *British Journal of Psychiatry* 190 (2007), 27–35. DOI: 10.1192/bjp.bp.106.022483.

Countries and their Cultures. "Jamaica." Accessed January 14, 2012. http://www.everyculture.com/Ja-Ma/Jamaica.html.

Countries and Their Cultures. "Southern Paiute—Religion and Expressive Culture." Accessed December 30, 2011. http://www.everyculture.com/North-America/Southern-Paiute-and-Chemehuevi-Religion-and-Expressive-Culture.html.

Crawford, S.J. and D.F. Kelley. *American Indian Religious Traditions*. Santa Barbara, CA: ABC-CLIO, Inc., 2005.

Crawshaw, M. and M. Balen, eds. *Adopting After Infertility*. Philadelphia, PA: Jessica Kingsley Publishers, 2010.

Crofoot Graham, T.L. "Using Reasons for Living to Connect to American Indian Healing Traditions." *Journal of Sociology and Social Welfare* 29, no.1 (March 2002): 55. http://heinonline.org/HOL/LandingPage?collection= journals&handle=hein.journals/jrlsasw29&div=7&id=&page=.

Culture and Religion. "Sikhism Fact Sheet." Accessed December 15, 2011. http://www.omi.wa.gov.au /resources/ publications/cr_diversity/sikh.pdf.

Cumella, S., N. Ransford, J. Lyons, and H. Burnham. "Needs for Oral Care Among People with Intellectual Disability Not in Contact with Community Dental Services." *Journal of Intellectual Disability Research* 44, no. 1 (Feb. 2000): 45–52. DOI: 10.1046/j.1365-2788.2000.00252.x.

The Curious Jew. "The Sanctity of Life: A Jewish Approach to End of Life Challenges." Updated September 14, 2008. http:// curiousjew.blogspot.com/2008/09/sanctity-of-life-jewish-approach-to-end.html.

Daily Word of Life. "Favorite Catholic Prayers." Accessed December 15, 2011. http://www.daily-word-of-life.com/catholic_ prayers.htm.

Daniel, A. "Religions in India." Accessed December 5, 2011. http://adaniel.tripod.com/religions.htm.

Danis, S.J. "The Gypsy Culture in South Florida." *Florida Nurse* 44, no. 7 (August 1996): 17. http://www.ncbi.nlm.nih.gov/ pubmed/8945166.

D'Avanzo, C. *Pocket Guide to Cultural Health Assessment*. St. Louis, MO: Elsevier Mosby, 2008.

Davies, N. "Learning Disabilities." *Nursing Standard* 20, no. 44 (July 2006): 67. http://www.ncbi.nlm.nih.gov/ pubmed/16872121.

Deaf Info.org. "Health and Well-Being: Physical Health." Accessed January 16, 2012. http://www.deafinfo.org.uk/wellbeing/ physical.html .

Death with Dignity National Center. "Religion and Spirituality." Accessed December 14, 2011. http://www.deathwithdignity. org/historyfacts/religion/.

Dell, D.D., M. Feleccia, L. Hicks, E. Longstreth-Papsun, S. Politsky, and C. Trommer. "Care of Patients with Autism Spectrum Disorder Undergoing Surgery for Cancer." *Oncology Nursing Forum* 35, no. 2 (March 2008): 177–182. DOI: 10.1188/08.ONF.177-182.

Department of Health and Human Services National Institutes of Health National Center for Complementary and Alternative Medicine. "National Advisory Council For Complementary and Alternative Medicine Minutes of the Seventeenth Meeting." Updated June 4, 2004. http://nccam.nih.gov/about/naccam /minutes/2004junemin.pdf.

Deutsch Smith, D. "Physical Impairments and Special Health Care Needs." IDEA Update. *Introduction to Special Education: Teaching in an Age of Opportunity*. Boston, MA: Allyn and Bacon, 2004. http://www.csus.edu/indiv/l/ lillyf/EDS100/smith%20physical%20and%20health%20issues.pdf.

Di Martino, A., G. Melis, C. Cianchetti, and A. Zuddas. "Methylphenidate for Pervasive Developmental Disorders: Safety and Efficacy of Acute Single Dose Test and Ongoing Therapy: An Open-Pilot Study." *Journal of Child and Adolescent Psychopharmacology* 14, no. 2 (Aug. 25, 2004): 207–218. DOI:10.1089/1044546041649011.

Doheny, D.O., D. de Leon, and D. Raymond. "Genetic Testing and Genetic Counseling" in *Dystonia: Etiology, Clinical Features and Treatment*. Philadelphia, PA: Lippincott Williams & Wilkins, 2004.

Dominguez-Ruvalcaba, H. and I. Corona, eds. *Gender Violence at the U.S.–Mexico Border*. Arizona: University of Arizona Press, 2010.

Donaldson, H., J. Kratzer, S. Okoturo-Ketter, and P. Tung. "Breastfeeding Among Chinese Immigrants in the United States." *Journal of Midwifery and Women's Health* 55, no. 3 (2010), 277–81. http://www.medscape.com/viewarticle/721460 .

Donate Life NM.org. "Religious Views on Organ, Tissue, and Blood Donation." Accessed December 20, 2011. http://www. donatelifenm.org/religiousviews.htm#sda.

Donovan, J. "Learning Disability Nurses' Experiences of Being with Clients Who May be in Pain." *Journal of Advanced Nursing* 38, no. 5 (June 2002): 458–466. DOI: 10.1046/j.1365-2648.2002.02207.x.

Dossey, L. *Healing Words: The Power of Prayer and the Practice of Medicine*. San Francisco, CA: Harper Collins, 1993.

DuBose, E.R., P.D. Numrich, D. Harris-Abbott, R.P. Hamel, eds. The Park Ridge Center for the Study of Health, Faith, and Ethics. *Religious Beliefs & Health Care Decisions—A Quick Reference to 15 Religious Traditions and their Application in Health Care*. n.p. Chicago?: The Center In Chicago, 1995.

Dummer Clark, M.J. *Community Health Nursing: Caring for Populations*. Upper Saddle River, NJ: Prentice Hall, 2003.

Dummies.com. "The Catholic Worship Service." Accessed December 15, 2011. http://www.dummies.com/how-to/content/the-catholic-worship-service-the-mass.html.

Earle Baum Center. "Guidelines for Medical Professionals." Updated April 2004. http://earlebaum.org/guidelines-and-information/guidelies-for-medical-professionals/.

Eddy, M.B. *Science and Health*. Boston, MA: Christian Science Publishing Society, 1902.

Editors of Hinduism Today Magazine. *What is Hinduism? Modern Adventures Into a Profound Global Faith*. Kapaa, HI: Himalayan Academy, 2007.

eHow.com. "How to Be Baptized in the Presbyterian Church." Accessed December 14, 2011. http://www.ehow.com/how_2214836_be-baptized-presbyterian-church.html.

eHow.com. "How to Decide When a Baby Should Be Baptized." Accessed December 14, 2011. http://www.ehow.com/how_2214669_decide-baby-should-be-baptized.html.

eHow.com Health. "How to Care for a Blind Person." Updated March 7, 2011. http://www.ehow.com/how_2040980_care-blind-person.html.

Eisenberg, D. Jewish Law Articles. "Medical Informed Consent in Jewish Law—from the Patient's Side." Accessed December 8, 2011. http://www.jlaw.com/Articles/MedConsent.html.

ElGindy, G. "Death and Dying Across Cultures," *Minority Nurse* (Spring 2004). http://www.minoritynurse.com/hospice-end-life-care/death-and-dying-across-cultures.

Ellis, R. NBC Nightly News. "As They Age, Baby Boomers Seek Spirituality." Updated November 8, 2005. http://www.msnbc.msn.com/id/9971428/ns/nightly_news_with_brian_williams.

Emerson, E. "Poverty and People with Intellectual Disabilities." *Mental Retardation and Developmental Disabilities Research Reviews* 13, no. 2 (2007), 107–13. DOI: 10.1002/mrdd.20144.

Encyclopedia of Death and Dying. "Islam." Accessed January 31, 2012. http://www.deathreference.com/Ho-Ka/Islam.html.

Engerman, S.L. "A Population History of the Caribbean." In *A Population History of North America*, ed. M.R. Haines and R.H. Steckel, 483–528. New York: Cambridge University Press, 2000.

EnsignMessage.com. "What Leaves the Body at Death?" Accessed December 15, 2011. http://www.ensignmessage.com/archives/leavesbody.html.

The Episcopal Church. "Evangelism." Accessed December 27, 2011. http://www.episcopalchurch.org /congdev/2020home.html.

The Episcopal Church Visitors' Center. "The Creeds." Accessed December 26, 2011. http://www.episcopalchurch.org/visitors_11838_ENG_HTM.htm.

The Episcopal Church Visitors' Center. "God the Father." Accessed December 26, 2011. http://www.episcopalchurch.org/visitors_11773_ENG_HTM.htm.

The Episcopal Church Visitors' Center. "Holy Baptism." Accessed December 26, 2011. http://www.episcopalchurch.org/visitors_11674_ENG_HTM.htm.

The Episcopal Church Visitors' Center. "The Holy Scriptures." Accessed December 26, 2011. http://www.episcopalchurch.org/visitors_11564_ENG_HTM.htm.

The Episcopal Church Visitors' Center. "The Ministry." Accessed December 26, 2011. http://www.episcopalchurch.org/visitors_11748_ENG_HTM.htm.

The Episcopal Church Visitors' Center. "The Sacraments." Accessed December 26, 2011. http://www.episcopalchurch.org/visitors_10850_ENG_HTM.htm

The Episcopal Church Visitors' Center. "What is the Episcopal Church About?" Accessed December 27, 2011. http://www.episcopalchurch.org/visitors_16976_ENG_HTM.htm?menupage=49678.

Episcopal Diocese of Michigan. "Advance Directives." Accessed December 27, 2011. http://edomi.org/index.php/resources/people-resources/advance-directives.

Episcopal Diocese of New York. "Positions on Social Issues: Birth Control, Death Penalty, Children." Accessed December 27, 2011. http://www.dioceseny.org/pages/322.

Episcopal News Service Archive. "Episcopal Church Offers Resources for End-of-Life Issues." Accessed December 27, 2011. http://www.episcopalchurch.org/3577_60370_ENG_HTM.htm.

Ethnicity Online—Cultural Awareness in Healthcare. "Hindus: Birth, Babies, and Motherhood." Accessed December 6, 2011. http://www.ethnicityonline.net/hindu_birth.htm.

Ethnicity Online—Cultural Awareness in Healthcare. "Hindus: Dietary Guidelines." Accessed December 5, 2011. http://www.ethnicityonline.net/hindu_diet.htm.

Ethnicity Online—Cultural Awareness in Healthcare. "Hindus—Physical Examinations." Accessed December 5, 2011. http://www.ethnicityonline.net/hindu_examinations.htm.

Ethnicity Online—Cultural Awareness in Healthcare. "Jews: Dietary Guidelines." Accessed December 8, 2011. http://www.ethnicityonline.net/judaism_diet.htm.

Ethnicity Online—Cultural Awareness in Healthcare. "Muslims: Birth, Babies, and Motherhood." Accessed December 6, 2011. http://www.ethnicityonline.net/islam_birth.htm.

Ethnicity Online—Cultural Awareness in Healthcare. "Muslims-Dietary Guidelines." Accessed December 6, 2011. http://www.ethnicityonline.net/islam_diet.htm.

Ethnicity Online—Cultural Awareness in Healthcare. "Sikhs: Birth, Babies, and Motherhood." Accessed December 15, 2011. http://www.ethnicityonline.net/sikh_birth.htm.

Ethnicity Online—Cultural Awareness in Healthcare. "Sikhs: Death and the Dead." Accessed December 15, 2011. http://www.ethnicityonline.net/sikh_death.htm.

Etiquette International. "Taboo Table Offerings." Accessed December 6, 2011. http://www.etiquetteinternational.com/Articles/TableOfferings.aspx.

Evangelical Church in America. "Abortion." Updated September 4, 1991. http://www.elca.org/What-We-Believe/Social-Issues/Social-Statements/Abortion.aspx.

Evangelical Lutheran Church in America. "Prayer: Fasting." Accessed January 31, 2012. http://www2.elca.org/prayer/resources/fasting.html.

Evangelical Lutheran Church of America. "End of Life Decisions." Accessed December 12, 2011. http://www.elca.org/What-We-Believe/Social-Issues/Messages/End-of-Life-Decisions.aspx.

Evangelical Lutheran Church of America. "Funerals." Accessed December 12, 2011. https://www.elca.org/Growing-In-Faith/Worship/Learning-Center/FAQs/Funerals.aspx.

Evangelical Lutheran Church of America. "How Can We Provide for Communion of the Ill, Homebound, and the Imprisoned?" Accessed December 8, 2011. https://www.elca.org/Growing-In-Faith/Worship/Learning-Center/FAQs/Communion-Distribution-Outside.aspx.

Evangelical Lutheran Church of America. "Organ Donation." Accessed December 12, 2011. http://www.elca.org/What-We-Believe/Social-Issues/Resolutions/1989/CA89,-p-,07,-p-,72-Organ-Donation.aspx.

Exploring Religions. "Life Cycle Observances in Islam." Accessed December 6, 2011. http://uwacadweb.uwyo.edu/religionet/er/islam/islife.htm.

Faqs.org. "Jewish Childrearing Related Questions." Last updated April 10, 1996. http://www.faqs.org /faqs/judaism/FAQ/12-Kids/.

Ferrell, B.R. and N. Coyle, eds. *Oxford Textbook of Palliative Nursing*. New York: Oxford University Press, 2010.

Ferris-Taylor, R. "Communication," in *Learning Disabilities: Toward Inclusion*, 5th ed., edited by B. Gates. Oxford, UK: Churchill Livingstone, 2003.

Fina, D.K. "The Spiritual Needs of Pediatric Patients and Their Families." *AORN* 62, no. 4 (October 1995): 556–58, 560, 562, 564. http://dx.doi.org/10.1016/S0001-2092(06)63497-2.

Find Your Fate. "Things To Do Before You Die—Christianity." Accessed December 14, 2011. http://death.findyourfate.com/christianity.html.

Finkbeiner, W.E., P.C. Ursell, and R.L. Davis. *Autopsy Pathology: A Manual and Atlas*. Philadelphia, PA: Saunders Elsevier, 2009.

First United Methodist Church. "What United Methodists Believe." Accessed December 12, 2011. http://www.siouxcityfirst.com/283125.

Firth, S. *Dying, Death and Bereavement in a British Hindu Community*. n.p. Belgium? Peeters, Bondgenotenlaan, Leuven, 1997.

Fisheaters.com. "The Catholic Way of Dying." Accessed January 18, 2012. http://fisheaters.com/dying.html.

Fisher, N.L. *Cultural and Ethnic Diversity: A Guide for Genetics Professionals*. Baltimore, MD: Johns Hopkins University Press, 1996.

Fletcher, D.C. "Low Vision: The Physician's Role in Rehabilitation and Referral." *Geriatrics* 49, no. 5 (May 1994): 50–53. http://www.ncbi.nlm.nih.gov/pubmed/8174941.

Flint, W. *Alabama Baptists: Southern Baptists in the Heart of Dixie*. Tuscaloosa, AL: University of Alabama Press, 1998.

Fowler, M., S. Reimer-Kirkham, R. Sawatzky, and E.J. Taylor. *Religion, Religious Ethics, and Nursing*. New York: Springer Publishing Company, 2012.

Francoeur, R.T. and R.J. Noonan, eds. *The Continuum Complete International Encyclopedia of Sexuality*. New York: Continuum International Publishing Group, Inc., 2004.

Frankel, W. *World Jewish Congress, Survey of Jewish Affairs*. Cranbury, NJ: Associated University Presses, 1988.

FreeRepublic.com. "Fetal Personhood Law Has Radical Implications For Freedom of Religion Says Religious Coalition." April 1, 2004. http://www.freerepublic.com/focus/f-news/1109601/posts.

From the Minister's Study. "What Good is Baptism?" Updated March 26, 1999. http://archive.uua.org/CONG/column75.html.

Funeral_Rites_website.doc. "Funeral Rites Across Different Cultures." Accessed December 6, 2011. www.egfl.org.uk/export/sites/egfl/.../Furneral_Rites_website.doc.

Gabbard, G.O., L.W. Roberts, H. Crisp-Han, V. Ball, G. Hobday, and F. Rachal. *Professionalism in Psychiatry*. Arlington, VA: American Psychiatric Publishing, 2012.

Galanti, G.A. *Caring for Patients From Different Cultures*, 4th ed. Philadelphia, PA: University of Pennsylvania Press, 2008.

Gassmann, G. and S.H. Hendrix. *Fortress Introduction to the Lutheran Confessions*. Minneapolis, MN: Augsburg Fortress, 1999.

Gates-Williams, J., M.N. Jackson, V. Jenkins-Monroe, and L.R. Williams. "The Business of Preventing African-American Infant Mortality." *Western Journal of Medicine* 157, no.3 (1992): 350–56. http://www.ncbi.nlm.nih.gov/pmc/articles/PMC1011293/.

Gatrad, A.R. "Muslim Customs Surrounding Death, Bereavement, Postmortem Examinations, and Organ Transplants." *British Medical Journal* 309 (August 1994): 521–23. DOI: 10.1136/bmj.309.6953.521.

Gatrad, R., J. Jhutti-Johal, P.S. Gill, and A. Sheikh. "Sikh birth customs." *Archives of Disease in Childhood* 90, no. 6 (June 2005): 560–63. DOI:10.1136/adc.2004.064378.

Gatrad, R., S.S. Panesar, E. Brown, H. Notta, and A. Sheikh. "Palliative care for Sikhs." *International Journal of Palliative Nursing* 9, no.11 (November 2003): 496–98. http://www.ncbi.nlm.nih.gov/pubmed/14676727.

Gellar, S. "Religious Attitudes and the Autopsy." *Archives of Pathology & Laboratory Medicine* 108 (1984): 494–96. http://ukpmc.ac.uk/abstract/MED/6547302.

General Board of the American Baptist Churches. "American Baptist Policy Statement on Health, Healing, and Wholeness." Updated June 1991. http://www.abc-usa.org/LinkClick.aspx?fileticket-kA7NkRgFPIE %3D&tabid=199.

Geyman, J. "Societal Blind Spots as Barriers to Health Care Reform." Physicians for a National Health Program. Updated July 15, 2009. http://pnhp.org/blog/2009/07/15/societal-blind-spots-as-barriers-to-health-care-reform/ .

The Gift of a Lifetime. "Religion and Organ and Tissue Donation." Accessed December 12, 2011. http://www.organtransplants.org/understanding/religion/.

Giger, J.N., and R.E. Davidhizar. *Transcultural Nursing, Assessment and Intervention*. St. Louis, MO: Elsevier Mosby, 2008.

Gill, B.K. "Nursing with Dignity: Part 6: Sikhism." *Nursing Times* 98, no. 14 (April 2002): 39–41.

Global Anabaptist Mennonite Encyclopedia Online. "Baptism, Age at." Accessed December 12, 2011. http://www.gameo.org/encyclopedia/contents/B369ME.html.

Goepp, J.G. "Autism: A Nutraceutical Approach." *Life Extension Magazine*. December 2007, 53–60. http://www.lef.org/magazine/mag2007/dec2007_report_autism_02.html.

Good, M. and P. Good. *20 Most Asked Questions About the Amish and Mennonites*, rev. ed. Intercourse, PA: Good Books, 1995.

Granju, K.A. CityPages. "The Culture of Childbirth." May 1, 1999. http://www.citypages.com/1999-05-01/feature/the-culture-of-childbirth/.

Gravett, L. and R. Throckmorton. *Bridging the Generation Gap: How to Get Radio Babies, Boomers, Gen Xers, and Gen Yers to Work Together and Achieve More*. Franklin Lakes, NJ: Career Press, Inc., 2007.

Gypsy Vodou. "Gypsy Death Rituals and Customs." Accessed January 9, 2012. http://gypsyvodou.com/gypsies/875/.

Haas, J.G. *The Orange County Register*. "Final Goodbye Isn't as Hard as You Might Think." June 11, 2007. http://www.ocregister.com/articles/people-36253-dying-death.html.

Hale, W.D. and R.G. Bennett. *Building Healthy Communities Through Medical-Religious Partnerships*. Baltimore, MD: Johns Hopkins University Press, 2000.

Hamilton, E.H. *The Health and Wellness Ministry in the African American Church*. n.p.: Xulon Press, 2004.

Hammoud, M.M., C.B. White, and M.D. Fetters. "Opening Cultural Doors: Providing Culturally Sensitive Healthcare to Arab American and American Muslim Patients." *American Journal of Obstetrics & Gynecology* 193, no. 4 (October 2005): 1307–11. http://dx.doi.org/10.1016/j.ajog.2005.06.065.

Handen, B.L., C.R. Johnson, and M. Lubetsky. "Efficacy of Methylphenidate Among Children with Autism and Symptoms of Attention-Deficit Hyperactivity Disorder." *Journal of Autism and Developmental Disorders* 30, no. 3 (2000), 245–255. DOI: 10.1023/A:1005548619694.

Handen, B.L. and M. Lubetsky. "Pharmacotherapy in Autism and Related Disorders." *School Psychology Quarterly* 20, no. 2 (2005): 155–171. DOI: 10.1521/scpq.20.2.155.66514.

Harper, D.C. and J.S. Wadsworth. "Improving Health Care Communication for Persons with Mental Retardation." *Public Health Reports* 107, no. 3 (1992): 297–302. http://www.ncbi.nlm.nih.gov /pmc/articles/PMC1403650/.

Head and Brain Injuries. "Traumatic Brain Injury – The Medical Insurance Maze." Accessed January 16, 2012. http://www.headbraininjuries.com/brain-injury-medical-insurance.

Health Careers Journal. "A Guide for Nurses: Teaching Healthcare Effectively to Patients." Accessed December 16, 2011. http://www.healthcareersjournal.com/a-guide-for-nurses-teaching-healthcare-effectively-to-patients/.

"Healthcare for People with Physical Disabilities: Access Issues," *Medscape General Medicine* 3, no. 2 (2001), http://www.medscape.com/viewarticle/408122_4.

The Heart of the Healer Foundation. "Teachers; Apprenticeships." Accessed December 30, 2011. http://www.heartofthehealer.org/apprenticeships/Teachers.

Hedayat, K. "When the Spirit Leaves: Childhood Death, Grieving, and Bereavement in Islam." *Journal of Palliative Medicine* 9, no. 6 (2006), 1282–91. DOI:10.1089/jpm.2006.9.1282.

Hedayat, K.M. and R. Pirzadeh. "Issues in Islamic Biomedical Ethics: A Primer for the Pediatrician." *Pediatrics* 108, no. 4 (2001): 965–71. DOI: 10.1542/peds.108.4.965.

Hetherington, E.M., R.D. Parke, and V.O Locke. *Child Psychology: A Contemporary Viewpoint*. Boston, MA: McGraw-Hill, 2003.

History of Circumcision.net. "History of Circumcision." Accessed January 31, 2012. http://www.historyofcircumcision.net/.

Hoffman, S. *Mental Health, Psychotherapy and Judaism*. New York: Golden Sky, 2011.

Hollander, E., R. Dolgoff-Kaspar, C. Cartwright, R. Rawitt, and S. Novotny, "An Open Trial of Divalproex Sodium in Autism Spectrum Disorders," *Journal of Clinical Psychiatry* 62, no. 7 (July 2001): 530–534. http://psycnet.apa.org/psycinfo/2001-01982-006.

Honer, D. and P. Hoppie. "The Enigma of the Gypsy Patient." *Modern Medicine*. August 1, 2004. http://www.modernmedicine.com/modernmedicine/article/articleDetail.jsp?id=114152.

Humes, K.R., N.A. Jones, and R.R. Ramirez. "Overview of Race and Hispanic Origin: 2010; 2010 Census Briefs." Issued March 2011. http://www.census.gov/prod/cen2010/briefs/c2010br-02.pdf.

ICTMN Staff. Indian Country Today Media Network. "New Bill Would Authorize Federally Funded Abortions for Servicewomen." June 7, 2011. http://indiancountrytodaymedianetwork.com/2011/06/07/new-bill-would-authorize-federally-funded-abortions-for-servicewomen-37282.

Iezzoni, L.I., R.B. Davis, J. Soukup, and B. O'Day. "Satisfaction with Quality and Access to Health Care Among People with Disabling Conditions." *International Journal for Quality in Health Care* 14, no. 5 (2002), 369–81. DOI: 10.1093/intqhc/14.5.369.

Iezzoni, L.I., B.L. O'Day, M. Killeen, and H. Harker. "Communicating About Health Care: Observations from Persons Who are Deaf or Hard of Hearing." *Annals of Internal Medicine* 140, no. 5. March 2,2004: 356–362. http://annals.ba0.biz/content/140/5/356.short.

IMANA Ethics Committee. "Islamic Medical Ethics." Accessed December 6, 2011. http://www.isna.net/Leadership/pages/Islamic-Medical-Ethics.aspx.

In Vitro Fertilization IVF. "IVF Concept in Different Religions." Accessed December 6, 2011. http://in-vitro-fertilization.eu/different-religious-concepts-in-vitro-fertilization-assisted-reproduction/.

IndiaCurry.com. "Beliefs and Facts About Foods During Pregnancy in India." Accessed December 6, 2011. http://www.indiacurry.com/women/pregnancytaboo.htm.

Info About Sikhs. "Sikh Ceremonies." Accessed December 15, 2011. http://www.infoaboutsikhs.com /sikh_ceremonies.htm.

Institute of Developing Economies. "Pakistani Migration to the US: An Economic Perspective." Accessed January 18, 2012. http://ir.ide.go.jp/dspace/bitstream/2344/839/1/196_oda.pdf.

Institute of Medicine. Committee on Quality of Health Care in America. *Crossing the Quality Chasm: A New Health System for the 21st Century*. Washington, DC: National Academy Press, 2001.

International Strategy and Policy Institute. "Guidelines for Health Care Providers Interacting with Muslim Patients and their Families." Last modified June 10, 2006. http://www.ispi--usa.org/guidelines.htm.

Islam for Children. "The Five Pillars of Wisdom." Accessed December 6, 2011. http://atschool.eduweb.co.uk/carolrb/islam/fivepillars.html.

IslamCan.com. "Prohibition of Free-Mixing Between Men and Women." Accessed December 6, 2011. http://www.islamcan.com/youth/prohibition-of-free-mixing-between-men-and-women.shtml.

Islamhelpline. "If Husband Can Be Present." Accessed December 6, 2011. http://www.islamhelpline.com/node/4425.

The Islamic Bulletin. "Islamic Dietary Laws and Practices." Accessed December 6, 2011. http://www.islamicbulletin.org/newsletters/issue_2/dietarylaws.aspx.

Islamic Forum; IslamicBoard.com. "Male Circumcision in Islam." September 22, 2008. http://www.islamicboard.com/health-science/134271551-male-circumcision-islam.html.

IslamWeb. "Using Alcohol or Gelatin Derived from Pork as Medicine." Accessed December 6, 2011. http://www.islamweb.net/emainpage/index.php?page=showfatwa&Option=FatwaId&Id=90894.

iValue. T.E. Track. "Defining Truths of the Assemblies of God: Divine Healing." Accessed January 31, 2012. http://agchurches.org/Sitefiles/Default/RSS/IValue/Resources/Divine%20Healing/Articles/Defining_DivineHealing.pdf.

ivf-worldwide. "In Vitro Fertilization." Accessed December 27, 2011. http://www.ivf-worldwide.com/Education/christianity.html.

Jamaica-Guide.info. "Religion in Jamaica." Accessed January 14, 2012. http://jamaica-guide.info/past.and.present/religion/.

Jeffery, D. "Adapting De-escalation Techniques with Deaf Service Users." *Nursing Standard* 19, no. 49 (2005): 41–47. http://cat.inist.fr/?aModele=afficheN&cpsidt=17066380.

Jehovah's Witness Official Web Site. "Infertility—The Choice, The Issues." Accessed December 7, 2011. http://www.watchtower.org/e/20040922/article_02.htm.

Jehovah's Witnesses Official Web Site. "What Do They Believe?" Accessed December 7, 2011. http://www.watchtower.org/e/jt/article_03.htm.

Jevon, P, *Advanced Cardiac Life Support: A Guide For Nurses*. Oxford, UK: Wiley-Blackwell, 2010.

Jewish Women's Health. "Childbirth in Jewish Law." Accessed December 0, 2011. http://www.jewishwomenshealth.org/article.php?article=20

Judaism101."Kashrut: Jewish Dietary Laws." Accessed December 8, 2011. http://www.jewfaq.org/kashrut.htm.

JVNA. "Judaism, Health, and Vegetarianism." Accessed December 8, 2011. http://jewishveg.com/jh.html.

Kadden, B.B. and B. Kadden. *Teaching Jewish Life Cycle: Traditions and Activities*. Denver, CO: A.R.F. Publishing, Inc. 1997.

Kauai's Hindu Monastery. "Four Facts of Hinduism." Accessed December 5, 2011. http://www.himalayanacademy.com/basics/fourf/.

Kauai's Hindu Monastery. "Glossary" Accessed December 5, 2011. http://www.himalayanacademy.com /resources/lexicon/.

Kauai's Hindu Monastery. "Nine Beliefs of Hinduism." Accessed December 5, 2011. http://www.himalayanacademy.com/basics/nineb/.

Kelly, E.B. *Gene Therapy.* Santa Barbara, CA: Greenwood Publishing Group.

Kennel-Shank, C. Mennonite Weekly Review. "Choices at the End of Life." Accessed December 12, 2011. http://www.mennoweekly.org/2011/1/24/choices-end-life/.

Khan, Mas'ud Ahmed's Home Page. "Etiquettes of Reading and Handling the Qur'an al-Kareem." Accessed December 6, 2011. http://www.themodernreligion.com/basic/quran/etiquette.html.

Khoda, B. *Islamic Duas: A Compilation of Prayers.* n.p.[Iran?]: A Duas Publishing Project. duas.org.

Kim, J.R., D. Elliott, and C. Hyde. "The Influence of Sociocultural Factors on Organ Donation and Transplantation in Korea: Findings From Key Informant Interviews." *Journal of Transcultural Nursing* 15, no. 2 (April 2004): 147–54. DOI: 10.1177/1043659603262485.

Kim, S.H., W.K. Kim, K.A. Lee, Y.S. Song, and S.Y. Oh. "Breastfeeding in Korea." *World Review of Nutrition and Dietetics* 78 (1995): 114–27. http://www.ncbi.nlm.nih.gov/pubmed/7495140.

Klessig, J. "Cross-Cultural Medicine a Decade Later: The Effect of Values and Culture on Life-Support Decisions." *Western Journal of Medicine* 157, no. 3 (September 1992): 316–22. http://www.ncbi.nlm.nih.gov /pmc/articles/PMC1011285/.

Kohli, S.S. *The Sikh and Sikhism.* New Delhi: Atlantic Publishers & Distributors, 1993.

Komoto, J., S. Usui, and J. Hirata. "Infantile Autism and Affective Disorder." *Journal of Autism and Developmental Disorders* 14, no. 1 (1984), 81–84. DOI: 10.1007/BF02408557.

Dr. Kornhaber. "Grandparents Raising Grandchildren." Accessed January 17, 2012. http://www.grandparenting.org/Grandparents_Raising_Grandchildren.htm.

Kramer, B.J. "Health and Aging of Urban American Indians." *Western Journal of Medicine* 157, no. 3 (September 1992): 281–85. http://www.ncbi.nlm.nih.gov/pmc/articles/PMC1011277/.

Kraybill, D.B., S.M. Nolt, and D.L. Weaver-Zercher. *The Amish Way: Patient Faith in a Perilous World.* San Francisco: John Wiley & Sons, Inc., 2010.

Kriegman-Chin, M. "A Japanese Birth." *Midwifery Today* 26 (1993), 32–3, 40. http://www.ncbi.nlm.nih.gov /pubmed/8369855.

Krohm, C. and S.K. Summers. *Advance Health Care Directives: A Handbook for Professionals.* Chicago: American Bar Association, 2002.

Kwintessential. "India—Language, Culture, Customs and Etiquette." Accessed December 5, 2011. http://www.kwintessential.co.uk/resources/global-etiquette/india-country-profile.html.

Lamb, J. "The Basics on Advance Directives—Thy Will Be Done." May 26, 2010. http://www.lutheransforlife.org/article/the-basics-on-advance-directives-thy-will-be-done/.

Lassiter, S.M. *Multicultural Clients: A Professional Handbook for Health Care Providers and Social Workers.* Westport, CT: Greenwood Publishing Group, 1995.

LDS.net. "Abortion." Accessed December 12, 2011. http://mormon.lds.net/abortion.

LDS.net. "Birth Control." Accessed December 12, 2011. http://mormon.lds.net/birth-control.

Learning Disabilities Association of America. "For Teachers: Understanding Learning Disabilities and ADHD." Accessed January 16, 2012. http://www.ldanatl.org/aboutld/teachers/index.asp.

Lee, D.J., B.L. Lam, S. Arora, K.L. Arheart, K.E. McCollister, D.D. Zheng, S.L. Christ, and E.P. Davila. "Reported Eye Care Utilization and Health Insurance Status Among US Adults." *Archives of Ophthalmology* 127, no. 3 (March 2009): 303–310. http://archopht.ama-assn.org/cgi/content/abstract/127/3/303.

Leichter, J. "Lactose Tolerance in a Jewish Population." *Digestive Diseases and Sciences* 16, no. 12: 1123–1126. http://www.springerlink.com/content/lh25036588434651/.

Leininger, M.M. and M.R. McFarland. *Culture Care Diversity and Universality: A Worldwide Nursing Theory.* Sudbury, MA: Jones and Bartlett Publishers, 2006.

Leming, M.R. and G.E. Dickinson. *Understanding Dying, Death, and Bereavement.* Belmont, CA: Wadsworth, 2011.

Liégeois, J.P. *Roma, Gypsies, Travellers.* The Netherlands. Council of Europe, 1994.

LifeCenter Northwest. "Religion and Donation." Accessed January 31, 2012. http://www.lcnw.org/understanding-donation/religion-and-donation/.

Lipson, J. and S. Dibble, eds. *Culture and Clinical Care*. San Francisco, CA: UCSF Nursing Press, 2005.

Lipson, J.G., S. Dibble, and P.A. Minarik, eds., *Culture and Nursing Care: A Pocket Guide*. San Francisco, CA: UCSF Nursing Press, 1996.

Livestrong.com. "What Foods Are On the 7th Day Adventist Diet?" Accessed December 20, 2011. http://www.livestrong.com/article/441583-what-foods-are-on-the-7th-day-adventist-diet/.

Loeb, G. The Philadelphia Jewish Voice. "Living Judaism: Judaism's Perspective on Organ Donation After Death." Accessed December 8, 2011. http://www.pjvoice.com/v38/38700judaism.aspx.

Luce, J.M. and T.A. Raffin. "Withholding and Withdrawal of Life Support From Critically Ill Patients." *Western Journal of Medicine* 167, no. 6 (December 1997): 411–416. http://ukpmc.ac.uk/abstract/MED/3409745.

Lutherans for Life. "Life Thoughts in the Church Year." Accessed December 9, 2011. http://www.lutheransforlife.org/media/life-thoughts-in-the-church/.

Macdonald, E. *Difficult Conversations in Medicine*. New York: Oxford, 2004.

Maguire, D.C. "Contraception and Abortion in Islam." Accessed December 6, 2011. http://www.religiousconsultation.org/islam_contraception_abortion_in_SacredChoices.htm.

Marty, M.E. *Health and Medicine in the Lutheran Tradition*. New York: Crossroad Publishing Co., 1986.

Matlins, S. and A. Magida, eds. *How to Be a Perfect Stranger: A Guide to Etiquette in Other People's Religious Ceremonies*. Woodstock, VT: SkyLight Paths Publishing, 2011.

Matsumura, S., S. Bito, H. Liu, K. Kahn, S. Fukuhara, M. Kagawa-Singer, and N. M. Wenger. "Acculturation of Attitudes Toward End-of-Life Care: A Cross-Cultural Survey of Japanese Americans and Japanese." *Journal of General Internal Medicine* 17, no. 7 (July 2002), 531–539.

Mauk, K.L. and N.K. Schmidt. *Spiritual Care in Nursing Practice*. Philadelphia, PA: Lippincott Williams & Wilkins, 2004.

Mayell, J.S. *Universality of the Sikh Religion*. Columbia, MO: Mayell Publishers, 2006.

Mayo Clinic.org. "Diabetes Diet: Create Your Healthy-Eating Plan." Accessed January 15, 2012. http://www.mayoclinic.com/health/diabetes-diet/DA00027.

McAleer, M. "Communicating Effectively with Deaf Patients." *Nursing Standard* 20, no. 19 (2006): 51–54. http://cat.inist.fr/?aModele=afficheN&cpsidt=17466038.

McClure, J. "Finding Faith, Hope, and Love." Last updated February 27, 2011. http://rss.ag.org/articles/detail.cfm?RSS_RSSContentID=18592&RSS_OriginatingChannelID=global&RSS_OriginatingRSSFeedID=global&RSS_Source=search.

McKennis, A. "Caring for the Islamic Patient," *AORN Journal* 69, no. 6 (June 1999): 1185–96. DOI:10.1016/S0001-2092(06)61885-1.

Mead, F.S., S.S. Hill, and C.D. Atwood. *Handbook of Denominations in the United States*, 13th ed. Nashville, TN: Abingdon Press, 2010.

Melville, C.A., J. Morrison, L. Allan, E. Smiley, and A. Williamson. "The Prevalence and Determinants of Obesity in Adults with Intellectual Disabilities." *Journal of Applied Research in Intellectual Disabilities* 21, no. 5 (Sept. 2008): 425–37. DOI: 10.1111/j.1468-3148.2007.00412.x.

A Memory Tree. "Customs and Religious Protocols." Accessed December 7, 2011. http://www.amemorytree.co.nz/customs.php.

Michael C. Carlos Museum of Emory University, Odyssey Online Africa. "Death and Burial." Accessed December 28, 2011. http://www.carlos.emory.edu/ODYSSEY/AFRICA/AF_death.html.

Midwest Orthopaedics at Rush. "Physical Medicine/Pain Management." Accessed January 16, 2012. http://www.rushortho.com/pain_management.cfm.

Migration Policy Institute. "Why Immigrants Lack Adequate Access to Health Care and Health Insurance." updated September 2006. http://www.migrationinformation.org/Feature/display.cfm?ID=417.

Milestones. "Checklist for Learning Disabilities." Accessed January 16, 2012. http://www.advancingmilestones.com/PDFs/m_resources_LD-checklist.pdf.

Mingkok Buddhist News. "Buddhism and Organ Donation." Last modified August 31, 2011. http://mingkok.buddhistdoor.com/en/news/d/22456.

Ministerial Association, General Conference of Seventh-day Adventists. *Adventists Believe... A Biblical Exposition of 27 Fundamental Doctrines*. Hagerstown, MD: Review & Herald Publishing Association, 1988.

Moltmann, J. *God in Creation: A New Theology of Creation and the Spirit of God*. Minneapolis, MN: Augsburg Fortress, 1993.

Monti, D.A. and E.J.S. Kunkel. "Practical Geriatrics: Management of Chronic Pain Among Elderly Patients." *Psychiatric Services* 49, no. 12 (1998), 1537–1539. http://www.ps.psychiatryonline.org/article.aspx?articleid =82193&RelatedWidget Articles=true.

MormonBeliefs.org. "Do Mormons Believe in the Resurrection?" Accessed December 12, 2011. http://www.mormonbeliefs. org/mormon_beliefs/mormon-doctrine-salvation/do-mormons-believe-in-the-resurrection.

MormonBeliefs.org. "Fasting." Accessed December 12, 2011. http://www.mormonbeliefs.org/mormon_beliefs/mormon-beliefs-culture/fasting.

MormonBeliefs.org. "Laws of Health." Accessed December 12, 2011. http://www.mormonbeliefs.org/mormon_beliefs/mormon-beliefs-laws-of-health.

MormonBeliefs.org. "A Lay Clergy: The Value of Service." Accessed December 12, 2011. http://www.mormonbeliefs.org/mormon_beliefs/mormon-beliefs-culture/a-lay-clergy-the-value-of-service.

MormonBeliefs.org. "Mormon Beliefs." Accessed December 12, 2011. http://www.mormonbeliefs.org/.

MormonBeliefs.org. "Mormon Missionaries." Accessed December 12, 2011. http://www.mormonbeliefs.org/mormon_ missionaries.

MormonBeliefs.org. "Mormon Rites" Accessed December 12, 2011. http://www.mormonbeliefs.org /mormon_beliefs/mormon-beliefs-culture/mormon-rites.

MormonBeliefs.org. "Mormon Underwear." Accessed December 12, 2011. http://www.mormonbeliefs.org/mormon_ temples/mormon-underwear.

MormonBeliefs.org. "Prayer." Accessed December 12, 2011. http://www.mormonbeliefs.org /mormon_beliefs/mormon-doctrine-salvation/mormon-beliefs-prayer.

MormonBeliefs.org. "Spiritual Gifts in the Mormon Church." Accessed December 12, 2011. http://www.mormonbeliefs.org/mormon_beliefs/thoughts-mormon-beliefs/spiritual-gifts-the-mormon-church.

Mull, D.S., N. Nguyen, and J.D. Mull. "Vietnamese Diabetic Patients and Their Physicians: What Ethnography Can Teach Us." *Western Journal of Medicine* 175, no. 5 (November 2001): 307–11. http://www.ncbi.nlm.nih.gov/pmc/articles/PMC1071603/.

Muller, J.H. and B. Desmond. "Ethical Dilemmas in a Cross-Cultural Context. A Chinese Example." *Western Journal of Medicine* 157, no.3 (September 1992): 323–27. http://www.ncbi.nlm.nih.gov/pmc/articles /PMC1011287/.

Munoz-Baell, I.M. and M.T. Ruiz. "Empowering the Deaf. Let the Deaf be Deaf." *Journal of Epidemiology and Community Health* 54, no. 1 (2000): 40–44. DOI:10.1136/jech.54.1.40.

Murray, M.L. and G.M. Huelsmann. *Labor and Delivery Nursing: A Guide to Evidence-Based Practice*. New York: Springer Publishing Company, Inc., 2009.

Muslim Population.com ."Muslim Population in the World." Accessed January 17, 2012. http://www.islamicpopulation.com/.

My Jewish Learning. "Dying." Accessed December 8, 2011. http://www.myjewishlearning.com/life /Life_Events/Death_and_Mourning/Dying.shtml.

National Dissemination Center for Children with Disabilities. "Categories of Disability Under IDEA." Updated April 2009. http://nichcy.org/disability/categories/.

National Institute on Aging. *A Clinician's Handbook: Talking with Your Older Patient*. Bethesda, MD: National Institutes of Health, Department of Health and Human Services, 2008.

National Oceanographic and Atmospheric Association Office of Diversity. "Tips to Improve Communication Across Generations." Accessed January 17, 2012. http://honolulu.hawaii.edu/intranet /committees/FacDevCom/guidebk/teachtip/intergencomm.htm.

Nelson, C.P., R. Dunn, J. Wan, and J. Wei. "The Increasing Incidence of Newborn Circumcision: Data from the Nationwide Inpatient Sample." *Journal of Urology* 173, no.3 (March 2005): 978–981.

Nelson, D. and K. Amplo. "Care of the Autistic Patient in the Perioperative Area." *AORN Journal* 89, no. 2 (February 2009): 391–397. DOI:10.1016/j aorn.2000.01.018.

Nelson, P.C. *Bible Doctrines*. Springfield, MO: Gospel Publishing House, 1998.

New York Presbyterian Hospital. "Circumcision." Accessed December 14, 2011. http://nyp.org/health /pediatrics_ circumcision.html.

New York Presbyterian Hospital. "Contraception/Birth Control." Accessed December 14, 2011. http://nyp.org/health/ women-contra.html.

New York Presbyterian Hospital. "Food for Thought." Accessed December 14, 2011. http://nyp.org/nutrition/resources/ index.html.

New York-Presbyterian Hospital. "Office of External Relations." Accessed December 14, 2011. http://nyp.org/oer/.

New York-Presbyterian Hospital. "Ten Thousand Dreams Come True Through New York-Presbyterian/Weill Cornell's IVF Program." Accessed December 14, 2011. http://nyp.org/news/hospital/crmi-ivf-milestone.html.

New York-Presbyterian Morgan Stanley Children's Hospital. "Blood and Organ Donation." Accessed December 14, 2011. http://childrensnyp.org/mschony/patients/blood-organ-donation.html.

Nichols, A.D., R.L. Ward, R.I. Freedman, and L.V. Sarkissian. The Boston Foundation. "Left Out in the Cold: Healthcare Experiences of Adults with Intellectual and Developmental Disabilities in Massachusetts." Updated December 2008. http://www.arcmass.org/Portals/0/TheArcofMassHealthCareFullReport_12.08.pdf.

Nunn, J., R. Freeman, E. Anderson, L.C. Carneiro, M.S.A. Carneiro, and A. Formicola et al. "Inequalities in Access to Education and Healthcare," special issue "Global Congress on Dental Education" in *European Journal of Dental Education* 12 (Feb. 2008), 30–39. DOI: 10.1111/j.1600-0579.2007.00478.x.

Nurses Neighborhood. "Filipino Culture Paper; Nursing Culture Class." Accessed January 6, 2012. http://www.nurses-neighborhood.com/filipino-culture.html.

Obernberger, S. "When Love and Abuse are not Mutually Exclusive." *Issues in Law and Medicine* 355 (Spring 1997). http://heinonline.org/HOL/LandingPage?collection=journals&handle=hein.journals /ilmed12&div=42&id=&page=.

O'Brien, M.E. *A Nurse's Handbook of Spiritual Care: Standing on Holy Ground*. Sudbury, MA: Jones and Bartlett, 2004.

O'Brien, S. About.Com. "Multigenerational Households are Growing." Accessed January 17, 2012. http://seniorliving.about.com/od/boomerscaringforparents/a/multigeneration-household.htm.

Ochsner. "Religious Views." Accessed January 9, 2012. http://www.ochsner.org/services /multi_organ_transplant/ transplant_organ_donation_religious_views/#GYP.

The Office of the Stated Clerk of the General Assembly of the Presbyterian Church in America. *The Book of Church Order of the Presbyterian Church in America*, 5th ed. (2010).

Ohlhoff, E.L. National Right to Life. "Abortion: Where Do the Churches Stand?" Updated September 12, 2000. http://www.pregnantpause.org/people/wherchur.htm.

Ong, A. and N.N. Chen, eds. *Asian Biotech: Ethics and Communities of Fate*. Durham, NC: Duke University Press, 2010.

Oppapers.com. "Hinduism vs. Buddhism." Accessed December 6, 2011. http://www.oppapers.com/essays /Hinduism-Vs-Buddhism/141221.

Ott, B.B., J. Al-Khaduri, and S. Al-Junaibi. "Preventing Ethical Dilemmas: Understanding Islamic Health Care Practices." *Pediatric Nursing* 29, no. 3 (2003). http://www.medscape.com/viewarticle/457485.

Our Catholic Faith. "Healing Prayers." Accessed December 15, 2011. http://www.ourcatholicfaith.org /prayer/p-healing.html.

Pakistan Red Crescent Society. "Blood Transfusion Service." Accessed January 7, 2012. http://prcs.org.pk/blood.asp.

Paris, J.J. and A. Bell. "Ethical Issues in Perinatology: Guarantee My Child Will Be 'Normal' or Stop All Treatment." *Journal of Perinatology* 13, no.6 (1993), 469.

Patheos.com. "Anglican Afterlife and Salvation." Accessed December 27, 2011. http://www.patheos.com/Library/Anglican/ Beliefs/Afterlife-and-Salvation?offset=0&max=1.

Patheos.com. "Baptist." Accessed December 26, 2011. http://www.patheos.com/Library/Baptist.html.

Patheos.com. "Jehovah's Witnesses." Accessed December 7, 2011. http://www.patheos.com/Library /Jehovahs-Witnesses.html.

Patja, K., P. Eero, and M. Iivanlainen. "Cancer Incidence Among People with Intellectual Disability." *Journal of Intellectual Disability Research* 45, no. 4 (Aug. 2001): 300–07. DOI: 10.1046/j.1365-2788.2001.00322.x.

Peel, R. *Health and Medicine in the Christian Science Tradition*. New York: Crossroad Publications, 1986.

Peelman, A. *Christ is a Native American*. Toronto, Ontario, Canada, Novalis-Saint Paul University, 1995.

Penn Medicine. "Jehovah's Witnesses—Position Overview—Bloodless Medicine & Surgery." Accessed December 7, 2011. http://www.pennmedicine.org/health_info/bloodless/000206.html.

Pennsylvania Medical Society. "Advance Health Care Directives and Health Care Decision-making for Incompetent Patients: A Guide to Act 169 of 2006 for Physicians and Other Health Care Professionals." Accessed January 18, 2012. http://www.pcacc.org/advance_health_directives.pdf.

Pennsylvania Medicine Pastoral Care and Education. "Faith Traditions and Health Care." Revised June 2003. http://www.uphs.upenn.edu/pastoral/pubs/traditions.html.

People of the United Methodist Church. "Abortion." Accessed January 31, 2012. http://archives.umc.org/interior.asp?mid=1732.

People of the United Methodist Church. "What Happens after a Person Dies?" Accessed January 18, 2012. http://www.umc.org/site/apps/nlnet/content3.aspx?c=lwL4KnN1LtH&b=4746357&ct=3008067.

Peron, J.E. "Christian Parents and the Circumcision Issue." Many Blessings 3 (Spring 2000). Accessed December 12, 2011. http://www.cirp.org/pages/cultural/peron1/.

Pew Forum on Religion & Public Life. "Religious Composition of the U.S.—U.S. Religious Landscape Survey." Accessed January 17, 2012. http://religions.pewforum.org/pdf/affiliations-all-traditions.pdf.

Pew Research Center. "The Millennials: Confident. Connected. Open to Change." Accessed January 17, 2012. http://pewresearch.org/pubs/1501/millennials-new-survey-generational-personality-upbeat-open-new-ideas-technology-bound?src=prc-latest&proj=peoplepress.

Pew Research Center. "U.S. Religious Landscape Survey." Accessed January 17, 2012. http://religions.pewforum.org/reports.

Phelan, S. "Generational Issues in the ob-gyn Workplace: 'Marcus Welby, MD' versus 'Scrubs.'" *Obstetrics and Gynecology* 116, no. 3 (Sept. 2010), 568–69. DOI: 10.1097/AOG.0b013e3181f086b9.

Phipps, E.J., G. True, and G.F. Murray. "Community Perspectives on Advance Care Planning: Report from the Community Ethics Program." *Journal of Cultural Diversity* 10, no.4 (Winter 2003): 118–23.

Poloma, M.M. and J.C. Green. *The Assemblies of God*. New York: New York University Press, 2010.

Potts, N.L. and B.L. Mandleco. *Pediatric Nursing: Caring for Children and Their Families*. Clifton Park, NY: Delmar Publishing, 2012.

Prentice, D.A. and D.T. Miller, eds. *Cultural Divides: Understanding and Overcoming Group Conflict*. New York: Russell Sage Foundation, 1999.

Presbyterian Church USA. "What Do Presbyterians Believe About Life After Death?" Accessed December 14, 2011. http://gamc.pcusa.org/ministries/today/life-after-death/.

Presbyterian Elders in Prayer. "Who We Are." Accessed December 14, 2011. http://presbypray.org/.

Presbyterian Healthcare Decisions. "Presbyterian: Advance Directives." Accessed December 14, 2011. http://www.phs.org/PHS/Chaplaincy/Patient_Education/Advance/index.htm.

PubMed Health. "Lactose Intolerance." Last updated July 7, 2010. http://www.ncbi.nlm.nih.gov /pubmedhealth/PMH0001321/.

Purnell, L.D. and B.J. Paulanka. *Guide to Culturally Competent Health Care*. Philadelphia, PA: F. A. Davis Company, 2009.

Queensland Government. "Health Care Providers' Handbook on Sikh Patients." Accessed December 15, 2011. http://www.health.qld.gov.au/multicultural/health_workers/hbook-sikh.asp.

Qul.org. "Tayammum / Dry Ablution." Accessed January 31, 2012. http://www.qul.org.au/library/a-guide-on-praying/conducting-tayammum.

Ramakrishna, J. and M.J. Weiss. "Health, Illness, and Immigration—East Indians in the United States," in "Cross-cultural Medicine a Decade Later." J. Barker and M.M. Clark, eds., special issue, *Western Journal of Medicine*, 157, no.3 (1992): 267. http://www.ncbi.nlm.nih.gov/pmc/articles/PMC1011274/?page=1.

Randall-David, E. *Strategies for Working with Culturally Diverse Communities and Clients*. Washington, DC: Association for the Care of Children's Health, 1989.

Ray-Mihm, R. "Autism: Part 1. Deficits, Prevalence, Symptoms, and Environmental Factors." *Journal of Continuing Education in Nursing* 39, no. 2 (February 2008): 55–56. http://www.slackjournals.com /article.aspx?rid=26239.

Real Sikhism. "Five Articles of Faith." Accessed January 31, 2012. http://www.realsikhism.com /index.php?subaction=show full&id=1193703788&ucat=5.

RedOrbit. "Thomson Reuters Study Finds Baby Boomers and Generation X Face Healthcare Cost Hurdles." Updated June 22, 2009. http://www.redorbit.com/news/health/1708934/thomson_reuters_study_finds _baby_boomers_and_ generation_x_face/.

Reeb, R.M. and S.T. McFarland. "Emergency Baptism." *Journal of Christian Nursing:* 12, no. 2 (Spring 1995), 26–27. http://journals.lww.com/journalofchristiannursing/Citation/1995/12020 /Emergency_Baptism.10.aspx.

Reier, J. *McGraw-Hill's GED Language Arts, Reading.* New York: McGraw-Hill, 2003.

ReligionFacts. "Beliefs and Doctrines of Sikhism." Accessed December 15, 2011. http://www.religionfacts.com/sikhism/ beliefs.htm.

ReligionFacts. "Church of Christ, Scientist." Accessed December 26, 2011. http://www.religionfacts.com /a-z-religion-index/christian_science.htm.

ReligionFacts. "History of Sikhism." Accessed December 15, 2011. http://www.religionfacts.com /sikhism/history.htm.

ReligionFacts. "Presbyterian Practices." Accessed December 14, 2011. http://www.religionfacts.com /christianity/ denominations/presbyterian/practices.htm.

Religion Link. "Spirituality Emerges as Point of Debate in Mind-Body Movement." Updated Feb. 13, 2006. http://www. religionlink.com/tip_060213.php.

Religious Portal—All About Hinduism. "Rituals Related to Death in Hindu Family." Accessed December 5, 2011. http://www. religiousportal.com/HinduDeathRituals.html.

Religious Tolerance.org. "Judaism—Beliefs and Practices." Accessed December 8, 2011. http://www.religioustolerance. org/judaism.htm.

Religious Tolerance.org. "Native American Spirituality, Beliefs of Native Americans from the Arctic to the Southwest." Accessed December 30, 2011. http://www.religioustolerance.org/nataspir3.htm.

Religious Tolerance.org. "The Roma: Their Beliefs and Practices." Accessed January 9, 2012. http://www. religioustolerance.org/roma2.htm.

Religious Tolerance.org. "Sikhism, Its Beliefs, Practices, Symbol, and Names." Accessed December 15, 2011. http://www. religioustolerance.org/sikhism2.htm.

Riordan, J. *Breastfeeding and Human Lactation.* Sudbury, MA: Jones and Bartlett Publishers, 2005.

Ritter, L.A. and N.A. Hoffman. *Multicultural Health.* Sudbury, MA: Jones and Bartlett Publishers, 2010.

Riverwood Presbyterian Church blog. "Prayer for the Sick." August 26, 2006. http://www.riverwoodchurch.org/ blog/2006/08/26/prayer-for-the-sick/.

Rizvi, S.M. Islamic-Laws. "Taharat and Najasat." Accessed December 6, 2011. http://www.islam-laws.com/ taharatandnajasat.htm.

Roberson, C.M. "ASNA Independent Study Activity – Cultural Assessment of Koreans." *Alabama Nurse* 30, no. 3 (Sep–Nov 2003): 13–16. http://www.ncbi.nlm.nih.gov/pubmed/14596143.

Robinson, G. InterfaithFamily. "Planning a Brit Milah: What to Do Besides Calling the Mohel." Accessed December 8, 2011. http://www.interfaithfamily.com/life_cycle/pregnancy_and_birth_ceremonies /Planning_a_Brit_Milah_What_To_Do_ Besides_Calling_the_Mohel.shtml.

Rodriguez, R. Pacific News Service. "A Cultural Identity." June 18, 1997. http://www.pbs.org /newshour/essays/june97/ rodriguez_6-18.html.

Roger, J. *Presbyterian Creeds: A Guide to the Book of Confessions.* Louisville, KY: Louisville John Knox Press, 1991.

Rosdahl, C.B. and M.T. Kowalski. *Textbook of Basic Nursing.* Philadelphia, PA: Lippincott Williams & Wilkins, 2008.

Rosenberg, E.A. and L.C. Sperazza. "The Visually Impaired Patient." *American Family Physician* 77, no. 10 (2008): 1431–1436, 1437–38. Available from www.aafp.org/afp. http://journals.dev.aafp.org/XML-journal-files/afp/2008/0515/ afp20080515p1431.pdf.

Rucker, W.C. *The River Flows On: Black Resistance, Culture, and Identity Formation in Early America.* (Baton Rouge, LA: LSU Press, 2006).

Rugino, T.A. and T.C. Samsock. "Levetiracetam in Autistic Children: An Open-Label Study." *Journal of Developmental & Behavioral Pediatrics* 23, no. 4 (August 2002): 225–230. http://journals.lww.com/jrnldbp /Abstract/2002/08000/Levetiracetam_in_Autistic_Children__An_Open_Label.6.aspx.

Salimbene, S. *What Language Does Your Patient Hurt In?*, 2nd ed. Amherst, MA: Diversity Resources, Inc., 2005.

Salkowitz, R. *Generation Blend: Managing Across the Technology Age Gap*. Hoboken, NJ: John Wiley & Sons, Inc., 2008.

Samovar, L.A., R.E. Porter, and E.R. McDaniel. *Intercultural Communication: A Reader*, 13th ed. Boston, MA: Wadsworth, 2012.

Sarhill, N., S. LeGrand, R. Islambouli, M.P. Davis, and D. Walsh. "The Terminally Ill Muslim: Death and Dying from the Muslim Perspective." *American Journal of Hospice & Palliative Medicine* 18, no. 4 (July/August, 2001): 252. DOI: 10.1177/104990910101800409.

Sarker, A. *Understand My Muslim People*. Newberg, OR: Barclay Press, 2004.

Scheib, A. Jewish Virtual Library. "Autopsy." Accessed December 8, 2011. http://www.jewishvirtuallibrary.org/jsource/Judaism/autopsy.html.

Scheiman, M., M. Scheiman, and S.G. Whittaker. *Low Vision Rehabilitation: A Practical Guide for Occupational Therapists*. Thorofare, NJ: Slack Incorporated, 2007.

Seale, J. and M. Nind, eds. *Understanding and Promoting Access for People with Learning Disabilities*. New York: Routledge, 2010.

The Secretariat, General Counsel of Seventh-day Adventists. *Seventh-day Adventist Church Manual*. Hagerstown, MD: Review and Herald Publishing Association, 2010.

Seitz, R.H. *Amish Values: Wisdom that Works*. Harrisburg, PA: RB Books, Seitz and Seitz, Inc., 1995.

Selin, H. and P.K. Stone. *Childbirth Across Cultures: Ideas and Practices of Pregnancy, Childbirth, and the Postpartum*. New York: Springer, 2009.

Seventh-day Adventist Church. "Birth Control: A Seventh-day Adventist Statement of Consensus." Accessed December 20, 2011. http://adventist.org/beliefs/statements/main-stat6.html.

Seventh-day Adventist Church. "Considerations on Assisted Human Reproduction." Accessed December 20, 2011. http://adventist.org/beliefs/other-documents/other-doc10.html.

Seventh-day Adventist Church. "Fundamental Beliefs." Accessed December 20, 2011. http://www.adventist.org/beliefs/fundamental/index.html.

Seventh-day Adventist Church. "Guidelines for Sabbath Observance." Accessed December 20, 2011. http://www.adventist.org/beliefs/other-documents/other-doc6.html.

Seventh-day Adventist Church. "Guidelines on Abortion." Accessed December 20, 2011. http://www.adventist.org/beliefs/guidelines/main-guide1.html.

Seventh-day Adventist Church. "Health." Accessed December 20, 2011. http://www.adventist.org /mission-and-service/health.html.

Seventh-day Adventist Church. "A Statement of Consensus on Care for the Dying." Accessed December 20, 2011. http://adventist.org/beliefs/statements/main-stat6.html.

Sewell, P. "Respecting a Patient's Care Needs After Death." *Nursing Times.net* 98, no. 39 (September 24, 2002), 36–37. http://www.ncbi.nlm.nih.gov/pubmed/12374010.

Shah, M.A. *Transcultural Aspects of Perinatal Health Care: A Resource Guide*. Tampa, FL: National Perinatal Association, 2004.

Shah, P.C. and B. Sanwal. "Death: Hindu Rites, Rituals, and Preparations for Funerals." Accessed December 5, 2011. http://www.hcclondon.ca/Hindu%20Death%20Rites%20&%20Rituals.pdf.

Sheikh, A. and A. Gatrad. *Caring for Muslim Patients: Death and Bereavement*. Abingdon, Oxon: Radcliffe Medical Press, 2000.

Shelly, J.A. *Spiritual Care: A Guide for Caregivers*. Downers Grove, IL: InterVarsity Press, 2000.

Sherman, J. MedPage Today's KevinMD.com. "Patient Gender Preferences for Medical Care." Accessed December 30, 2011. http://www.kevinmd.com/blog/2010/11/patient-gender-preferences-medical-care.html.

Sigelman, C.K. *Communicating with Mentally Retarded Persons: Asking Questions and Getting Answers.* Lubbock, TX: Texas Tech University, 1983.

Sikhi Wiki. "Talk: Sikhism and Circumcision." Accessed December 15, 2011. http://www.sikhiwiki.org /index.php/ Talk:Sikhism_and_Circumcision.

Sikhism. "Your Role as a Sikh Minister at the Time of Death." Accessed December 15, 2011. http://fateh.sikhnet.com/ sikhnet/sikhism.nsf/d22e910786b2d7a98725658f0002790d/b9334fece71488a0872565b7007b339b!OpenDocument.

Singh, S., A. Karafin, A. Karlin, A. Mahapatra, A. Thomas, and R. Wlodarski. *South India.* Melbourne: Lonely Planet, 2007.

Slice and Dice Data.com. "Learning About America ...Through US Census Data." Accessed January 30, 2012. http://www. sliceanddicedata.com/detfil16.htm.

Something Jewish. "Sick Visiting," Last updated March 23, 2007. http://www.somethingjewish.co.uk /articles/2257_sick_ visiting.htm.

Sorajjakool, S., M.F. Carr, and J.J. Nam. *World Religions for Healthcare Professionals.* New York: Routledge, 2010.

Sowney, M., M. Brown, and O. Barr. "Caring for People with Learning Disabilities in Emergency Care." *Emergency Nurse* 14, no. 2 (May 2006): 23–30. http://www.ncbi.nlm.nih.gov/pubmed/16739444.

Spector, R.E. *Cultural Diversity in Health & Illness.* New York: Appleton & Lange, 1996.

Star of David Memorial Chapels, Inc. "Jewish Burial Customs." Accessed December 8, 2011. http://jewish-funeral-home. com/Jewish-burial-customs.html.

Steinberg, A. and F. Rosner. *Encyclopedia of Jewish Medical Ethics: A Compilation of Jewish Medical Law.* Jerusalem, Israel: Feldheim Publishers, 2003.

Steinberg, A.G., S. Barnett, H.E. Meador, E. Wiggins, and P. Zazove. "Health Care System Accessibility. Experiences and Perceptions of Deaf People." *Journal of General Internal Medicine* 21, no. 3 (March 2006), 260–66. DOI: 10.1111/j.1525-1497.2006.00340.x.

Storti, C. *Americans at Work: A Guide to the Can-Do People.* Yarmouth, ME: Intercultural Press, Inc., 2004.

Straight Dope Message Board. "Churchgoers – How Different Are Your Beliefs From the Next Church Over?" Last updated January 23, 2006. http://boards.straightdope.com/sdmb/archive/index.php/t-355383.html.

Strydom, A., G. Livingston, M. King, and A. Hassiotis. "Prevalence of Dementia in Intellectual Disability Using Different Diagnostic Criteria." *British Journal of Psychiatry* 191 (2007): 150–57. DOI: 10.1192 /bjp.bp.106.028845.

Suite 101.com. Sarah Tennant. "Amish Kapps, Traditional Head Coverings for Amish Women." Updated June 11, 2008. http:// sarah-tennant.suite101.com/amish-kapps-a56816.

Sukumaran, A. "Hinduism and Medicine." 1999. Accessed December 5, 2011. http://www.angelfire.com /az/ ambersukumaran/medicine.html.

Supportive Care Coalition. "Advance Care Planning—Catholic Perspective." Accessed December 15, 2011. http://www. supportivecarecoalition.org/AdvanceCarePlanning/Advance+Care+Planning+-+Catholics Perspective.php.

Sutherland, A. "Gypsies and Health Care." *Western Journal of Medicine* 157, no. 3 (September 1992): 276–80. http:// www.ncbi.nlm.nih.gov/pmc/articles/PMC1011276/.

Sutherland, A. *Gypsies, The Hidden Americans.* Prospect Heights, IL: Waveland Press, Inc., 1975.

SWAHS Pastoral Care and Chaplaincy Services. "After Death: Religious Needs of Patients in Sickness, Dying, and Death." Last updated December 21, 2011. http://www.wsahs.nsw.gov.au/services /pastoralcare/relneeds.htm.

Sysco. "Different Generations, Different Worlds." Accessed January 17, 2012. http://www.syscosf.com /about/ DECEMBER2009_GENERATIONS.pdf .

Takrouri, M.S.M. and T.M. Halwani. "An Islamic Medical and Legal Prospective of Do Not Resuscitate Order in Critical Care Medicine." *Internet Journal of Health* 7, no. 1 (2008). http://www.ispub.com/journal/the-internet-journal-of-health/ volume-7-number-1/an-islamic-medical-and-legal-prospective-of-do-not-resuscitate-order-in-critical-care-medicine.html.

Tangent Mennonite Church. "What We Believe." Accessed December 12, 2011. http://www.tangentmennonite.org/faith.html.

Taub, H.A., G.E. Kline, and M.T. Baker. "The Elderly and Informed Consent: Effects of Vocabulary Level and Corrected Feedback." *Experimental Aging Research* 7, no. 2 (1981), 137–146. DOI: 10.1080/03610738108259796.

Taylor, H.R. "Fred Hollows Lecture: Eye Care for the Community." *Clinical and Experimental Ophthalmology* 30, no. 3 (June 2002): 151–154. DOI: 10.1046/j.1442-9071.2002.00525.x.

TDL Cluster Blog. "Muslim Prayer Rugs and The Way They're Used." Accessed December 6, 2011. http://www.tdlcluster.org/shopping-and-product-reviews/muslim-prayer-rugs-and-the-way-theyre-used/.

Telushkin, J. Jewish Virtual Library. "Afterlife." Accessed December 8, 2011. http://www.jewishvirtuallibrary.org/jsource/Judaism/afterlife.html.

Thaindian News. "Balanced Diet Quadruples Survival Chances After Traumatic Brain Injury." Accessed January 16, 2012. http://www.thaindian.com/newsportal/lifestyle/balanced-diet-quadruples-survival-chances-after-traumatic-brain-injury_10066971.html.

Thakrar, D., R. Das, and A. Sheikh, eds. *Caring for Hindu Patients*. Abingdon, UK: Radcliffe Publishing, 2008.

Third Way Café. "Empty Arms." Accessed December 12, 2011. http://www.thirdway.com/AW /?Page=5668%7CEmpty+Arms.

Third Way Café. "What Do Mennonites Believe About Death and Dying?" Accessed December 12, 2011. http://www.thirdway.com/menno/faq.asp?f_id=7.

Thompson, A. *Feng Shui*. New York: St. Martin's Press, 1996.

Thompson, W. and J. Hickey. *Society in Focus*. Boston: Pearson, 2005.

Thrane, S. "Hindu End of Life: Death, Dying, Suffering, and Karma: Professional Care Issues." *Journal of Hospice and Palliative Nursing* 12, no. 6 (2010): 337–42. http://journals.lww.com/jhpn/Abstract/2010/11000 /Hindu_End_of_Life__Death,_Dying,_Suffering,_and.3.aspx.

Toews, J.B. *The Story of the Early Mennonite Brethren*. Fresno, CA: Centers for Mennonite Brethren Studies, 2002.

Tower Watch Ministries. "Highlights of the Beliefs of Jehovah's Witnesses." Accessed December 7, 2011. http://www.towerwatch.com/Witnesses/Beliefs/their_beliefs.htm.

Tripod. "Mennonite Patients." Accessed December 12, 2011. http://members.tripod.com /mattmiller_16/id44.htm.

Tseng, W.S. and J. Streltzer. *Cultural Competence in Health Care, Volume 877*. New York: Springer Science and Business Media, 2008.

Unitarian Universalist Association of Congregations. "Abortion: Right to Choose." Accessed December 16, 2011. http://www.uua.org/statements/statements/20271.shtml.

Unitarian Universalist Association of Congregations. "Baptism/Child Dedication." Accessed December 16, 2011. http://www.uua.org/beliefs/worship/ceremonies/6976.shtml.

Unitarian Universalist Association of Congregations. "Beliefs About Life and Death in Unitarian Universalism." Accessed December 16, 2011. http://www.uua.org/beliefs/welcome/183025.shtml.

Unitarian Universalist Association of Congregations. "Chalice." Accessed December 16, 2011. http://www.uua.org/worship/words/chalice/submissions/151521.shtml.

Unitarian Universalist Association of Congregations. "Faith without a Creed: Asking Questions as a Unitarian Universalist." Accessed December 16, 2011. www.uuabookstore.org/client/client_pages/3089.pdf.

Unitarian Universalist Association of Congregations. "Governance and Management of the Unitarian Universalist Association." Accessed December 16, 2011. http://www.uua.org/uuagovernance/.

Unitarian Universalist Association of Congregations. "Holidays." Accessed December 16, 2011. http://www.uua.org/beliefs/worship/holidays/index.shtml.

Unitarian Universalist Association of Congregations. "Membership." Accessed December 16, 2011. http://www.uua.org/beliefs/congregationallife/7004.shtml.

Unitarian Universalist Association of Congregations. "Our Unitarian Universalist Principles." Accessed December 16, 2011. http://www.uua.org/beliefs/principles/.

Unitarian Universalist Association of Congregations. "Sermons—Getting Serious About Unitarian Universalism." Accessed December 16, 2011. http://www.uua.org/worship/words/sermons /submissions/183412.shtml.

Unitarian Universalist Association of Congregations. "Sermons—How Shall We Be Healed?" Accessed December 16, 2011. http://www.uua.org/worship/words/sermons/submissions/183464.shtml.

Unitarian Universalist Association of Congregations. "Sermons—The Spiritual Imperative of Choice." Accessed December 16, 2011. http://www.uua.org/worship/words/sermons/submissions/8788.shtml.

Unitarian Universalist Association of Congregations. "Visiting the Ill or Hospitalized." Accessed December 16, 2011. http://www.uua.org/care/team/104543.shtml.

Unitarian Universalist Association of Congregations. "Worship." Accessed December 16, 2011. http://www.uua.org/beliefs/worship/index.shtml.

University of Virginia Children's Hospital. "Autism." Accessed January 15, 2012. http://uvahealth.com/services/childrens-hospital/conditions-treatments/12028/?searchterm=autism.

U.S. Census Bureau. "American Fact Finder." Accessed January 30, 2012. http://factfinder2.census.gov /faces/nav/jsf/pages/searchresults.xhtml?refresh=t.

U.S. Census Bureau. "State & County QuickFacts." Accessed January 18, 2012. http://quickfacts.census.gov/qfd/states/00000.html.

U.S. Department of Health and Human Services, National Institutes of Health. "Prayer and Spirituality in Health: Ancient Practices, Modern Science." *CAM at the NIH* XII, no. 1 (Dec. 2005). http://www.jpsych.com /pdfs/NCCAM%20-%20 Prayer%20and%20Spirituality%20in%20Health.pdf.

U.S. Department of Labor. "Communicating With and About People with Disabilities." Accessed January 18, 2012. http://www.dol.gov/odep/pubs/fact/comucate.htm.

U.S. Department of Commerce. "Profiles of General Demographic Characteristics 2000 Census of Population and Housing." Issued May 2001. http://www.census.gov/prod/cen2000/dp1/2kh00.pdf.

U.S. Equal Employment Opportunity Commission. *Communicating and Interacting with People Who Have Disabilities*. Upland, PA: DIANE Publishing Company, n.d.: 5–6.

UUs and the News. "Religions Ponder the Stem Cell Issue." Updated August 27, 2001. http://archive.uua.org/news/010827.html.

Value Options. "The Baby Boomer Generation [Born 1946–1964]." Accessed January 17, 2012. http://www.eapexpress.com/spotlight_YIW/baby_boomers.htm.

Value Options. "Generation X." Accessed January 17, 2012. http://www.valueoptions.com /spotlight_YIW/gen_x.htm.

Value Options. "Generation Y [Born 1980-1994]." Accessed January 17, 2012. http://www.valueoptions.com/spotlight_YIW/gen_y.htm.

Value Options. "The Traditional Generation [Born 1922–1945]." Accessed January 16, 2012. http://www.valueoptions.com/spotlight_YIW/traditional.htm.

Van Schrojenstein Lantman-de Valk, H., C. Linehan, M. Kerr, and P. Noonan-Walsh. "Developing Health Indicators for People with Intellectual Disabilities. The Method of the Pomona Project." *Journal of Intellectual Disability Research* 51, no. 6 (June 2007): 427–34. DOI: 10.1111/j.1365-2788.2006.00890.x.

Van Schrojenstein Lantman-De Valk, H.M., J.F. Metsemakers, J.M. Haveman, and H.F.J.M. Crebolder. "Health Problems in People with Intellectual Disability in General Practice: A Comparative Study." *Family Practice* 17, no. 5 (2000), 405–7. DOI: 10.1093/fampra/17.5.405.

Vivian, C. and L. Dundes. "The Crossroads of Culture and Health Among the Roma (Gypsies)." *Journal of Nursing Scholarship* 36, no.1 (March 2004): 86–91. DOI: 10.1111/j.1547-5069.2004.04018.x.

Wakau-Villagomez, L. Critical Multicultural Pavilion Research Room. "A Native American Approach to Teaching and Learning." Last updated September 2003. http://www.edchange.org/multicultural /papers/medicinewheel.html.

Watchtower Bible and Tract Society of Pennsylvania. International Bible Students Association. "Family Care and Medical Management for Jehovah's Witnesses." Brooklyn, NY: 1992.

Welner, S. and C. Hammond. Global Library of Women's Medicine. "Gynecologic and Obstetric Issues Confronting Women with Disabilities." Last updated August 2009. http://www.glowm.com /index.html?p=glowm.cml/section_view&articleid=76.

Wenger, J.C. *The Doctrines of the Mennonites*. Mennonite Publishing House, 1950.

White, E.G. *Counsels on Health*. Nama, ID: Pacific Press Publishing Association, 1951.

White, E.G. *The Ministry of Healing*. Nampa, ID: Pacific Press Publishing Association, 1942.

White, G.C. *Believers and Beliefs: A Practical Guide to Religious Etiquette for Business and Social Occasions*. New York: Berkley Publishing Group, 1997.

White, L. *Foundations of Nursing*. New York: Thomson Delmar, 2005.

Why Mormonism. "Sacrament Mormonism." Updated July 3, 2008. http://whymormonism.org /33/sacrament_mormonism.

Williams, N. *The Mexican American Family: Tradition and Change*. Walnut Creek, CA: AltaMira Press, 2003.

Witte, J. *God's Joust, God's Justice: Law and Religion in the Western Tradition*. Grand Rapids, MI: Eerdmans Publishing Co., 2006.

Wood, W.J. "Advance Directives: Religious, Moral, and Theological Aspects." *The Elder Law Journal* (1999). https://litigation-essentials.lexisnexis.com/webcd/app?action=DocumentDisplay&crawlid=1&srctype= smi&srcid=3B15&doctype=cite&docid=7+Elder+L.J.+457&key=bc39b2fabc06c96b649a1b0f65085b68.

Wu, A., R. Molteni, Z. Ying, and F. Gomez-Pinilla. "A Saturated-Fat Diet Aggravates the Outcome of Traumatic Brain Injury on Hippocampal Plasticity and Cognitive Function by Reducing Brain-derived Neurotrophic Factor." *Neuroscience* 119, no. 2 (June 2003): 365–75. http://dx.doi.org/10.1016/S0306-4522(03)00154-4.

Yahoo!Answers. "Are Most Lutherans Circumcised at Birth?" Accessed December 12, 2011. http://answers.yahoo.com/question/index?qid=20110426210543AAPEL05.

Yahoo!Answers. "Do Assembly of God Men Get Circumcised?" Accessed December 14, 2011. http://ph.answers.yahoo.com/question/index?qid=20100725030235AATDMXU.

Yahoo!Answers. "Do Jehovah's Witnesses Practice Circumcision?" Accessed December 6, 2011. http://answers.yahoo.com/question/index?qid=20080920181032AA82nwp.

Yehieli, M. and M.A. Grey. *Health Matters: A Pocket Guide for Working with Diverse Cultures and Underserved Populations*. Yarmouth, ME: Intercultural Press, Inc., 2005.

Young, C. and C. Koopsen. *Spirituality, Health, and Healing*. Sudbury, MA: Jones and Bartlett Publishers, 2006.

Yousif, A.F. "Muslim Medicine and Health Care. " Accessed December 6, 2011, http://www.truthandgrace.com/muslimmedicine.htm.

Zaidman-Zait, A. "Everyday Problems and Stress Faced by Parents of Children with Cochlear Implants." *Rehabilitation Psychology* 53, no. 2 (May 2008): 139–152. http://psycnet.apa.org/doi/10.1037/0090-5550.53.2.139.

Zavada, J. About.com Christianity. "Christian Science Church Beliefs and Practices." Accessed December 26, 2011. http://christianity.about.com/od/christianscience/a/christsciencebeliefs.htm.

Zavada, J. About.com Christianity. "Church of the Nazarene Beliefs and Practices." Accessed December 4, 2011. http://www.christianity.about.com/od/Nazarene-Church/a/Nazarene-Beliefs.htm.

Disclaimer and Legal Notice

Acknowledgements

I WISH TO THANK THE MEMBERS OF THE FLORIDA HOSPITAL BIOMEDICAL ETHICS AND Perinatal Ethics Committees for their support, comments, and suggestions. A special thanks to Louis R. Preston Jr., MDiv, CDM, Diversity and Inclusion Officer and Director, and Karen Marcarelli, RN, JD, MSN, BSN, Vice President for Risk Management and Patient Safety, for their vision and leadership on this project. I especially thank my Director, Louis Preston, Jr. for his belief in my abilities, which frees me up to do my best work. You have become an influential part of my journey and growth. I would also like to thank the Florida Hospital I-Extend and Web team, Darren Greene, Scott Denzio, Rick Mann, and Kevin Finley for their assistance in making the second edition of this guide available on I-Extend and InSite for all our caregivers and employees. Thanks to Sherrie Greenlee and David Posluszny with our E-learning team for creating a CBL available through Net Learning, and to Alice DeSantola for making it a part of required Nursing Education. Thanks also to Ann McDonald and Nancy Aldrich with the Florida Hospital Medical Library for their assistance in locating the many books and journal articles used in preparing this update.

Thank you to many Florida Hospital leaders who have extended their support and belief in this work including, Sheryl Dodds, John Guarneri, MD, Ted Hamilton, MD, Monica Reed, MD, Laurie Levin, Wanda Davis, Greg Ellis, Jay Perez and the FH Chaplains, the external and internal peer review team and numerous people that reviewed this guide and gave feedback. Great thanks to Todd Chobotar, Dr. David Biebel, and the rest of the Florida Hospital Publishing Team for their incredible support and efforts in publishing this edition – including Lillian Boyd, Laurel Dominesey, and Tim Brown. Thanks to Thank you to Sandy Santos, who has picked up many additional duties as my time was usurped in finishing this guide. I would like to extend a special appreciation to Marie Ruckstuhl, who served as co-editor in developing the second edition of this guide, which has been viewed and accessed over 35,000 times to date. Thanks also to Candice Ricketts, whose time and efforts have greatly assisted me in compiling the many suggestions we have received since the release of the second edition, and in researching new information to bring you our revised and expanded third edition. Thank you to Rogue Gallart and The Central Florida Disability Chamber for their contribution in the Disabilities section of this guide.

Finally, my most heartfelt thanks to God for leading me in this work and allowing me to share my passion with all of you. To my husband Chris, and my children, Christopher and Christian, for their support and patience during the long journey it took in completing this document. I couldn't have done it without any of you. You three are the greatest joy in my life.

I dedicate this book the late Steve Jeffers, PhD, founder of the Institute for Spirituality in Health at Shawnee Mission Medical Center, who provided tremendous assistance in developing our second edition, and to all caregivers who not only want to provide the best care for all the patients they serve, but also a better encounter by providing a more personal, culturally competent, patient care experience.

Aurora P. Realin, MBA, CDM
General Editor
Florida Hospital Diversity and Inclusion

About the Editorial Team

One of the strengths of *A Desk Reference to Personalizing Patient Care* is the combination of background, education, experience, and interests of the team of contributors who helped produce it. The range of professional training of the contributors include: healthcare, healthcare management, pastoral ministry, journalism, curriculum creation, editorial, diversity and inclusion. In addition to the team's professional experience, their diverse cultural roots and family history added perspective to the creation of the guide. The team members' diverse culture and family heritage includes: Hispanic, French, German, African American, Jamaican, Chinese, African, Scottish, and Filipino influences.

General Editor

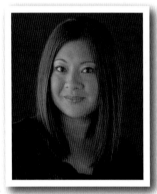

Aurora P. Realin, MBA, CDM, was born in the Philippines. She moved with her family to Queens, NY, when Aurora was thirteen years old. "In New York," she recalls, "I attended public school for the first time in my life. All my life, I had grown up with people who looked and acted like me. I wasn't used to seeing different people from all walks of life. Talk about culture shock! I also noticed that most of the students gravitated toward people of their own kind, or people they liked, and they could be quite unkind to others. Most of them weren't open to other views and ways of life. By contrast, I did my best to make friends with the 'outcasts,' partly because I thought of myself as different, so in essence I felt like we were in the same 'boat.' Even back then I dreamt of a world where differences between people would not be an issue, where everyone - no matter who they were, or where they came from - would all get along, and the word 'diversity' would no longer be an issue because accepting others would just be part of our everyday life."

Aurora grew up in a medical family with a physician for a grandfather, a pharmacist for a grandmother, and a brain injury rehab certified registered nurse for a mother. As a result of their experiences, she developed her own passion for helping others from all walks of life, especially within the context of healthcare. She earned a BS in Communicative Disorders (Speech Language Pathology) from the University of Central Florida and an MBA, with emphasis in Healthcare Administration, from Southern Adventist University. She also holds a Certificate in Diversity Management in Healthcare (CDM) from Simmons College.

Today, Aurora serves as the Manager for Diversity and Inclusion at Florida Hospital – the largest admitting hospital in America – where she has worked since 1998. She also serves as the Chairperson for The Beacon Network – a community organization whose focus is to promote diversity and inclusion in the Central Florida community, and is also an active board member in both her church and children's school. She is married to Chris, a Police Officer First Class for the City of Orlando, and they have two sons, Christopher and Christian.

Her mission in life is to accept, include, and love all people and help them to do the same for each other. She considers it truly a God-given privilege and honor to serve in her current role, which affords her the opportunity to help build relationships and further enhance the concept of inclusion at Florida Hospital and the larger community she serves.

Contributing Editors

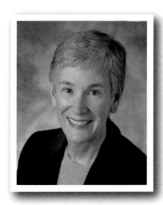

Marie C. Ruckstuhl, BSN, MBA, RN, CPHQ, CHRM, earned her BSN from Florida Southern College and her MBA from Florida Institute of Technology. She obtained certification in healthcare quality and became a certified healthcare risk manager with Florida Hospital. Marie worked in Progressive Care for six years before focusing in the quality arena in the Medical Quality Assessment Department, then Nursing Performance Improvement Department. She was elected to various leadership positions in the national, state, and local associations for Healthcare Quality. In 1997, 2003, and 2006 Marie was selected "Outstanding Quality Professional for the State of Florida" by the Florida Association for Healthcare Quality. Marie's interest in personalizing patient care in diverse populations grew naturally from her family background which includes extended family from various Latin American countries as well as Europe and Asia. With a strong interest in how multicultural ideas and manners, as well as religious background, affect interaction with others, Marie became involved as a Nursing committee chair and editor of the original nursing edition of this guide.

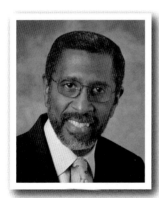

Louis R. Preston Jr., MDiv, CDM, is an ordained minister, third-generation pastor and church administrator. Diversity and inclusion have been part of his life since desegregating both his high school and college. In 1979, Preston was sent to quell racial tension within churches in England and Scotland. After ten years in Britain, he was called to develop financial stability for churches in eleven countries in Eastern Africa. Back in the United States, Preston again worked as church pastor and administrator with an emphasis on integrating various institutions. He currently serves as Diversity Officer for Florida Hospital. Under his leadership, Florida Hospital became a recipient of the Beacon Award's Corporate Advocate for Diversity. Preston is passionate about the integration of faith and healthcare for all God's children no matter their religion, culture, generation or background.

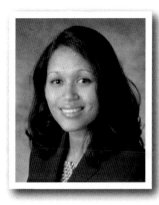

Candice Ricketts, BA, MBA (candidate) holds a Bachelors Degree in journalism from the University of Florida, and is earning her MBA from Stetson University. Ricketts has extensive experience in writing for both consumer and professional audiences. She currently serves as an e-Learning manager for a healthcare company where she develops content for online education. She has a passion for helping others understand diversity and how to improve human relations by incorporating our unique differences. A native of Jamaica, where their national slogan is "Out of Many...One People," her ethnic background is a melting pot - including Chinese, African, Scottish, and German ancestry.

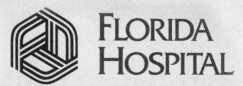

FLORIDA HOSPITAL

The skill to heal. The spirit to care.®

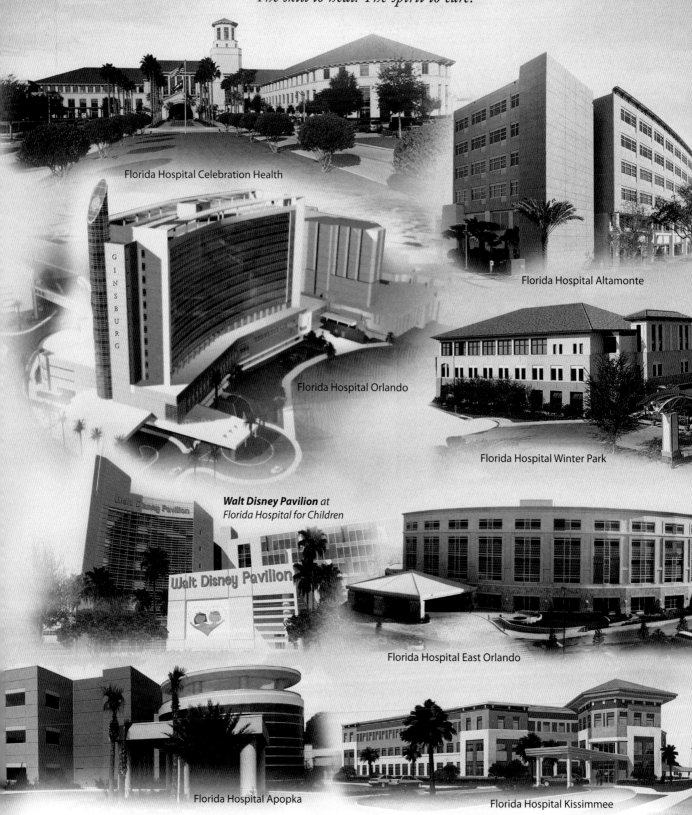

Florida Hospital Celebration Health

Florida Hospital Altamonte

Florida Hospital Orlando

Florida Hospital Winter Park

Walt Disney Pavilion *at*
Florida Hospital for Children

Florida Hospital East Orlando

Florida Hospital Apopka

Florida Hospital Kissimmee

About Florida Hospital

For over one hundred years the mission of Florida Hospital has been: *To extend the health and healing ministry of Christ.* Opened in 1908, Florida Hospital is comprised of eight hospital campuses housing over 2,200 beds and twenty walk-in medical centers. With over 17,000 employees—including 2,000 doctors and 4,000 nurses—Florida Hospital serves the residents and guests of Orlando, the No. 1 tourist destination in the world. Florida Hospital cares for over one million patients a year. Florida Hospital is a Christian, faith-based hospital that believes in providing Whole Person Care to all patients – mind, body and spirit. Hospital fast facts include:

- **LARGEST ADMITTING HOSPITAL IN AMERICA.** Ranked No. 1 in the nation for inpatient admissions by the *American Hospital Association.*

- **AMERICA'S HEART HOSPITAL.** Ranked No. 1 in the nation for number of heart procedures performed each year, averaging 15,000 cases annually. MSNBC named Florida Hospital "America's Heart Hospital" for being the No. 1 hospital fighting America's No. 1 killer—heart disease.

- **HOSPITAL OF THE FUTURE.** At the turn of the century, the *Wall Street Journal* named Florida Hospital the "Hospital of the Future."

- **ONE OF AMERICA'S BEST HOSPITALS.** Recognized by *U.S. News & World Report* as "One of America's Best Hospitals" for ten years. Clinical specialties recognized have included: Cardiology, Orthopaedics, Neurology & Neurosurgery, Urology, Gynecology, Digestive Disorders, Hormonal Disorders, Kidney Disease, Ear, Nose & Throat and Endocrinology.

- **LEADER IN SENIOR CARE.** Florida Hospital serves the largest number of seniors in America through Medicare with a goal for each patient to experience a "Century of Health" by living to a healthy hundred.

- **TOP BIRTHING CENTER.** *Fit Pregnancy* magazine named Florida Hospital one of the "Top 10 Best Places in the Country to have a Baby". As a result, *The Discovery Health Channel* struck a three-year production deal with Florida Hospital to host a live broadcast called "Birth Day Live." FH annually delivers over 8,000 babies.

- **CORPORATE ALLIANCES.** Florida Hospital maintains corporate alliance relationships with a select group of Fortune 500 companies including Disney, Nike, Johnson & Johnson, Philips, AGFA, and Stryker.

- **DISNEY PARTNERSHIP.** Florida Hospital is the Central Florida health & wellness resource of the *Walt Disney World* ® Resort. Florida Hospital also partnered with Disney to build the ground breaking health and wellness facility called Florida Hospital Celebration Health located in Disney's town of Celebration, Florida. Disney and Florida Hospital recently partnered to build a new state-of-the-art Children's Hospital.

- **HOSPITAL OF THE 21ST CENTURY.** Florida Hospital Celebration Health was awarded the *Premier Patient Services Innovator Award* as "The Model for Healthcare Delivery in the 21st Century."

- **SPORTS EXPERTS.** Florida Hospital is the official hospital of the Orlando Magic NBA basketball team. In addition, Florida Hospital has an enduring track record of providing exclusive medical care to many sports organizations. These organizations have included: Disney's Wide World of Sports, Walt Disney World's Marathon Weekend, the Capital One Bowl, and University of Central Florida Athletics. Florida Hospital has also provided comprehensive healthcare services for the World Cup and Olympics.

- **PRINT RECOGNITION.** Self magazine named Florida Hospital one of America's "Top 10 Hospitals for Women". Modern Healthcare magazine proclaimed it one of America's best hospitals for cardiac care.

- **CONSUMER CHOICE AWARD WINNER.** Florida Hospital has received the Consumer Choice Award from the National Research Corporation every year from 1996 to the present.

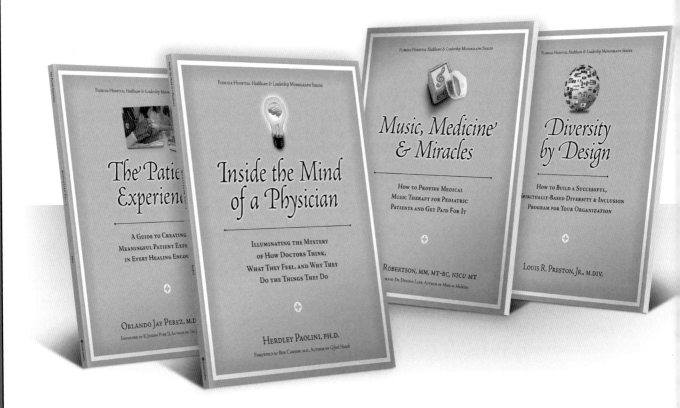

Florida Hospital Publishing presents the *Healthcare & Leadership* monograph series.

Building Bridges: A Guide to Optimizing Physician-Hospital Relationships, written by Dr. Ted Hamilton. In these pages you will find help not only in relating more effectively to physicians, but in developing initiatives that will build healthier relationships between hospitals and medical staff that will ultimately improve patient care. A valuable publication for leadership of mission-focused health care organizations and their physician partners.

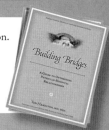

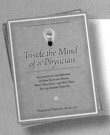

Inside the Mind of a Physician, written by Dr. Herdley Paolini, does a great service by opening the inner world of physicians and helping us understand them, how to relate to them, and how to support them in their critical role in health care. Her insights will be of great value to everyone from hospital administrators and clinical staff, to insurance providers, government agencies, and anyone who interacts with physicians.

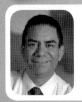

The Patient Experience, written by Jay Perez, offers simple solutions that everyone can do to create an exceptional patient experience. Hospitals are so clinically oriented they often overlook the emotional and relational aspects of patient care, which is how many patients judge their experience. When caregivers let patients know who they are, what they do, and why the care it creates a great sense of hope, trust, and belonging.

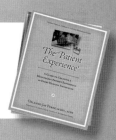

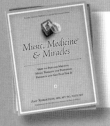

Music, Medicine & Miracles: How to Provide Medical Music Therapy for Pediatric Patients and Get Paid for It, written by Amy Robertson, founder of the Music Therapy program at *Florida Hospital for Children,* offers in-depth solutions for utilizing music to help pediatric patients heal in mind, body and spirit. Music Therapy is becoming an important part of the mission of many health care facilities.

Making History Together: How to Create Innovate Strategic Alliances to Fuel the Growth of Your Company, written by Keith Lowe, takes you through the steps of how Florida Hospital creates and cultivates outstanding strategic alliance relationships—and how you can, too. ***Have you ever wondered*** how Florida Hospital creates world-class partnerships with companies like Disney, Nike, GE, IBM, Philips, Johnson & Johnson, and Bayer? Now you can discover the secrets for yourself.

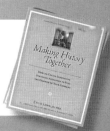

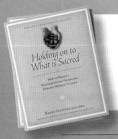

Holding on to What is Sacred, written by Dr. Randy Haffner, lays out a persuasive vision for how organizations can stay focused on their true values. The most intriguing aspect of the monograph is Dr. Haffner's concept of Confessional Identity. It seeks the spiritual heart of an organization's reason for being. Why? Because so much is at stake. Your employees need to know why you exist and why their efforts matter. Your customers need to know why you really care. Your leaders need to embrace your core convictions whole-heartedly or they will lose direction.

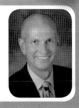

The *Florida Hospital Healthcare and Leadership Monograph* series are perfect for:
Hospitals | Clinicians | Music Therapists | Business Professionals | Chaplains | And many more!

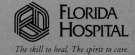

FLORIDA HOSPITAL
The skill to heal. The spirit to care.

LEAD YOUR COMMUNITY
TO HEALTHY LIVING

With C·R·E·A·T·I·O·N Health
Seminars, Books, & Resources

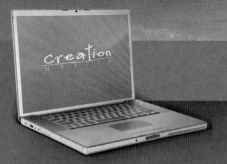

SHOP OUR ONLINE STORE AT:

CREATIONhealth.com

FOR MANY MORE RESOURCES

SEMINAR MATERIALS

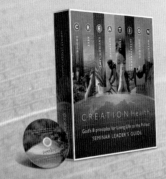
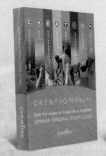
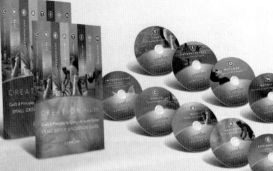

Leader Guide
Everything a leader needs to conduct this seminar successfully, including key questions to facilitate group discussion and PowerPoint presentations for each of the eight principles.

Participant Guide
A study guide with essential information from each of the eight lessons along with outlines, self assessments, and questions for people to fill-in as they follow along.

Small Group Kit
It's easy to lead a small group using the CREATION Health videos, the Small Group Leaders Guide and the Small Group Discussion Guide.

GUIDES AND ASSESSMENTS

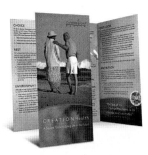

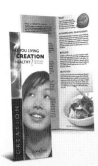

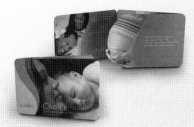

Senior Guide
Share the CREATION Health principles with seniors and help them be healthier and happier as they live life to the fullest.

Self-Assessment
This instrument raises awareness about how CREATION Healthy a person is in each of the eight major areas of wellness.

Pregnancy Guides
Expert advice on how to be CREATION Healthy while expecting.

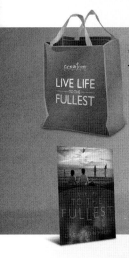

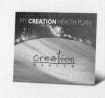

GET ORGANIZED!

Tote Bag
A convenient way for bringing CREATION Health materials to and from class.

Presentation Folder
Keep CREATION Health notes and resources organized and in one place.

Pocket Guide
A tool for keeping people committed to living all of the CREATION Health principles daily.

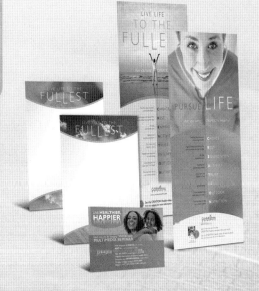

MARKETING MATERIALS

Postcards, Posters, Stationary, and more
You can effectively advertise and generate community excitement about your CREATION Health seminar with a wide range of available marketing materials such as enticing postcards, flyers, posters, and more.

CREATION HEALTH BOOKS

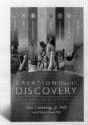

CREATION Health Discovery
Written by Des Cummings Jr., PhD and Monica Reed, MD, this wonderful companion resource introduces people to the CREATION Health philosophy and lifestyle.

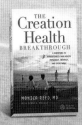

The CREATION Health Breakthrough
Written by Monica Reed, MD, this book guides you through a personal weekend retreat that will integrate healthy behaviors into your lifestyle and rejuvenate your life.

Healthy 100 Resources

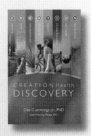

CREATION Health Discovery (Softcover)

CREATION Health Discovery takes the 8 essential principles of CREATION Health and melds them together to form the blueprint for the health we yearn for and the life we are intended to live.

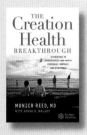

CREATION Health Breakthrough (Hardcover)

Blending science and lifestyle recommendations, Monica Reed, MD, prescribes eight essentials that will help reverse harmful health habits and prevent disease. Discover how intentional choices, rest, environment, activity, trust, relationships, outlook, and nutrition can put a person on the road to wellness. Features a three-day total body rejuvenation therapy and four-phase life transformation plan.

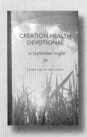

CREATION Health Devotional (English) (Hardcover)

Stories change lives. Stories can inspire health and healing. In this devotional you will discover stories about experiencing God's grace in the tough times, God's delight in triumphant times, and God's presence in peaceful times. Based on the eight timeless principles of wellness: Choice, Rest, Environment, Activity, Trust, Interpersonal relationships, Outlook, Nutrition.

CREATION Health Devotional (Spanish) (Softcover)

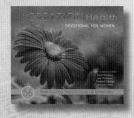

CREATION Health Devotional for Women (English)

Written for women by women, the CREATION Health Devotional for Women is based on the principles of whole-person wellness represented in CREATION Health. Spirits will be lifted and lives rejuvenated by the message of each unique chapter. This book is ideal for women's prayer groups, to give as a gift, or just to buy for your own edification and encouragement.

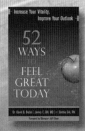

52 Ways to Feel Great Today (Softcover)

Wouldn't you love to feel great today? Changing your outlook and injecting energy into your day often begins with small steps. In 52 Ways to Feel Great Today, you'll discover an abundance of simple, inexpensive, fun things you can do to make a big difference in how you feel today and every day. Tight on time? No problem. Each chapter is written as a short, easy-to-implement idea. Every idea is supported by at least one true story showing how helpful implementing the idea has proven to someone a lot like you. The stories are also included to encourage you to be as inventive, imaginative, playful, creative, or adventuresome as you can.

Healthy 100 Resources

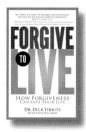

Forgive To Live *(English) (Hardcover)*

In *Forgive to Live* Dr. Tibbits presents the scientifically proven steps for forgiveness – taken from the first clinical study of its kind conducted by Stanford University and Florida Hospital.

Forgive To Live *(Spanish) (Softcover)*

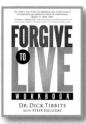

Forgive To Live Workbook *(Softcover)*

This interactive guide will show you how to forgive – insight by insight, step by step – in a workable plan that can effectively reduce your anger, improve your health, and put you in charge of your life again, no matter how deep your hurts.

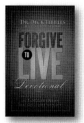

Forgive To Live Devotional *(Hardcover)*

In his powerful new devotional Dr. Dick Tibbits reveals the secret to forgiveness. This compassionate devotional is a stirring look at the true meaning of forgiveness. Each of the 56 spiritual insights includes motivational Scripture, an inspirational prayer, and two thought-provoking questions. The insights are designed to encourage your journey as you begin to Forgive to Live.

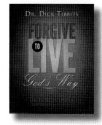

Forgive To Live God's Way *(Softcover)*

Forgiveness is so important that our very lives depend on it. Churches teach us that we should forgive, but how do you actually learn to forgive? In this spiritual workbook noted author, psychologist, and ordained minister Dr. Dick Tibbits takes you step-by-step through an eight-week forgiveness format that is easy to understand and follow.

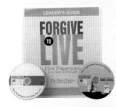

Forgive To Live Leader's Guide

Perfect for your community, church, small group or other settings.

The *Forgive to Live Leader's Guide* Includes:

- 8 Weeks of pre-designed PowerPoint™ presentations.
- Professionally designed customizable marketing materials and group handouts on CD-Rom.
- Training directly from author of *Forgive to Live* Dr. Dick Tibbits across 6 audio CDs.
- Media coverage DVD.
- CD-Rom containing all files in digital format for easy home or professional printing.
- A copy of the first study of its kind conducted by Stanford University and Florida Hospital showing a link between decreased blood pressure and forgiveness.
- Much more!

Healthy 100 Resources

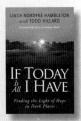

If Today Is All I Have *(Softcover)*

At its heart, Linda's captivating account chronicles the struggle to reconcile her three dreams of experiencing life as a "normal woman" with the tough realities of her medical condition. Her journey is punctuated with insights that are at times humorous, painful, provocative, and life-affirming.

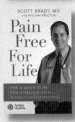

Pain Free For Life *(Hardcover)*

In *Pain Free For Life*, Scott C. Brady, MD, – founder of Florida Hospital's Brady Institute for Health – shares for the first time with the general public his dramatically successful solution for chronic back pain, Fibromyalgia, chronic headaches, Irritable bowel syndrome and other "impossible to cure" pains. Dr. Brady leads pain-racked readers to a pain-free life using powerful mind-body-spirit strategies used at the Brady Institute – where more than 80 percent of his chronic-pain patients have achieved 80-100 percent pain relief within weeks.

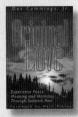

Original Love *(Softcover)*

Are you ready for: God's smile to affirm your worth? God's forgiveness to renew your relationship? God's courage to calm your fears? God's gifts to fulfill your dreams? The God who made you is ready to give you all this and so much more! Join Des Cummings Jr., PhD, as he unfolds God's love drama in the life stories of Old Testament heroes. He provides fresh, biblical light on the original day God made for love. His wife, Mary Lou, shares practical, creative ways to experience Sabbath peace, blessings, and joy!

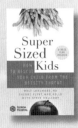

SuperSized Kids *(Hardcover)*

In *SuperSized Kids*, Walt Larimore, MD, and Sherri Flynt, MPH, RD, LD, show how the mushrooming childhood obesity epidemic is destroying children's lives, draining family resources, and pushing America dangerously close to a total healthcare collapse – while also explaining, step by step, how parents can work to avert the coming crisis by taking control of the weight challenges facing every member of their family.

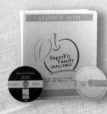

SuperFit Family Challenge - Leader's Guide

Perfect for your community, church, small group or other settings.

The *SuperFit Family Challenge Leader's Guide* Includes:

- 8 Weeks of pre-designed PowerPoint™ presentations.
- Professionally designed marketing materials and group handouts from direct mailers to reading guides.
- Training directly from Author Sherri Flynt, MPH, RD, LD, across 6 audio CDs.
- Media coverage and FAQ on DVD.
- Much more!

---

*"**Come near to God and he will come near to you...**" – James 4:8, NIV*

www.FloridaHospitalPublishing.com

f www.Facebook.com/FloridaHospitalPublishing

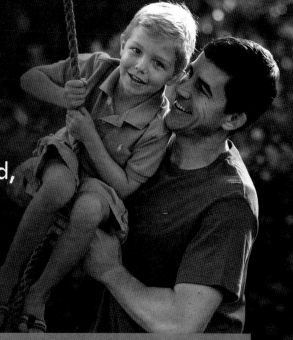

IMAGINE...

A body that is healthy and strong,

A spirit that is vibrant and refreshed,

A life that glorifies God,

Imagine living to a Healthy 100!

What is a Healthy 100 Church?

The goal of the Healthy 100 movement is simple: inspire individuals, families and communities to fill their days with God's power, passion and purpose, enabling them to live long and vibrant lives.

The Healthy 100 Church Ministry inspires, informs and equips churches, pastors, faith community nurses, health ministers and lay leaders to transform people through principles of whole-person health and healing. Our vision for Healthy 100 Churches is to partner with you while providing a health and healing platform full of incredible inspiration and practical implementation resources. This life-enhancing outreach of health ministry can help your church create a place where God's people live abundant lives full of physical, mental and spiritual health. After all, Jesus said: *"I have come that they may have life, and have it to the full."* John 10:10

Together we can:

▶ **Inspire Clergy** – Pastoral leaders are provided opportunities to learn how a health ministry can motivate their parishioners, revitalize families and invigorate their whole church. It may even inspire a commitment to improve their own health and wellness.

▶ **Equip Teams** – We provide health ministry training and tools that teach lay leaders how to start and grow a vibrant health ministry in their church. The training not only establishes the connections between faith and health, but gives instructions on how to sustain it in congregations.

▶ **Energize Congregations** – Would you like to energize your church's mission and vision? Why not start by energizing your people! Empower every individual in your congregation to live life to the fullest in body, mind, and spirit. By starting a church-based health ministry, you can engage people to be at their best for serving God and serving others.

Become a Healthy 100 church by visiting
www.Healthy100Churches.org

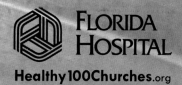

FLORIDA HOSPITAL

Healthy100Churches.org

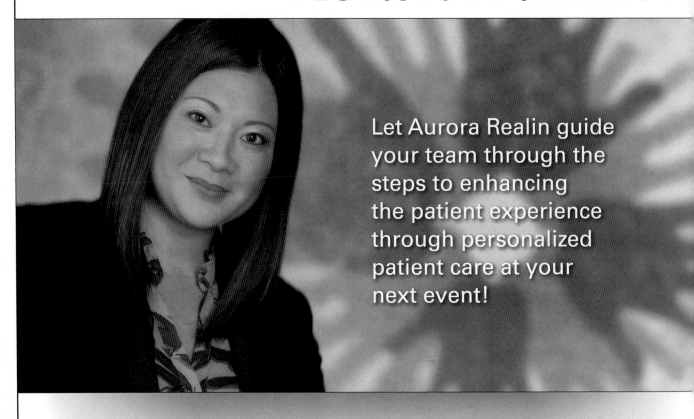